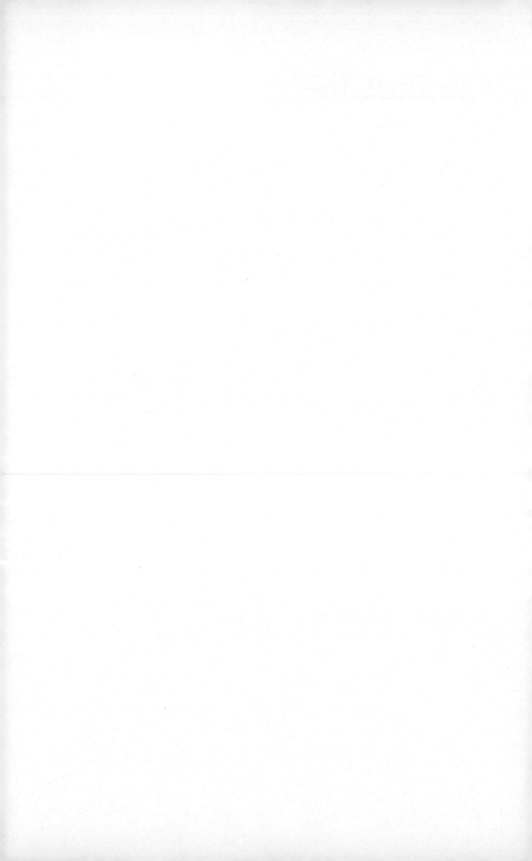

Clinical Veterinary Dentistry

Editor

STEVEN E. HOLMSTROM

VETERINARY CLINICS OF NORTH AMERICA: SMALL ANIMAL PRACTICE

www.vetsmall.theclinics.com

May 2013 • Volume 43 • Number 3

ELSEVIER

1600 John F. Kennedy Boulevard • Suite 1800 • Philadelphia, Pennsylvania, 19103-2899
http://www.vetsmall.theclinics.com

VETERINARY CLINICS OF NORTH AMERICA: SMALL ANIMAL PRACTICE Volume 43, Number 3
May 2013 ISSN 0195-5616, ISBN-13: 978-1-4557-7352-7

Editor: John Vassallo; j.vassallo@elsevier.com
Developmental Editor: Teia Stone

Veterinary Clinics of North America: Small Animal Practice (ISSN 0195-5616) is published bimonthly (For Post Office use only: volume 43 issue 3 of 6) by Elsevier Inc., 360 Park Avenue South, New York, NY 10010-1710. Months of issue are January, March, May, July, September, and November. Business and Editorial Offices: 1600 John F. Kennedy Blvd., Ste. 1800, Philadelphia, PA 19103-2899. Customer Service Office: 3251 Riverport Lane, Maryland Heights, MO 63043. Periodicals postage paid at New York, NY and additional mailing offices. Subscription prices are $294.00 per year (domestic individuals), $473.00 per year (domestic institutions), $143.00 per year (domestic students/residents), $390.00 per year (Canadian individuals), $580.00 per year (Canadian institutions), $433.00 per year (international individuals), $580.00 per year (international institutions), and $208.00 per year (international and Canadian students/residents). To receive student/resident rate, orders must be accompanied by name of affiliated institution, date of term, and the *signature* of program/residency coordinator on institution letterhead. Orders will be billed at individual rate until proof of status is received. Foreign air speed delivery is included in all *Clinics* subscription prices. All prices are subject to change without notice. **POSTMASTER:** Send address changes to *Veterinary Clinics of North America: Small Animal Practice*, Elsevier Health Sciences Division, Subscription Customer Service, 3251 Riverport Lane, Maryland Heights, MO 63043. Customer Service (orders, claims, online, change of address): Elsevier Periodicals Customer Service, Elsevier Health Sciences Division Subscription Customer Service 3251 Riverport Lane Maryland Heights, MO 63043. Tel: 1-800-654-2452 (U.S. and Canada); 314-447-8871 (outside U.S. and Canada). Fax: 314-447-8029. E-mail: journalscustomerservice-usa@elsevier.com (for print support); journalsonlinesupport-usa@elsevier.com (for online support).

Reprints. For copies of 100 or more of articles in this publication, please contact the Commercial Reprints Department, Elsevier Inc., 360 Park Avenue South, New York, NY 10010-1710. Tel.: 212-633-3812; Fax: 212-462-1935; E-mail: reprints@elsevier.com.

Veterinary Clinics of North America: Small Animal Practice is also published in Japanese by Inter Zoo Publishing Co., Ltd., Aoyama Crystal-Bldg 5F, 3-5-12 Kitaaoyama, Minato-ku, Tokyo 107-0061, Japan.

Veterinary Clinics of North America: Small Animal Practice is covered in *Current Contents/Agriculture, Biology and Environmental Sciences, Science Citation Index, ASCA, MEDLINE/PubMed (Index Medicus), Excerpta Medica,* and *BIOSIS.*

Printed and bound by CPI Group (UK) Ltd, Croydon, CR0 4YY
Transferred to digital print 2013

Contributors

EDITOR

STEVEN E. HOLMSTROM, DVM
Diplomate, American Veterinary Dental College; Animal Dental Clinic, San Carlos, California

AUTHORS

KRISTIN M. BANNON, DVM, FAVD
Diplomate, American Veterinary Dental College; Veterinary Dentistry and Oral Surgery of New Mexico, LLC, Santa Fe, New Mexico

BRETT BECKMAN, DVM, FAVD
Diplomate, American Veterinary Dental College; Diplomate, American Academy of Pain Management, Florida Veterinary Dentistry and Oral Surgery, Punta Gorda, Florida

JAN BELLOWS, DVM
Diplomate, American Veterinary Dental College; Diplomate, American Board of Veterinary Practitioners; All Pets Dental, Weston, Florida

GLENN M. BRIGDEN, DVM
Diplomate, American Veterinary Dental College; Arizona Veterinary Dental Specialists, PC, Scottsdale, Arizona

CURT R. COFFMAN, DVM, FAVD
Diplomate, American Veterinary Dental College; Arizona Veterinary Dental Specialists, PC, Scottsdale, Arizona

EDWARD R. EISNER, AB, DVM
Diplomate, American Veterinary Dental College; Chief of Dental Services, Dental Department, Animal Hospital Specialty Center, Highlands Ranch, Colorado

BILL GENGLER, DVM
Diplomate, American Veterinary Dental College; Emeritus Associate Dean for Clinical Affairs and Dentistry, Oral Surgery Section Head, School of Veterinary Medicine, University of Wisconsin, Middleton, Wisconsin

MATTHEW LEMMONS, DVM
Diplomate, American Veterinary Dental College; Circle City Veterinary Specialty and Emergency Hospital, Carmel, Indiana

JOHN R. LEWIS, VMD, FAVD
Diplomate, American Veterinary Dental College; Assistant Professor of Dentistry and Oral Surgery, Department of Clinical Studies, School of Veterinary Medicine, University of Pennsylvania, Philadelphia, Pennsylvania

MILINDA J. LOMMER, DVM
Diplomate, American Veterinary Dental College; Medical Director, Aggie Animal Dental Center, Mill Valley; Assistant Clinical Professor–Volunteer, Department of Surgical and Radiological Sciences, School of Veterinary Medicine, University of California, Davis, California

SANDRA MANFRA MARRETTA, DVM
Diplomate, American College of Veterinary Surgeons; Diplomate, American Veterinary Dental College; Professor of Small Animal Surgery and Dentistry, Section Head, Department of Veterinary Clinical Medicine, Veterinary Teaching Hospital, University of Illinois, Urbana, Illinois

ALEXANDER M. REITER, Dipl Tzt, Dr med vet
Diplomate, American Veterinary Dental College; Diplomate, European Veterinary Dental College; Associate Professor of Dentistry and Oral Surgery, Chief of the Dentistry and Oral Surgery Service, Department of Clinical Studies, School of Veterinary Medicine, University of Pennsylvania, Philadelphia, Pennsylvania

AMALIA M. ZACHER, DVM
Former Resident (2010–2012), Dentistry and Oral Surgery, Department of Veterinary Clinical Medicine, University of Illinois, Urbana, Illinois; Associate Veterinarian, VCA San Francisco Veterinary Specialists, San Francisco, California

Contents

Preface: Clinical Veterinary Dentistry   ix

Steven E. Holmstrom

Standard of Care in North American Small Animal Dental Service   447

Edward R. Eisner

> Veterinary standard of care is peer-regulated, measured as the level of care provided and acceptable among most veterinarians in a given geographic area. This article proposes that today it should be the responsibility of the guiding organization of each medical discipline, such as the American Veterinary Dental College for the veterinary dental profession, to provide guidance to ruling Medical Boards regarding a recommended standard of care, rather than being defined by geographic boundaries. Within each medical discipline, specialists should be held to a higher standard than generalists, with both operating to a standard of care commensurate with their training.

Therapeutic Decision Making and Planning in Veterinary Dentistry and Oral Surgery   471

John R. Lewis

> Veterinary dentistry is an exacting science, in which decisions are made not only for an individual patient, but also for individual teeth, which may vary in severity of disease. Multiple therapeutic decisions and treatment plans may be necessary for a single patient. Veterinary dental patients must be anesthetized to receive thorough treatment, which results in additional decisions that may not be necessary for human dental patients. This article discusses considerations and approaches toward therapeutic decision making and treatment planning in veterinary dentistry and oral surgery.

Oral and Dental Imaging Equipment and Techniques for Small Animals   489

Curt R. Coffman and Glenn M. Brigden

> In the diagnosis and treatment of oral and dental diseases in dogs and cats, digital intraoral radiography offers many advantages over the use of standard dental radiographic film, including rapid image generation, easier exposure correction, enhancement, and paperless storage. Digital image receptors can be divided into 2 main types, direct digital systems using charged coupled devices and complementary metal oxide semiconductor sensors, and indirect digital systems using phosphor plates with a computerized scanner. Each system is paired with a computer software system to allow handling, visualization, enhancement, sharing, and archiving of the images.

Clinical Canine Dental Radiography   507

Kristin M. Bannon

> The purpose of this article is to provide small animal veterinarians in private practice a guideline for interpretation of the most common findings in canine intraoral radiology. Normal oral and dental anatomy is presented. A brief review of variations of normal, common periodontal and endodontic pathology findings and developmental anomalies is provided.

Clinical Feline Dental Radiography   533

Matthew Lemmons

> Dental radiography is a necessary diagnostic modality in small animal practice. It is not possible to accurately assess and diagnose tooth resorption, periodontal disease, endodontic disease, neoplasia and injury without it. Dental radiography is also necessary for treatment and assessment of the patient postoperatively.

Oral Inflammation in Small Animals   555

Milinda J. Lommer

> The oral cavity can be affected by a wide variety of disorders characterized by inflammation of the gingiva and/or oral mucosa. In dogs and cats, differential diagnoses for generalized oral inflammatory disorders include plaque-reactive mucositis, chronic gingivostomatitis, eosinophilic granuloma complex, pemphigus and pemphigoid disorders, erythema multiforme, and systemic lupus erythematosus. In addition, endodontic or periodontal abscesses, infectious conditions, reactive lesions, and neoplastic conditions may initially present with localized or generalized inflammation of the oral mucosa. Determination of the underlying cause of an oral inflammatory condition relies on a thorough history, complete physical and oral examination, and incisional biopsy and histopathologic examination of lesions.

Exodontics: Extraction of Teeth in the Dog and Cat   573

Bill Gengler

> Dental disease can have a profound effect on the comfort and well-being of pets. Oral disease can be difficult to detect. Patients often hide their discomfort. The identification and treatment or removal of diseased teeth are the responsibility of the veterinarian. When diseased teeth cannot be saved by specialized care, extraction of teeth is necessary. Proper extraction of teeth in dogs and cats can be challenging and frustrating, but with review of the oral anatomy, proper instrumentation, and gentle tissue-handling techniques, this can be a rewarding part of clinical practice.

Equipment for Oral Surgery in Small Animals   587

Alexander M. Reiter

> This article provides an overview of equipment used for oral surgery. Specific instruments and materials used when performing relevant operative procedures are also mentioned in other articles in this issue.

Oral and Maxillofacial Surgery in Dogs and Cats   609

Amalia M. Zacher and Sandra Manfra Marretta

> Advancements in diagnostic and treatment modalities for oral and maxillofacial surgery have allowed veterinarians to offer clients a range of alternatives for their pets. Categories of oral and maxillofacial surgery reviewed in this article include jaw fracture management, management of palatal/oronasal defects, recognition and treatment of oral masses, and management of several miscellaneous pathologic conditions. Miscellaneous oral lesions discussed in this article include odontogenic cysts, osteonecrosis and osteomyelitis, and lesions of the tongue and lips.

Laser and Radiosurgery in Veterinary Dentistry   651

Jan Bellows

> Lasers and radiosurgery frequently used in human dentistry are rapidly entering veterinary dental use. The carbon dioxide, diode, and low-level therapy lasers have features including hemostasis control, access to difficult to reach areas, and decreased pain, that make them useful for oral surgery. Periodontal pocket surgery, gingivectomy, gingivoplasty, gingival hyperplasia, operculectomy, tongue surgery, oropharyngeal inflammation therapy, oral mass surgery, crown, and frenectomy laser surgeries are described, including images.

Anesthesia and Pain Management for Small Animals   669

Brett Beckman

> Anesthesia for oral surgery in dogs and cats requires special consideration and thorough planning to maximize patient safety. Well-trained technical staff capable of providing expedient delivery of quality dental radiographs and precision anesthesia monitoring are essential. Doctors need to be well versed in dental radiographic interpretation and competent and experienced in oral surgical techniques, particularly in surgical extractions. The work flow from patient induction to recovery involves estimate generation and client communication with multiple staff members. Knowledge of anesthetic and analgesic agents from premedication to postoperative pain management play an equally important role in patient safety.

Index   689

VETERINARY CLINICS OF NORTH AMERICA: SMALL ANIMAL PRACTICE

FORTHCOMING ISSUES

July 2013
Emergency Medicine
Justine A. Lee, DVM, DACVECC and
Lisa L. Powell, DVM, DACVECC, *Editors*

September 2013
Clinical Pharmacology and Therapeutics
Katrina L. Mealey, DVM, PhD, *Editor*

November 2013
Clinical Pathology and Diagnostic Testing
Mary Jo Burkhard, DVM, PhD and
Maxey Wellman, DVM, PhD, *Editors*

RECENT ISSUES

March 2013
Feline Diabetes
Jacquie S. Rand, BVSc, DVSc, MANZVS,
Editor

January 2013
Clinical Dermatology
Daniel O. Morris, DVM, MPH, DACVD and
Robert A. Kennis, DVM, MS, DACVD,
Editors

November 2012
Otology and Otic Disease
Bradley L. Njaa, DVM, MVSc and
Lynette K. Cole, DVM, MS, *Editors*

RELATED INTEREST

Veterinary Clinics of North America: Exotic Animal Practice
May 2013 (Vol. 16, No. 2)
New and Emerging Diseases
Sue Chen, DVM and Nicole Wyre, DVM, *Editors*

THE CLINICS ARE NOW AVAILABLE ONLINE!
Access your subscription at:
www.theclinics.com

Preface

Clinical Veterinary Dentistry

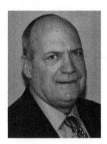

Steven E. Holmstrom, DVM, DAVDC
Editor

Most recently, small animal dental editions of *Veterinary Clinics of North America* have been published in 1986, 1992 (feline), 1998 (canine), and 2005. This issue of *Veterinary Clinics of North America* serves as a clinically oriented update on veterinary dentistry. Veterinary dentistry is best practiced as an annual renewable service of every dog and cat every year of their life. It is our goal to aid the day-to-day practitioner in their practice of providing quality dental service for their clients and their patients.

Oral care is essential for optimum health and quality of life. There is a standard of care that must be provided for veterinary services; this standard is documented in the first article. Many therapeutic and decision-making skills are used in planning and executing this standard of care, as covered in the second article.

Arguably the most important advancement in veterinary dentistry in the past decade is the addition of digital intraoral radiography. Three articles are devoted to this very important area in veterinary dentistry. The articles include oral and dental imaging equipment and techniques to get good intraoral radiographs, and the interpretation of these radiographs for dogs and cats.

Oral inflammation in both the dog and the cat continues to be a challenge to the practitioner. The reality is that many problems can be solved by extraction of the teeth; therefore, an article has been devoted to simple and surgical exodontia. The veterinarian is often called on to surgically treat maxillofacial disease and one article has been devoted to equipment, whereas another article has been devoted to the surgical treatment of various oral conditions. The article includes congenital malformation, fractures, and neoplasia.

An article has been devoted to the technologies of laser and electro/radiosurgery. And last, but not least, a clinical update on anesthesia and pain management has been included. The understanding of pain and its control has gone hand in hand with the development of veterinary dentistry.

It is hoped that this edition will aid the day-to-day practitioner in the practice of this discipline. It is a compilation of work by veterinary dentists involved both in private

Vet Clin Small Anim 43 (2013) ix–x
http://dx.doi.org/10.1016/j.cvsm.2013.02.013
0195-5616/13/$ – see front matter © 2013 Published by Elsevier Inc.

vetsmall.theclinics.com

practice and at universities. I would like to thank the veterinary dental community for their generosity in the sharing of knowledge that has taken place on almost a daily basis over the Internet and on a yearly basis at such meetings as the Veterinary Dental Forum (www.veterinarydentalforum.com). Such sharing, as well as the individual contributions herein, helped to make this issue possible.

Steven E. Holmstrom, DVM, DAVDC
Animal Dental Clinic
987 Laurel Street
San Carlos, CA 94070, USA

E-mail address:
steve@toothvet.info

Standard of Care in North American Small Animal Dental Service

Edward R. Eisner, AB, DVM

KEYWORDS

- Dental guidelines • American Veterinary Dental College (AVDC) position statement
- General practitioner standard of care • Specialist standard of care

KEY POINTS

- *The continually increasing dynamic of standard of care.* Technological developments such as facsimiles and electronic mail that transmit laboratory information, Federal Express and similar overnight couriers for transportation of laboratory specimens, and telemedical consultations for diagnostic information and therapeutic advice are now in widespread use. It is important to realize that rural practices today have the ability to practice at a much higher clinical level than in former years, and should be expected to do so.
- *Standard of care.* The standard of care can be elusive. It actually refers to an abstract standard, generally controlled jurisdictionally by State or Provincial Boards of Veterinary Medicine that have the power to administer their regional, legal Practice Act. The state and provincial Practice Acts consist of the Act itself as well as associated rules and regulations.
- *Standard of care for general practitioners.* Standard of care in general practice is peer-regulated, and is measured as the level of care provided and acceptable among most veterinarians in a given geographic area.
- *Standard of care for specialists.* In the case of specialists, very specific parameters of competence make up their minimum acceptable standard of care.
- *American Animal Hospital Association dental guidelines.* The guidelines provide advice for the practice of companion animal dentistry at a general practice level.
- *Future guidance to ruling medical boards.* Guidance to ruling medical boards in the not too distant future may well be given by the specialty organization of each medical discipline, such as The American Veterinary Dental College for the veterinary dental profession. The specialty organization will provide guidance to ruling medical boards regarding a recommended standard of care, rather than such standards being defined by geographic boundaries.

Dental Department, Animal Hospital Specialty Center, 5640 County Line Place, Suite One, Highlands Ranch, CO 80121-3924, USA
E-mail address: dog2thdoc@gmail.com

Vet Clin Small Anim 43 (2013) 447–469
http://dx.doi.org/10.1016/j.cvsm.2013.02.002
0195-5616/13/$ – see front matter © 2013 Elsevier Inc. All rights reserved.

INTRODUCTION

Standard of care in veterinary medicine can be very elusive to specifically identify and regulate. It is described as the level of practice performance that is customarily acceptable by peers for a given geographic area. Guidelines for appropriate level of small animal practice in North America have changed over time. An acceptable standard of care has been rising on a parallel track that can be associated with continual urbanization, educational advances, technological improvements, and consumer demand.

HISTORY OF VETERINARY DENTAL ADVANCEMENT
General Considerations

Dentistry for animals has been performed since 600 BCE (Before Common Era) on equines by the Chinese, and in 333 BCE Aristotle gave an account of periodontal disease. Understandably its first popular service in a current era was for horses, as they were ubiquitous for transportation, agricultural work, and pleasure throughout Europe and the Americas. The first veterinary dental text was published in 1889, followed by books in 1905 and 1938. Small animal dentistry has been a part of general practice since the 1930s. In the first 75 years of the twentieth century veterinary dentistry consisted mostly of tooth extractions and dental cleanings, and then usually only in the cases of fulminating abscesses or overwhelming infection. In the mid-1970s a veterinary dental evolution emerged, mostly in the United States, and to a limited level in Europe. In the 1980s and 1990s dental disciplines of endodontic, periodontal, restorative, and orthodontic care were developed by an emerging small cadre of new dental specialists, board-certified veterinarians recognized by the American Veterinary Medical Association (AVMA) as dental experts. The technology developed because of increasing consumer demand, a phenomenon that promotes many technological advances. Services appear when people are both willing to pay for them and are dissatisfied with lesser service.

Standard of care in general practice differs from that at the expert level. To become an entry-level expert, also referred to as a specialist, one must meet demanding standards set by the American Veterinary Board of Specialists (ABVS), a registered arm of the AVMA. Becoming an entry-level expert in a specialty organization implies that the individual awarded this recognition has passed rigorous credential requirements and has passed a multipart qualifying examination that satisfies both the ABVS and the individual specialty organization (SO). In the case of dentistry, the SO is the American Veterinary Dental College (AVDC). The AVDC qualifying examination consists of 3 parts: a written examination testing knowledge of the literature, a clinically oriented examination testing specific knowledge of clinical aspects of practice, and a practical examination that demonstrates expert skill in performing dental procedures. All 3 portions of the examination must be passed and an individual's redacted examination performance approved by an examination committee. Their committee report must then be approved by the AVDC Board of Directors before an individual is identified and declared a veterinary dental specialist. So in the case of specialists, very specific parameters of competence make up their minimum acceptable standard of care.

In general practice dental guidelines, such as the ones prepared by the American Animal Hospital Association (AAHA), help define an expected goal for the standard of care. The AAHA dental care guidelines are built on the premise that "dental care is necessary to provide optimum health and quality of life (Appendix I: Dental Guidelines)."[1] Diseases of the oral cavity, if left untreated, are often painful and can contribute to other local or systemic diseases. The purpose of the AAHA dental guidelines is "to provide advice for the practice of companion animal dentistry"[1] at a general practice level. This article refers to these guidelines from time to time, because the credibility of AAHA is very high and the task force that created them included both dental specialists and veterinary generalists (see guidelines in Appendix I).

The standard of care can be elusive. It actually refers to an abstract, dynamic standard, generally controlled jurisdictionally by state or provincial boards of veterinary medicine that have the power to administer their regional, legal Practice Act. The state and provincial Practice Acts consist of the Act itself as well as associated rules and regulations. Standard of care is thus peer-regulated, and is measured as the level of care provided and acceptable among the majority of veterinarians in a given geographic area. The state or provincial boards of veterinary medicine, through the Act and its rules and regulations, approve professional licensing, make rulings, and deliver discipline when the Act is violated. The medical boards in the United States are made up of a small group of gubernatorially appointed members, both veterinarians and consumers. These appointments are political, providing peer representation that is neither especially above average nor below average: simply peer veterinarians and consumers actively involved in animal organizations or production, such as being breeders or representatives of cattle associations, and so forth. The function of a Board of Veterinary Medicine is to process licensing and discipline cases of violation of their Practice Act. The Board of Medicine has a consumer-protection role, differing somewhat from a State Veterinary Medical Association, the role of which is to function as a veterinarian's advocate. In the United States, oversight for the board itself falls under the realm of the state legislatures. Membership of the Board of Medicine is term-limited. Usually board structure is such that a small percentage of each board membership is refreshed at regular intervals so as to maintain continuity, as well as to gain new and contemporary perspective regarding medicine as it is being practiced during any given time.

At present, technological developments such as facsimiles and electronic mail that transmit laboratory information, Federal Express and similar overnight couriers for transportation of laboratory specimens, and telemedical consultations for diagnostic information and therapeutic advice are in widespread use. Rural practices today have the ability to practice at much higher clinical levels than in former years, and should be expected to do so.

Medical Board license requirements have relaxed their formerly more restrictive covenants for residents with licensees from out-of-state who desire to move their practice across state borders. Interstate license endorsement predominates for veterinarians with active licenses who are unencumbered by disciplinary actions.

The author's thesis is that determining the future standard of care will become the responsibility of the guiding organization of each medical discipline, such as the AVDC for the veterinary dental profession, to provide guidance to ruling medical boards regarding a recommended standard of care, rather than such standards being defined by geographic boundaries. Within each medical discipline it becomes appropriate that specialists, or people who hold themselves out to be specialists, be held to a higher standard than generalists. Generalists and specialists each operate to an acceptable standard of care commensurate with their training.

The veterinary profession operates within a peer-policing format. Veterinarians who perform veterinary dentistry, as with other veterinary disciplines, are expected by their peers to perform as patient advocates and watchdogs, protecting naïve consumers, and establishing and maintaining within the veterinarian's discipline what have become the generally accepted standards of care. As technology and consumer demand increase, even today's acceptable standard of care will be gradually elevated to new levels of practice performance in the future.

In this article the author shares his thoughts, as well as the thoughts of others in the field of state veterinary advocates (State Veterinary Medical Associations), disciplinary specialists (members of State Medical Boards), and veterinary dentistry (Diplomates of the AVDC, as well as general practitioners performing dentistry in veterinary practice situations). First, what is expected at the specialist level is described, because it is more precise and quantified, having been defined by successfully passing a qualifying examination in the field. Second, the author explains what sensibly, in today's marketplace, should be the standard of care in veterinary practice performed by general practitioners whose licenses proclaim that they are qualified to practice medicine, surgery, and dentistry in their defined geographic confines. Included is information drawn from the AVDC Position Statement on Dental Health Care Providers (Appendix II: Dental Health Care Providers),[2] and the AVDC Position Statement on Nonprofessional Dental Scaling (Appendix III: Dental Scaling Without Anesthesia).[3,4]

Specialty Practice Dental Standard of Care, 2013

Specialty organization and client expectations
Specialist expected level of practice

- *Anesthesia and pain management.* Although this is not really dentistry, it is an important consideration when performing dentistry. It is expected that a dental specialist will, first and foremost, do no harm and will cause as little discomfort for his patients as is necessary to accomplish the dental service being performed. Anesthesia makes a patient compliant, but often does not provide pain relief. A dental specialist should be skilled in providing local and general injectable anesthesia appropriate for the procedure at hand. His or her knowledge and skills should also include providing inhalant general anesthesia and perioperative pain control in a timely fashion to prevent "pain wind-up." In other words, pain management should be used before painful procedures are begun, continued during the procedure, and be extended not only to the anesthetic recovery period but also postoperatively in the form of dispensed or prescribed medication to be administered by the animal owner for a sufficient period of time to ensure patient comfort. The protocol for ensuring comfort should be at the discretion of the clinician, and adjusted intraoperatively, if patient pain is observed.
- *Oral anatomy.* A specialist should possess knowledge of normal anatomy, as well as developmental, genetic, and acquired abnormalities.
- *Diagnostics.* A higher level of diagnostics, including a greater variety of case assessment, is expected of a specialist. These techniques include, but are not limited to, being competent in performing intraoral imaging and its assessment by means of intraoral radiography. Awareness of the value of computed axial tomography and magnetic resonance imaging techniques is expected. These modalities or the referral of these modalities should be offered appropriately, in accordance with individual case parameters.
- *Orthodontics and interceptive orthodontics.* A specialist should be able to recognize abnormal conditions and implement breeding and therapeutic advice and treatment, including appropriate extraction(s), according to his or her personal philosophy and professional judgment.
- *Prophylactic dental hygiene.* A dental expert should be able to show proficiency and familiarity with dental prophylaxis, and home hygiene techniques and products.
- *Periodontics.* A dental specialist is expected to be proficient in identifying and treating the most frequently encountered conditions. He or she should have moderate surgical tissue skills, and the ability to perform simple and surgical extractions on dogs and cats.

- *Tooth erosions in dogs and cats.* A dental Diplomate should be able to provide accurate assessment and therapeutic recommendations and treatment in line with current scientific thought, in concert with acceptable classification of stage and type of abnormality encountered.
- *Endodontics.* Veterinary dentists should be able to identify and classify fractured teeth, determine tooth vitality and health, and be able to effectively counsel animal owners and provide appropriate endodontic therapy or extraction.
- *Maxillofacial surgery.* A dental expert should be able to identify and assess injury, and be competent to treat or refer for therapy to satisfy the level of the client's wishes.
- *Restorative procedures.* A dental specialist should be able to identify pathologic conditions in need of restorative treatment, and be competent to place direct or indirect restorations, in accordance with the level of abnormality and satisfaction of the client's wishes.

Legal concerns

A board-certified veterinary dentist does not always have to be right. A specialist is expected to have an above-average level of knowledge and to apply that knowledge in a scientific evidence-based method. Difficulties may occur because some cases are difficult. Some clients are guilty of neglect or do not comply with instructions. A general practitioner, the source of specialist referral, may be guilty of neglect or practicing beyond his or her level of competence. A specialist may also be guilty of neglect. Some patients do not comply with owners' attempts at treatment aftercare. Consequently, the prognosis is not always "excellent," and not every case ends successfully. Some clients can accept this, and some cannot. A client does not have to be correct in an accusation to have either the right or the justification to complain to the ruling Board of Medicine, or to sue a veterinarian in a court of law. However, legality remains in the realm of the attorneys and the courts; standard of care, on the other hand is determined by peer review.

General Practice Standard of Care in Dentistry, 2013

Client and peer expectations

Client expectations Professionalism is what clients want. Clients want understandable explanations, an examination that is thorough and accompanied by an accurate assessment, a written therapeutic plan with a written fee estimate, treatments or procedures competently delivered, timely service, a prognosis, and a follow-up plan.

General practitioner peer (Board of Medicine) expected level of practice AAHA dental guidelines are different from the AAHA standards for accreditation. The Standards are AAHA requirements that must be met in order for a hospital to be accepted as an AAHA member hospital; the extent to which the standards are met determines the level of AAHA accreditation that is awarded. On the other hand, there are no hoops for a practitioner to jump through, no absolutes to be met, no specific requirements or membership that must be reached to be grouped under the umbrella of AAHA dental guidelines; these are guidelines provided in the interest of ensuring reasonable patient management in general practice (see Appendix I).[1]

The AAHA Guidelines express it well. "The veterinarian is obligated to practice within the scope of his or her education, training, and experience."[1]

- *Anesthesia and pain management.* The generalist veterinarian, like the specialist, should cause no harm and as little pain as possible, before, during, and after a dental procedure. Like the dental specialist, anesthetic protocol and pain management is subject to professional discretion, but should be provided within the guidelines of humane procedure management for any given case. The one modality that is substandard for the dental generalist and specialist alike is what is commonly referred to as "anesthesia-free" dentistry, because neither the patient nor its teeth are well served (see Appendix III).[3] With anesthesia-free dentistry, intraoral radiographs cannot be taken, while performing routine dental prophylaxis the distal (caudal) teeth (which typically accumulate the heaviest dental deposits) cannot be adequately cleaned, and the palatal/lingual surfaces of the teeth cannot be cleaned appropriately. In addition, subgingival curettage, so important in reducing oral malodor and infection, cannot be performed.[1–3]

- *Oral anatomy.* As a licensed, graduate veterinarian, an individual is expected to have knowledge of normal anatomy, and conversely be able to identify that there is a pathologic condition present when the anatomy is abnormal.
- *Diagnostics.* A veterinarian licensed to practice dentistry should be able to provide accurate dental charting in his or her medical records, and perform diagnostic quality dental radiography.
- *Orthodontics.* Having knowledge of normal anatomy, a general practitioner should be able to recognize an abnormal occlusion and to triage necessary treatment, including performing appropriate extraction(s).
- *Prophylactic dental hygiene.* Veterinarians in general practice should be able to demonstrate proficiency and familiarity with dental prophylaxis, home hygiene techniques, and oral hygiene products.
- *Periodontics.* General practitioners should be able to demonstrate competency in identifying and treating the most frequently encountered conditions; they should have moderate surgical tissue skills, and the ability to perform simple and surgical extractions on dogs and cats.
- *Tooth erosions in dogs and cats.* General practitioners should be able to identify and classify tooth erosions and classify them for stage and type of abnormality, and recommend treatment or refer to a specialist for treatment.
- *Endodontics.* A general practitioner should be able to identify fractured, infected, or nonvital teeth, and determine client wishes regarding salvage or removal of traumatically or atraumatically affected teeth. General practitioners should be familiar with the value of treatment by root canal therapy compared with that of extraction. Practitioners should be able to treat or be willing and able to recommend referral to a specialist for treatment, if so desired by a client.
- *Maxillofacial surgery.* General practitioners, licensed to practice medicine, surgery, and dentistry, should be able to identify injury and be able to competently treat or refer to a specialist for therapy, to satisfy the level of the client's wishes and the needs of the patient.
- *Restorative procedures.* General practitioners should be able to identify pathologic disorder in need of treatment. The practitioner should be able to treat or be willing to refer to a specialist for therapy, to satisfy the level of the client's wishes and the patient's needs.

Legal concerns

Practicing veterinarians who have active licenses are expected to not only practice within their level of competence but also to have general knowledge of a source of higher knowledge and competence in their field. If there is a better way to treat a condition than at their facility, they are expected to apprise their client of such services and, should the client wish to avail themselves of these services, facilitate a referral to a specialist.

SUMMARY

At present, technological developments, such as facsimiles and electronic mail that transmit laboratory information, Federal Express and similar overnight couriers for transportation of laboratory specimen, and telemedical consultations for diagnostic information and therapeutic advice are in widespread use. Because of these dynamics, it is important to realize that rural practices today have the ability to practice at a much higher clinical level than in former years, and should be expected to do so. Therefore, in the future it should become the burden of the guiding organization of each medical discipline, such as the AVDC for the veterinary dental profession, to provide guidance to ruling medical boards regarding a recommended standard of care, rather than such standards being defined by geographic boundaries.

REFERENCES

1. American Animal Hospital Association guidelines for dental care, 2012. American Veterinary Dental College position statement on dental health care providers. Available at: www.aaha.org. Accessed date Mar 29, 2013.
2. American Veterinary Dental College position statement on dental health care providers. Adopted by the Board of Directors, April 2004. Available at: www.avdc.org (follow link first to information for animal owners, then to position statements). Accessed date March 28, 2013.
3. American Veterinary Dental College position statement on nonprofessional dental scaling. Available at: www.avdc.org (follow link first to information for animal owners, then on the left sidebar to dental scaling without anesthesia). Accessed Mar 28, 2013.
4. Eisner ER. Colorado Veterinary Medical Association quarterly newsletter. Dental radiographs are becoming the standard of care. CVMA Voice 2012;2:28–9.

APPENDIX I: 2013 AAHA DENTAL CARE GUIDELINES FOR DOGS AND CATS[a]

Steven E. Holmstrom, DVM, DAVDC*, Jan Bellows, DVM, DAVDC, DABVP,
Stephen Juriga, DVM, DAVDC, Kate Knutson, DVM,
Brook A. Niemiec, DVM, DAVDC, Jeanne Perrone, CVT, VTS (Dentistry)

---

[a] This document is intended as a guideline only. Evidence-based support for specific recommendations has been cited whenever possible and appropriate. Other recommendations are based on practical clinical experience and a consensus of expert opinion. Further research is needed to document some of these recommendations. Because each case is different, veterinarians must base their decisions and actions on the best available scientific evidence, in conjunction with their own expertise, knowledge, and experience. These guidelines are supported by generous educational grants from Hill's Pet Nutrition, Merial, Ltd., Virbac Animal Health, and PDx BioTech, and are endorsed by the American Veterinary Dental College.
From the Animal Dental Clinic, San Carlos, CA (S.H.); All Pets Dental Clinic, Weston, FL (J.B.); Veterinary Dental Center, River Heights Veterinary Hospital, Oswego, IL (S.J.); Pet Crossing Animal Hospital & Dental Clinic, Bloomington, MN (K.K.); California Veterinary Dental Specialties, San Diego, CA (B.N.); and Tampa Bay Veterinary Dentistry, Largo, FL (J.P.).
* Corresponding author.
E-mail address: Toothvet@sbcglobal.net

ABSTRACT

Veterinary dentistry is constantly progressing. The purpose of this document is to provide guidelines for the practice of companion animal dentistry for the veterinary profession. Dental care is necessary to provide optimum health and optimize quality of life. Untreated diseases of the oral cavity are painful and can contribute to local and systemic diseases. This article includes guidelines for preventive oral health care, client communication, evaluation, dental cleaning, and treatment. In addition, materials and equipment necessary to perform a medically appropriate procedure are described. (J Am Anim Hosp Assoc 2005;41:277–283. http://dx.doi.org/10.5326/JAAHA-MS-4013).

INTRODUCTION

Veterinary medical dental care is an essential component of a preventive health care plan. Quality dental care is necessary to provide optimum health and quality of life. If left untreated, diseases of the oral cavity are painful and can contribute to other local or systemic diseases.[1,2] The purpose of this document is to provide guidelines for the practice of companion animal dentistry. A list of definitions to enhance the understanding of this article is provided in **Table 1**.

The dental health care team is obligated to practice within the scope of their respective education, training, and experience. It is imperative that the dental health care team remains current with regard to oral care, operative procedures, materials, equipment, and products. The team members must attain appropriate continuing education through courses such as those offered by the American Animal Hospital Association, the American Veterinary Medical Association, the annual Veterinary Dental Forum, industry and private facilities; by reading the Journal of Veterinary Dentistry; and by reading other appropriate journals and medical texts.[3–7]

FACILITY REQUIREMENTS

Dental procedures result in aerosolized bacteria and particulate matter. Using a dedicated space is recommended for nonsterile dental procedures. The dedicated dental space must be separate from the sterile surgical suite and needs to be placed in a low-traffic area. New practices and those planning on remodeling should incorporate a separate dental suite into the blueprint.

Appropriate ventilation and anesthetic scavenging systems must also be used. Low-heat, high-intensity lighting, and equipment for magnifying the target area are required to adequately and safely visualize the oral cavity and its structures. The operating table must allow for drainage and be constructed of impervious, cleanable material.

MATERIALS, INSTRUMENTS, AND EQUIPMENT

As with dental techniques, it is important to keep the dental materials up-to-date and veterinarians must be aware of what materials are considered appropriate for the treatment of dental conditions. Commonly used materials can be found by consulting a dental text and attending continuing education programs presented by a dental specialist.

Instruments and dental equipment require routine and frequent maintenance. Maintenance information can be found in some dental texts and through the manufacturer. Instruments must be sharp and properly stored, and instruments in poor condition need to be replaced. A written protocol needs to be established and followed for equipment and instrument care. As with human dentistry, instruments that enter the oral cavity should be sterilized. Packets organized by dental procedure (e.g., examination, extraction, periodontal surgery) should be prepared and sterilized before use.

Table 1
Definitions that pertain to dental guidelines[a]

Term	Definition
Dental chart	A written and graphical representation of the mouth, with adequate space to indicate pathology and procedures (see **Table 5** for included items)
Dental prophylaxis	A procedure performed on a healthy mouth that includes oral hygiene care, a complete oral examination, and techniques to prevent disease and to remove plaque and calculus from the teeth above and beneath the gum line before periodontitis has developed
Dentistry	The evaluation, diagnosis, prevention, and/or treatment of abnormalities in the oral cavity, maxillofacial area, and/or associated structures. Nonsurgical, surgical, or related procedures may be included
Endodontics	The treatment and therapy of diseases of the pulp canal system
Exodontia (extraction)	A surgical procedure performed to remove a tooth
Gingivitis	Inflammation of the gingiva without loss of the supporting structure(s) shown with X-ray
Oral surgery	The surgical invasion and manipulation of hard and soft tissue to improve/restore oral health and comfort
Orthodontics	The evaluation and treatment of malpositioned teeth for the purposes of improving occlusion and patient comfort and enhancing the quality of life
Periodontal disease	A disease process that begins with gingivitis and progresses to periodontitis when left untreated
Periodontitis	A destructive process involving the loss of supportive structures of the teeth, including the periodontium, gingiva, periodontal ligament, cementum, and/or alveolar bone
Periodontal surgery	The surgical treatment of periodontal disease. This is indicated for patients with pockets . 5 mm, class II or III furcation exposure, or inaccessible areas
Periodontal therapy	Treatment of tooth-supporting structures where periodontal disease exists. This involves the nonsurgical removal of plaque, calculus, and debris in pockets; and the local application of antimicrobials
Periodontium	The supporting structures of the teeth, including the periodontal ligament, gingiva, cementum, and alveolar and supporting bone
Pocket	A pathologic space between supporting structures and the tooth, extending apically from the normal site of the gingival epithelial attachment

[a] Some of these definitions were derived from descriptions in Holmstrom et al. (2004).[3]

Recommended materials, instruments, and equipment for performing dental procedures are listed in **Tables 2** and **3**. Consult the reference list associated with these guidelines for recommendations and information on ordering equipment.[3–7]

OPERATOR PROTECTION

Pathogens and debris such as calculus, tooth fragments, and prophy paste are aerosolized during dental procedures. Irrigating the oral cavity with a 0.12% chlorhexidine solution before dental scaling decreases bacterial aerosolization.[8]

Table 2
Materials needed for the practice of veterinary dentistry[a]

Necessary materials
  Antiseptic rinse
  Prophy paste/pumice
  Prophy angle and cups
  Hemostatic agents
  Sealant
  Needles and syringes
  Intraoral digital system or radiographic film
  Measures to prevent hypothermia (e.g., conductive blanket, hot air blanket, circulating
    water blanket, towels, blankets)
  Gauze and sponges
  Antimicrobial agent for local application
  Suture material (4-0 and smaller)
  Bone augmentation material
  Local anesthetic drugs
Necessary equipment
  Equipment to expose and process intraoral digital radiograph system orintraoral films
  Suction
  A high- and low-speed delivery system for air and water
  Fiber optic light source
  Equipment for sterilizing instruments
  Low- and high-speed hand pieces (minimum two of each)
  Various sizes of round/diamond and cross cut fissure burrs
  Powered scaler with tips for gross and subgingival scaling (ultrasonic, subsonic, or
    piezoelectric)
  Head or eye loupes for magnification

[a] Please note that disposable items are for single use only.

The safety of the operator must be ensured during dental procedures by using radiographic, oral, respiratory, skin, eye, and ear protective devices (**Table 4**). Ergonomic considerations include proper seating, fatigue mats for standing, and proper positioning of both the patient and materials to minimize immediate and chronic operator injuries. Provide the operator with instruction on proper instrument handling techniques.

Table 3
Instruments to include in the dental surgical pack[a]

Scalers
Curettes
Probes/explorer
Sharpening materials
Scalpel
Extraction equipment (e.g., periosteal elevators, luxating elevators, periodontal elevators,
  extraction forceps, root tip picks, root tip forceps)
Thumb forceps
Hemostats
Iris, LaGrange, Mayo, or Metzenbaum scissors
Needle holders
Mouth mirror
Retraction aid (e.g., University of Minnesota retractor)

[a] Instruments must be sterilized by accepted techniques prior to each use. Hand instruments must by properly sharpened and cared for.

Table 4
Minimum protective devices to be used during dental procedures
Cap or hair bonnet
Mask
Goggles, surgical spectacles, or face shield
Smock
Gloves
Earplugs
Dosimeter
Protection from radiation (e.g., lead shield)

PATIENT ASSESSMENT
History and Physical Examination

The history must include prior home dental hygiene delivered by the client; diet; access to treats and chews; chewing habits; current and previous dental care and procedures; prior and current diseases, including any behavioral issues and allergies; and medications or supplements currently administered. Perform a physical examination of all body systems based on the species, age, health status, and temperament of the animal. If the patient is presented for a complaint not related to dentistry, give due consideration to the primary complaint, performing the diagnostic tests and treatments indicated. Establish priorities if multiple procedures are indicated.

Assessment by Life Stage

Focus on age-related dental conditions and common abnormalities in the dog and cat. From birth to 9 mo of age, evaluate the patient for problems related to the deciduous teeth, missing or extra teeth, swellings, juvenile diseases (such as feline juvenile onset periodontitis), occlusion, and oral development. From 5 mo to 2 yr of age, evaluate the patient for problems related to developmental anomalies, permanent dentition, and the accumulation of plaque and calculus. Periodontal diseases may begin during that time period, especially in cats and small-breed dogs. The onset and severity of periodontal diseases varies widely depending on breed, diet, and home dental care. In a small-breed dog without home dental care, periodontal diseases can start as early as 9 mo of age. In a large-breed dog, periodontal diseases may not start until later. Many small-breed dogs have periodontal diseases by 3 yr of age.[9–12] Beyond 2 yr of age, evaluate the progression of periodontal diseases, damage to tooth structures, occurrence of oral masses, and the existence and adequacy of preventive home dental care. As the animal ages, continue to evaluate the patient for progressive periodontal diseases, oral tumors, and other aspects of dental pathology.[13]

Oral/Dental Examination in the Conscious Patient

Record all findings in the medical record (**Table 5**). Evaluate the head and oral cavity both visually and by palpation. Changes in body weight, eating habits, or other behaviors can indicate dental disease. Specific abnormal signs to look for may include pain; halitosis; drooling; dysphagia; asymmetry; tooth resorption; discolored, fractured, mobile, missing, or extra teeth; inflammation and bleeding; loss of gingiva and bone; and changes in the range of motion or pain in the temporomandibular joint. In addition, the practitioner should assess the patient's occlusion to ensure it is normal, or at least atraumatic. Evaluate the patient's eyes, lymph nodes, nose, lips, teeth, mucous membranes, gingiva, vestibule (i.e., the area between the gum tissue and

Table 5
Items to include in the dental chart and/or medical record
Signalment
Physical examination, medical, and dental history findings
Oral examination findings
Anesthesia and surgery monitoring log and surgical findings
Any dental, oral, or other disease(s) currently present in the animal
Abnormal probing depths (described for each affected tooth)
Dentition chart with specific abnormalities noted, such as discoloration; worn areas; missing, malpositioned, or fractured teeth; supernumerary, tooth resorption; and soft-tissue masses
Current and future treatment plan, addressing all abnormalities found. This includes information regarding initial decisions, decision-making algorithm, and changes based on subsequent findings
Recommendations for home dental care
Any recommendations declined by the client
Prognosis

cheeks), palatal and lingual surfaces of the mouth, dorsal and ventral aspects of the tongue, tonsils, and salivary glands and ducts. Note all abnormalities such as oral tumors, ulcers, or wounds. A diagnostic test strip for the measurement of dissolved thiol levels can be used as an exam room indicator of gingival health and periodontal status.[14]

The oral examination performed on a conscious patient allows the practitioner to design a preliminary diagnostic plan. Take into consideration potential patient pain. Do not offend the patient by probing unnecessarily when such manipulations can be better achieved under anesthesia. Also, realize in many instances that the examiner will underestimate the conditions present because it is impossible to visualize all oral structures when the patient is awake. It is only when the patient has been anesthetized that a complete and thorough oral evaluation can be accomplished successfully. The complete examination includes a tooth-by-tooth visual examination, probing, and radiographic examination. Only then can a precise treatment plan and fees for proposed services be tabulated and discussed with the pet owner(s).

MAKING RECOMMENDATIONS AND CLIENT EDUCATION

Discuss the findings of the initial examination and additional diagnostic and/or therapeutic plans with the client. Those plans will vary depending on the patient; the initial findings; the client's ability to proceed with the recommendations; as well as the client's ability to provide necessary, lifelong plaque prevention.

When either an anesthetic examination or procedure is not planned in a healthy patient, discuss preventive health care, oral health, and home oral hygiene. Options include brushing and the use of dentifrices, oral rinses, gels and sprays, water additives, and dental diets and chews. Discourage any dental chew or device that does not bend or break easily (e.g., bones, cow/horse hooves, antlers, hard nylon products). The Veterinary Oral Health Council lists products that meet its preset standard for the retardation of plaque and calculus accumulation.[15] Illustrate to the owner how to perform oral hygiene, such as brushing, wiping teeth, application of teeth-coating materials, and the use of oral rinses and gels. Allow the client to practice so they will be able to perform the agreed-upon procedure(s) at home.

All home oral hygiene options, from diet to the gold standard of brushing, along with any of their potential limitations need to be discussed with the client. It is essential that the oral health medical plan is patient-individualized to attain the greatest level of client compliance. For example, "dental" diets and chews can be used until the client is comfortable either brushing or applying an antiplaque gel, rinse, or spray with a wipe. The gold standard is brushing the pet's teeth using a brush with soft bristles either once or twice daily. If the client is either unable or unwilling to persevere with brushing, use any of the other oral hygiene options that the patient will tolerate.

Explain the two-part process involved in a diagnostic dental cleaning and patient evaluation to the client. It is critical that he/she understand the hospital protocol to minimize miscommunication and frustration. The procedure involves both an awake component and an anesthetized component for a complete evaluation. It is not until the oral radiographs have been evaluated that a full treatment plan including costs of the anticipated procedure(s) can be successfully made with any degree of accuracy.

Evaluation of a patient for dental disease involves the awake procedure as the first step. This is where an initial assessment is made. Although many problems may be seen at this point of the evaluation, a thorough diagnosis and treatment plan cannot be determined until charting, tooth-by-tooth examination of the anesthetized patient, and dental radiographs have been taken and evaluated. Studies have demonstrated that much of the pathology in a patient's oral cavity cannot be appreciated until dental radiographs are taken and assessed; therefore, have protocols in place within the practice to give clients ample time to make an informed decision on how they want to proceed with the proposed treatment plan.[16]

Some hospitals may want to do the awake examination and the anesthetic component (charting, cleaning, and dental radiographs) as the first procedure. They can then stage the treatment plan as a second procedure. This will give the hospital staff adequate time to explain to the client the treatment plan, including giving educational information on the diagnosis, reviewing radiographic findings, and going over costs. Other hospitals may want to perform the treatment plan during the first anesthetic event so everything is done at that procedure. Whichever way the hospital chooses, there must be a client communication plan in place so the client is involved and feels comfortable going forward with the proposed treatment plan.

Perform the anesthetized portion of the dental evaluation of charting, cleaning, and radiographs when abnormalities are seen on the awake exam (such plaque or tartar at the free gingival surface of the maxillary canines or fourth premolars) or at least on an annual basis starting at 1 yr of age for cats and small- to medium-breed dogs and at 2 yr of age for large-breed dogs. Details on the recommended frequency of examinations are discussed under Progress or Follow-Up Evaluation (below).

PLANNING THE DENTAL CLEANING AND PATIENT EVALUATION

Use well-monitored, inhalation anesthesia with cuffed intubation when performing dental cleanings. Such techniques increase safety, reduce stress, decrease the chances of adverse sequelae (e.g., inhalation pneumonia), and are essential for thorough and efficient evaluation and treatment of the patient. Attempting to perform procedures on an awake patient that is struggling, under sedation, or injectable anesthesia reduces the ability to make an accurate diagnosis, does not allow adequate treatment, and increases stress and risks to the patient.

Prior to Anesthesia

Preoperative evaluation includes a preanesthetic physical examination. It is crucial to follow the most up-to-date recommendations for preoperative laboratory testing based on the patient's life stage and any existing disease. Preoperative care includes

IV catheterization to facilitate administration of IV fluid therapy, preemptive pain management, and antibiotics (when indicated). Review the most up-to-date guidelines on anesthesia, antimicrobial use, fluid therapy, feline life stage, canine life stage, preventive health care, pain management, and referral for specific recommendations.[17–25]

Anesthesia

General anesthesia with intubation is necessary to properly assess and treat the companion animal dental patient. It is essential that aspiration of water and debris by the patient is prevented through endotracheal intubation. Cleaning a companion animal's teeth without general anesthesia is considered unacceptable and below the standard of care. Techniques such as necessary immobilization without discomfort, periodontal probing, intraoral radiology, and the removal of plaque and tartar above and below the gum line that ensure patient health and safety cannot be achieved without general anesthesia.[26]

During anesthesia, one trained person is dedicated to continuously monitoring and recording vital parameters, such as body temperature, heart rate and rhythm, respiration, oxygen saturation via pulse oximetry, systemic blood pressure, and end-tidal CO_2 levels q 5 min (or more frequently if sudden changes are noted).[27,28] IV fluid therapy is essential for circulatory maintenance. Customize the type and rate of fluids administered according to the patient's needs.[29,30]

Prevention of hypothermia with warming devices is essential because the patient may become wet, and dental procedures can be lengthy.[31,32] Additionally, suction and packing the caudal oral cavity with gauze can prevent aspiration and decrease hypothermia. If packing materials are used, steps must be taken to ensure there is no chance of the material being left behind following extubation. Regardless of whether packing is used, the last step prior to extubation is an examination of the caudal oral cavity to make certain no foreign material is left behind. Proper positioning of the patient by placing them in lateral recumbency can also help prevent aspiration. Provide safe immobilization of the head.

If oral surgery is planned, the institution of an intraoral local anesthetic is warranted in conjunction with the general anesthesia. This decreases the amount of general anesthetic needed and reduces the amount of systemic pain medication required postoperatively.[1,27,33] Local anesthetic blocks can last up to 8 hr, and they decrease hypotension and hypoventilation caused with inhalant anesthetics by reducing the amount of gas needed to maintain a safe anesthetic plane.[3,6,34,35]

DENTAL PROCEDURES

The terms prophy, prophylaxis, and dental are often misused in veterinary medicine. A professional dental cleaning is performed on a patient with plaque and calculus adhered to some of the teeth, but otherwise has an essentially healthy mouth or mild gingivitis only. The intent of dental cleaning is to prevent periodontitis. Patients with existing disease undergo periodontal therapy in addition to professional dental cleaning. Dental procedures must be performed by a licensed veterinarian, a credentialed technician, or a trained veterinary assistant under the supervision of a veterinarian in accordance with state or provincial practice acts. Practice acts vary from jurisdiction to jurisdiction, and the veterinarian must be familiar with those laws. Surgical extractions are to be performed only by trained, licensed veterinarians. All extractions need to have postextraction, intraoral radiographs. All dental procedures need to be described properly (see **Table 1**), and a consistent method should be used to record findings in the medical record (see **Table 5**).

Positioning and safety of the patient is important. Manually stabilize the head and neck when forces are being applied in the mouth. Avoid using mouth gags because they can cause myalgia, neuralgia, and/or trauma to the temporomandibular joint. If a mouth gag is necessary, do not fully open the mouth or overextend the temporomandibular joint. Never use spring-loaded mouth gags. Do not overinflate the endotracheal tube. Always disconnect the endotracheal tube when repositioning the patient to prevent trauma to the trachea.

Essential Steps for Professional Dental Cleaning

The essential steps for a professional dental cleaning and periodontal therapy are described in the following list:

1. Perform an oral evaluation, as described above, for the conscious patient.
2. Radiograph the entire mouth, using either intraoral or digital radiographic systems. Radiographs are necessary for accurate evaluation and diagnosis. In one published report, intraoral radiographs revealed clinically important pathology in 27.8% of dogs and 41.7% of cats when no abnormal findings were noted on the initial examination.[16] In patients with abnormal findings, radiography revealed additional pathology in 50% of dogs and 53.9% of cats.[16] Standard views of the skull are inadequate when evaluating dental pathology. If full mouth films are not taken, the client must be informed that they were not done.
3. Scale the teeth supra- and, most importantly, subgingivally using either a hand scaler or appropriate powered device followed by a hand instrument (i.e., scaler, curette). Do not use a rotary scaler, which excessively roughens the tooth enamel.[36]
4. Polish the teeth using a low-speed hand piece running at no more than 300 revolutions/min with prophy paste that is measured and loaded on a disposable prophy cup for each patient (to avoid cross-contamination).
5. Perform subgingival irrigation to remove debris and polishing paste and to inspect the crown and subgingival areas.
6. Apply antiplaque substances, such as sealants.
7. Provide instructions to the owner regarding home oral hygiene.

Additional Steps for Periodontal Therapy and Other Conditions

8. Evaluate the patient for abnormal periodontal pocket depths using a periodontal probe. The depth that is considered abnormal varies depending on the tooth and size of the dog or cat.[3,4,6,37] In medium-sized dogs, the probing depth should not be >2 mm, and in the mid-sized cats, the depth should not be >1 mm.
9. Perform periodontal therapy (see **Table 1**) based on radiographic findings and probing.[38–40]
10. Administer perioperative antibiotics when indicated, either parenterally or locally.[41,42]
11. Perform periodontal surgery to remove deep debris, eliminate pockets, and/or extract teeth. When either pockets or gingival recession is >50% of the root support, extraction or periodontal surgery is indicated and should be performed by trained veterinarians or referred to a specialist.
12. Biopsy all abnormal masses that are visualized grossly or noted on radiographs. Submit all samples for histopathology to be analyzed by a pathologist qualified in oral tissues analysis.[43]
13. Take postoperative radiographs to evaluate the treatment applied. This is especially important in extraction cases.

14. Examine and rinse the oral cavity. Remove any packing or foreign debris.
15. Recommend referral to a specialist when the primary veterinary practitioner does not have the skills, knowledge, equipment, or facilities to perform a specific procedure or treatment.

POSTOPERATIVE MANAGEMENT

Maintain an open airway via intubation until the animal is either swallowing or in sternal recumbency. Maintain body temperature and continue IV fluid support as needed. Continuously monitor and record vital signs until the patient is awake. Assess and record pain scores throughout the recovery period, continuing pain management while the pet is in the hospital and upon discharge.[34,44]

CLIENT EDUCATION AND FOLLOW-UP
Postoperative Communication

Client communication is fundamental to the maintenance of oral health. At the time of discharge, discuss all operative procedures and existing/potential complications (e.g., sedation, vocalization, bleeding, coughing, dehiscence, infection, neurologic signs, halitosis, vomiting, diarrhea, anorexia, signs of pain). Discuss immediate postoperative home oral hygiene, including medications and their side effects. Provide antibiotics and medication for inflammation and pain as indicated.[41,42] Discuss any change in diet that might be necessary, such as a change to either soft or premoistened food or to a prescription dental diet. Also indicate the duration of those changes. Provide individualized oral and written instructions at the time of discharge. Establish an appointment for a follow-up examination and further discussion.

Home Oral Hygiene

Home oral hygiene is vital for disease control. Telephone the client the day after the procedure to inquire about the pet's condition, to determine the client's ability to implement the medication and home oral hygiene plan, to answer questions, and address any concerns the client might have. The home oral hygiene plan includes the frequency, duration, and method of rinsing and brushing; applying sealants; and the use of dental diets and dental chews.[45] The Veterinary Oral Health Council has a list of products that are reportedly effective in retarding the accumulation of dental plaque and/or calculus.[46] Some of the details regarding the home oral hygiene plan might best be left for discussion with the client at the first postoperative follow-up evaluation.

PROGRESS OR FOLLOW-UP EVALUATION

With each follow-up examination and telephone communication, repeat the home dental care instructions and recommendations to the client. Set the number and timing of regular follow-up visits based on the disease severity. Although few studies have been performed in dogs and cats, extrapolation from the human literature and guidelines about aging in dogs and cats leads to the following recommendations[14]:

- Dental health care needs to be part of the preventive health care examination discussion and should begin at the first appointment at which the patient is seen and continue routinely throughout subsequent exams.
- Examinations q 6 mo can help ensure optimal home oral hygiene. At a minimum, evaluate animals with a healthy mouth at least q 12 mo.
- Evaluate pets with gingivitis at least q 6 mo.

- Evaluate pets with periodontitis at least q 3–6 mo.
- Advanced periodontal disease requires examinations q 1 mo until the disease is controlled.

Evaluate disease status, such as periodontal disease, on the conscious patient with products that allow an assessment of periodontal health without placing the patient under anesthesia.[14] During subsequent examinations, evaluate client compliance, revise the treatment plan as needed, and redefine the prognosis.

NUTRITION

Nutrition plays an important role in oral health; therefore, it is important for the health care team to have an understanding of the impact of nutrition on their patients. A properly balanced diet is essential for good general health, including health of oral tissues. For good oral health, it is the form of the diet, not the nutritional content, that is critical for good oral health. A diet that provides mechanical cleansing of the teeth is an excellent way of retarding the accumulation of dental plaque and calculus. Dental diets and chews can be very effective if the owner is unable to brush the teeth. Dental diets work either by "brushing" the crowns of the teeth as the animal chews or by coating an anti-calculus agent on the surface of the teeth. Nutrition becomes even more critical in dental health when the client is unable to provide home oral hygiene by brushing.[47] During subsequent examinations, evaluate client compliance, revise the treatment plan as needed, and redefine the prognosis.

SUMMARY

Pets can live more comfortable lives if oral health care is managed and maintained. All members of the veterinary team must strive to increase the quality of dental care delivered. Clients must be given options for the optimal care and treatment available for their pets. Dentistry is becoming more specialized, and referral to a veterinary dental specialist or a general practitioner with advanced training and proper equipment is recommended if the necessary expertise and/or equipment are unavailable at the primary veterinarian's office.

REFERENCES

1. Beckman BW. Pathophysiology and management of surgical and chronic oral pain in dogs and cats. J Vet Dent 2006;23(1):50–60.
2. Carpenter RE, Manfra Maretta S. Dental patients. In: Tranquilli WT, Grimm KA, Thurmon J, editors. Lumb and Jones' veterinary anesthesia and analgesia. 4th edition. Philadelphia: Wiley-Blackwell; 2007. p. 993–5.
3. Holmstrom SE, Frost-Fitch P, Eisner ER. Veterinary dental techniques for the small animal practitioner. 3rd edition. Philadelphia: WB Saunders; 2004.
4. Holmstrom SE. Veterinary dentistry: a team approach. 2nd edition. St Louis (MO): Elsevier; 2012.
5. Wiggs RB, Lobprise HB. Veterinary dentistry: principles and practice. Philadelphia: Lippincott-Raven; 1997.
6. Bellows J. Small animal dental equipment, materials and techniques. 1st edition. Ames (IA): Blackwell; 2004.
7. Mulligan T, Aller MS, Williams CA. Atlas of canine and feline dental radiography. Trenton (NJ): Veterinary Learning Systems; 1998.
8. Logothetis DD, Martinez-Welles JM. Reducing bacterial aerosol contamination with a chlorhexidine gluconate pre-rinse. J Am Dent Assoc 1995;126(12):1634–9.

9. Grove TK. Periodontal disease. In: Harvey C, editor. Veterinary dentistry. Philadelphia: WB Saunders; 1985. p. 59–78.

10. Harvey CE, Emily PP. Small animal dentistry. St Louis (MO): Mosby Year Book; 1993. p. 89–144.

11. Hennet PR, Harvey CE. Natural development of periodontal disease in the dog: a review of clinical, anatomical and histological features. J Vet Dent 1992;9(3):13–9.

12. Harvey CE, Shofer FS, Laster L. Association of age and body weight with periodontal disease in North American dogs. J Vet Dent 1994;11(3):94–105.

13. Niemiec BA. Systemic manifestations of periodontal disease. In: Niemiec BA, editor. Veterinary periodontology. Ames (IA): Wiley-Blackwell; 2012. p. 81–90.

14. Manfra Marretta S, Leesman M, Burgess-Cassler A, et al. Pilot evaluation of a novel test strip for the assessment of dissolved thiol levels, as an indicator of canine gingival health and periodontal status. Can Vet J 2012;1260.

15. Veterinary Oral Health Council. Available at: www.vohc.com. Accessed January 24, 2013.

16. Verstraete FJ, Kass PH, Terpak CH. Diagnostic value of full-mouth radiography in cats. Am J Vet Res 1998;59(6):692–5.

17. Epstein M, Kuehn N, Landsberg G, et al. AAHA senior care guidelines for dogs and cats. J Am Anim Hosp Assoc 2005;41(2):81–91. Available at: www.aahanet. org/Library/Guidelines.aspx. Accessed January 24, 2013.

18. Bednarski R, Grimm K, Harvey R, et al. AAHA anesthesia guidelines for dogs and cats. J Am Anim Hosp Assoc 2011;47(6):377–85. Available at: www.aahanet.org/ Library/Guidelines.aspx. Accessed January 24, 2013.

19. AAHA/AAFP Basic guidelines of judicious therapeutic use of antimicrobials. Available at: www.aahanet.org/Library/Guidelines.aspx. Accessed January 24, 2013.

20. Bartges J, Boynton B, Vogt AH, et al. AAHA canine life stages guidelines. J Am Anim Hosp Assoc 2012;48(1):1–11. Available at: www.aahanet.org/Library/ Guidelines.aspx. Accessed January 24, 2013.

21. Hoyumpa Vogt A, Rodan I, Brown M, et al. AAFP-AAHA feline life stages guidelines. J Feline Med Surg 2010;12(1):43–54. Available at: www.aahanet.org/ Library/Guidelines.aspx. Accessed January 24, 2013.

22. AAHA/AAFP Fluid Therapy Guidelines. in press.

23. Hellyer P, Rodan I, Brunt J, et al. AAHA/AAFP pain management guidelines for dogs and cats. J Am Anim Hosp Assoc 2007;43(5):235–48. Available at: www. aahanet.org/Library/Guidelines.aspx. Accessed January 24, 2013.

24. American Animal Hospital Association-American Veterinary Medical Association Preventive Healthcare Guidelines Task Force. Development of new canine and feline preventive healthcare guidelines designed to improve pet health. J Am Anim Hosp Assoc. 2011;47(5):306–11.

25. AAHA referral guidelines. Available at: www.aahanet.org/Library/Guidelines. aspx. Accessed January 24, 2013.

26. American Veterinary Dental College. American Veterinary Dental College position statement: companion animal dental scaling without anesthesia. Available at: http:// avdc.org/Dental_Scaling_Without_Anesthesia.pdf. Accessed January 24, 2013.

27. Pascoe P. Anesthesia and pain management. In: Verstraete F, Lommer M, editors. Oral and maxillofacial surgery in dogs and cats. WB Saunders; 2012. p. 26–7.

28. Stepaniuk K, Brock N. Anesthesia monitoring in the dental and oral surgery patient. J Vet Dent 2008;25(2):143–9.

29. Thurmon JC, et al. Acid-base balance and fluid therapy. In: Essentials of small animal anesthesia and analgesia. Philadelphia: Lippincott, Williams & Wilkins; 1999. p. 339–74.

30. Seeler D. Fluid, electrolyte, and blood component therapy. In: Veterinary anesthesia and analgesia. Blackwell Publishing; 2007. p. 185–96.
31. Hale FA, Anthony JM. Prevention of hypothermia in cats during routine oral hygiene procedures. Can Vet J 1997;38(5):297–9.
32. Stepaniuk K, Brock N. Hypothermia and thermoregulation during anesthesia for the dental and oral surgery patient. J Vet Dent 2008;25(4):279–83.
33. Chapman PJ, Ganendran A. Prolonged analgesia following preoperative bupivacaine neural blockade for oral surgery performed under general anesthesia. J Oral Maxillofac Surg 1987;45(3):233–5.
34. Tranquilli WJ, Grimm KA, Lamont LA. Pain management for the small animal practitioner. Jackson (WY): Teton New Media; 2000. p. 13–30.
35. Lantz GC. Regional anesthesia for dentistry and oral surgery. J Vet Dent 2003; 20(3):181–6.
36. Brine EJ, Marretta SM, Pijanowski GJ, et al. Comparison of the effects of four different power scalers on enamel tooth surface in the dog. J Vet Dent 2000; 17(1):17–21.
37. Niemiec BA. Veterinary periodontology. Ames (IA): Wiley-Blackwell; 2012.
38. Beckman BW. Patient management for periodontal therapy. In: Niemiec BA, editor. Veterinary periodontology. Ames (IA): Wiley-Blackwell; 2012. p. 305–12.
39. Niemiec BA. Advanced non-surgical therapy. In: Niemiec BA, editor. Veterinary periodontology. Ames (IA): Wiley-Blackwell; 2012. p. 154–69.
40. Niemiec BA. The complete dental cleaning. In: Niemiec BA, editor. Veterinary periodontology. Ames (IA): Wiley-Blackwell; 2012. p. 129–53.
41. Hennet P. Periodontal disease and oral microbiology. In: Crossley DA, Penman S, editors. Manual of small animal dentistry. 2nd edition. Shurdington (England): British Small Animal Veterinary Association; 1995. p. 105–13.
42. Sarkiala E, Harvey C. Systemic antimicrobials in the treatment of periodontitis in dogs. Semin Vet Med Surg (Small Anim) 1993;8(3):197–203.
43. Huffman LJ. Oral examination. In: Niemiec BA, editor. Small animal dental, oral and maxillofacial disease: a color handbook. London: Manson; 2010. p. 39–61.
44. Quality of Care. Pain management. Lakewood (CO): American Animal Hospital Association Standards of Accreditation; 2003.
45. Niemiec BA. Home plaque control. In: Niemiec BA, editor. Veterinary periodontology. Ames (IA): Wiley-Blackwell; 2012. p. 175–85.
46. Veterinary Oral Health Council. Available at: www.vohc.org/accepted_products. htm. Accessed January 24, 2013.
47. Jensen L, Logan E, Finney O, et al. Reduction in accumulation of plaque, stain, and calculus in dogs by dietary means. J Vet Dent 1995;12(4):161–3.

SUPPLEMENTARY REFERENCES

Bellows J. Feline dentistry. Ames (IA): Wiley; 2010.
Dupont GA, DeBowes LJ. Atlas of dental radiography in dogs and cats. St Louis (MO): WB Saunders; 2009.

APPENDIX II: AMERICAN VETERINARY DENTAL COLLEGE POSITION STATEMENT ON DENTAL HEALTH CARE PROVIDERS
Veterinary Dental Health Care Providers

This article can be downloaded from http://avdc.org/Dental_Health_Care_Providers. pdf

The AVDC developed this position statement as a means to safeguard the veterinary dental patient and to ensure the qualifications of persons performing veterinary dental procedures.

Primary responsibility for veterinary dental care

The AVDC defines veterinary dentistry as the art and practice of oral health care in animals other than man. It is a discipline of veterinary medicine and surgery. The diagnosis, treatment, and management of veterinary oral health care is to be provided and supervised by licensed veterinarians or by veterinarians working within a university or industry.

Who may provide veterinarian-supervised dental care

The AVDC accepts that the following health care workers may assist the responsible veterinarian in dental procedures or actually perform dental prophylactic services while under direct, in the room supervision by a veterinarian if permitted by local law: licensed, certified or registered veterinary technician or a veterinary assistant with advanced dental training, dentist, or registered dental hygienist.

Operative dentistry and oral surgery

The AVDC considers operative dentistry to be any dental procedure which invades the hard or soft oral tissue including, but not limited to, a procedure that alters the structure of one or more teeth or repairs damaged and diseased teeth. A veterinarian should perform operative dentistry and oral surgery.

Extraction of teeth

The AVDC considers the extraction of teeth to be included in the practice of veterinary dentistry. Decision making is the responsibility of the veterinarian, with the consent of the pet owner, when electing to extract teeth. Only veterinarians shall determine which teeth are to be extracted and perform extraction procedures.

Dental tasks performed by veterinary technicians

The AVDC considers it appropriate for a veterinarian to delegate maintenance dental care and certain dental tasks to a veterinary technician. Tasks appropriately performed by a technician include dental prophylaxis and certain procedures that do not result in altering the shape, structure, or positional location of teeth in the dental arch. The veterinarian may direct an appropriately trained technician to perform these tasks providing that the veterinarian is physically present and supervising the treatment.

Veterinary technician dental training

The AVDC supports the advanced training of veterinary technicians to perform additional ancillary dental services: taking impressions, making models, charting veterinary dental pathology, taking and developing dental radiographs, performing nonsurgical subgingival root scaling and debridement, providing that they do not alter the structure of the tooth.

Tasks that may be performed by veterinary assistants (not registered, certified, or licensed). The AVDC supports the appropriate training of veterinary assistants to perform the following dental services: supragingival scaling and polishing, taking and developing dental radiographs, making impressions and making models.

Tasks that may be performed by dentists, registered dental hygienists, and other dental health care providers. The AVDC recognizes that dentists, registered dental hygienists and other dental health care providers in good standing may perform those procedures for which they have been qualified under the direct supervision of the veterinarian. The supervising veterinarian will be responsible for the welfare of the patient and any treatment performed on the patient.

The AVDC understands that individual states have regulations that govern the practice of veterinary medicine. This position statement is intended to be a model for veterinary dental practice and does not replace existing law.

(Adopted by the Board of Directors April 1998; revised October 1999 and September 2006.)

Companion Animal Dental Scaling Without Anesthesia

This article can be downloaded from http://avdc.org/Dental_Scaling_Without_Anesthesia.pdf

In the United States and Canada, only licensed veterinarians can practice veterinary medicine. Veterinary medicine includes veterinary surgery, medicine, and dentistry. Anyone providing dental services other than a licensed veterinarian, or a supervised and trained veterinary technician, is practicing veterinary medicine without a license and shall be subject to criminal charges.

This position statement addresses dental scaling procedures performed on pets without anesthesia, often by individuals untrained in veterinary dental techniques. Although the term Anesthesia-Free Dentistry has been used in this context, AVDC prefers to use the more accurate term Nonprofessional Dental Scaling (NPDS) to describe this combination.

Owners of pets naturally are concerned when anesthesia is required for their pet. However, performing NPDS on an unanesthetized pet is inappropriate for the following reasons:

1. Dental tartar is firmly adhered to the surface of the teeth. Scaling to remove tartar is accomplished using ultrasonic and sonic power scalers, plus hand instruments that must have a sharp working edge to be used effectively. Even slight head movement by the patient could result in injury to the oral tissues of the patient, and the operator may be bitten when the patient reacts.
2. Professional dental scaling includes scaling the surfaces of the teeth both above and below the gingival margin (gum line), followed by dental polishing. The most critical part of a dental scaling procedure is scaling the tooth surfaces that are within the gingival pocket (the subgingival space between the gum and the root), where periodontal disease is active. Because the patient cooperates, dental scaling of human teeth performed by a professional trained in the procedures can be completed successfully without anesthesia. However, access to the subgingival area of every tooth is impossible in an unanesthetized canine or feline patient. Removal of dental tartar on the visible surfaces of the teeth has little effect on a pet's health, and provides a false sense of accomplishment. The effect is purely cosmetic.
3. Inhalation anesthesia using a cuffed endotracheal tube provides 3 important advantages—the cooperation of the patient with a procedure it does not understand, elimination of pain resulting from examination and treatment of affected dental tissues during the procedure, and protection of the airway and lungs from accidental aspiration.
4. A complete oral examination, which is an important part of a professional dental scaling procedure, is not possible in an unanesthetized patient. The surfaces of the teeth facing the tongue cannot be examined, and areas of disease and discomfort are likely to be missed.

Safe use of an anesthetic or sedative in a dog or cat requires evaluation of the general health and size of the patient to determine the appropriate drug and dose, and continual monitoring of the patient. Veterinarians are trained in all of these procedures. Prescribing or administering anesthetic or sedative drugs by a nonveterinarian can be very dangerous, and is illegal. Although anesthesia will never be 100% risk-free, modern anesthetic and patient evaluation techniques used in veterinary hospitals minimize the risks, and millions of dental scaling procedures are safely performed each year in veterinary hospitals.

To minimize the need for professional dental scaling procedures and to maintain optimal oral health, the AVDC recommends daily dental home care from an early age. This should include brushing or use of other effective techniques to retard accumulation of dental plaque, such as dental diets and chew materials. This, combined with periodic examination of the patient by a veterinarian and with dental scaling under anesthesia when indicated, will optimize life-long oral health for dogs and cats.

For general information on performance of dental procedures on veterinary patients, please read the AVDC Position Statement on Veterinary Dental Healthcare Providers, which is available on the AVDC Web site (www.AVDC.org). For information on effective oral hygiene products for dogs and cats, visit the Veterinary Oral Health Council Web site (www.VOHC.org).

For further information, send an e-mail message to the AVDC Executive Secretary (ExecSec@AVDC.org).

(Adopted by the Board of Directors, April 2004.)

APPENDIX III: AMERICAN VETERINARY DENTAL COLLEGE POSITION STATEMENT ON NONPROFESSIONAL DENTAL SCALING
Dental Scaling Without Anesthesia

In the United States and Canada, only licensed veterinarians can practice veterinary medicine. Veterinary medicine includes veterinary surgery, medicine, and dentistry. Anyone providing dental services other than a licensed veterinarian, or a supervised and trained veterinary technician, is practicing veterinary medicine without a license and is subject to criminal charges.

This document addresses dental scaling procedures performed on pets without anesthesia, often by individuals untrained in veterinary dental techniques. Although the term Anesthesia-Free Dentistry has been used in this context, AVDC prefers to use the more accurate term Nonprofessional Dental Scaling (NPDS) to describe this combination.

Owners of pets naturally are concerned when anesthesia is required for their pet. However, performing NPDS on an unanesthetized pet is inappropriate for the following reasons:

1. Dental tartar is firmly adhered to the surface of the teeth. Scaling to remove tartar is accomplished using ultrasonic and sonic power scalers, plus hand instruments that must have a sharp working edge to be used effectively. Even slight head movement by the patient could result in injury to the oral tissues of the patient, and the operator may be bitten when the patient reacts.
2. Professional dental scaling includes scaling the surfaces of the teeth both above and below the gingival margin (gum line), followed by dental polishing. The most critical part of a dental scaling procedure is scaling the tooth surfaces that are within the gingival pocket (the subgingival space between the gum and the root), where periodontal disease is active. Because the patient cooperates, dental scaling of human teeth performed by a professional trained in the procedures can be completed successfully without anesthesia. However, access to the subgingival area of every tooth is impossible in an unanesthetized canine or feline patient. Removal of dental tartar on the visible surfaces of the teeth has little effect on a pet's health, and provides a false sense of accomplishment. The effect is purely cosmetic.

3. Inhalation anesthesia using a cuffed endotracheal tube provides 3 important advantages—the cooperation of the patient with a procedure it does not understand, elimination of pain resulting from examination and treatment of affected dental tissues during the procedure, and protection of the airway and lungs from accidental aspiration.
4. A complete oral examination, which is an important part of a professional dental scaling procedure, is not possible in an unanesthetized patient. The surfaces of the teeth facing the tongue cannot be examined, and areas of disease and discomfort are likely to be missed.

Safe use of an anesthetic or sedative in a dog or cat requires evaluation of the general health and size of the patient to determine the appropriate drug and dose, and continual monitoring of the patient.

Veterinarians are trained in all of these procedures. Prescribing or administering anesthetic or sedative drugs by a nonveterinarian can be very dangerous, and is illegal. Although anesthesia will never be 100% risk-free, modern anesthetic and patient evaluation techniques used in veterinary hospitals minimize the risks, and millions of dental scaling procedures are safely performed each year in veterinary hospitals.

To minimize the need for professional dental scaling procedures and to maintain optimal oral health, AVDC recommends daily dental home care from an early age in dogs and cats. This should include brushing or use of other effective techniques to retard accumulation of dental plaque, such as dental diets and chew materials. This, combined with periodic examination of the patient by a veterinarian and with dental scaling under anesthesia when indicated, will optimize life-long oral health for dogs and cats. For information on effective oral hygiene products for dogs and cats, visit the Veterinary Oral Health Council Web site (www.VOHC.org).

For general information on performance of dental procedures on veterinary patients, read the AVDC Position Statement on Veterinary Dental Healthcare Providers.

Therapeutic Decision Making and Planning in Veterinary Dentistry and Oral Surgery

John R. Lewis, VMD, FAVD, DAVDC

KEYWORDS

- Clinical decision making • Treatment planning • Evidence-based veterinary dentistry
- Evidence-based practice • Evidence-based medicine

KEY POINTS

- There is no substitute for individual clinical expertise. Evidence-based veterinary dentistry aims to integrate individual clinical expertise with the best available external information about specific dental and maxillofacial conditions.
- To take advantage of one's own individual clinical expertise, one must be able to recall details of previous patients, procedures, and outcomes. This emphasizes the importance of a detailed dental record, well-archived dental radiography, and clear, retrievable photographs or video of prior procedures.
- The history and physical examination are of key importance in obtaining a correct diagnosis and assessing risks versus benefits of elective dental procedures.
- Performing "dry run" procedures on cadavers under the supervision of knowledgeable instructors may improve outcomes and relieve operator stress when done before clinical procedures.
- Patients with severe oral pathology may require decisions about prioritization and staging of procedures.
- Some dental procedures are elective in nature. Anesthetic and procedural risks sometimes outweigh the benefits of a procedure. It is important to accrue evidence in these cases to provide the clinician and the pet owner with as much information as possible regarding risks and benefits, so together they can decide on a course of action.

INTRODUCTION

A 13-year-old Yorkshire terrier is presented due to severe halitosis. The patient has no known concurrent medical conditions and was anesthetized only once previously at 6 months of age for ovariohysterectomy. An open-ended question of "What brings Guinevere to see us today?" reveals a worsening of her long-standing halitosis. Her

Previous Funding Sources: Nestle Purina, Academy of Veterinary Dentistry, MBF Therapeutics, Lankenau Institute for Medical Research, Waltham.
Conflicts of Interest: Nil.
Department of Clinical Studies, School of Veterinary Medicine, University of Pennsylvania, 3111 MJR VHUP, 3900 Delancey Street, Philadelphia, PA 19104-6010, USA
E-mail address: jrlewis@vet.upenn.edu

Vet Clin Small Anim 43 (2013) 471–487
http://dx.doi.org/10.1016/j.cvsm.2013.02.009
0195-5616/13/$ – see front matter © 2013 Elsevier Inc. All rights reserved.

appetite is good, although Guinevere does not chew on toys like she did in the past, and occasionally she approaches the food bowl to eat but then turns away, which is new for her. Guinevere has always sneezed and coughed occasionally, but both have increased recently.

The word "clinician" is derived from a Greek word meaning "bed." "Patient" is a term derived from the Latin "*pati,*" which means "to suffer." The clinician is the doctor at the bedside of the sufferer, accepting responsibility for the life entrusted to him or her and developing a plan for therapeutic care.[1] Although patient care is not usually envisioned as hard science, the truth is clinicians, knowingly or unknowingly, perform clinical experiments on patients every day. Well-designed therapeutic plans are created, performed, and appraised with the same intellectual approaches used in a well-designed scientific experiment.[1] This approach provides the opportunity to learn from every case, even if the therapeutic plan consists entirely of routine and accepted standards of care.

Therapeutic decision making is rarely taught didactically in veterinary school. Instead, skills in this arena are honed in the examination room during school and well beyond. This article discusses basic tenets of therapeutic decision making and highlights examples of therapeutic approaches to common oral conditions. Although algorithms are used in these examples, it is important to emphasize that algorithms are meant to be useful reminders of diagnostic and therapeutic considerations. Algorithms are not a replacement for the thought process required for each individual patient.

Therapeutics that work in the hands of one clinician may not work for every clinician, and therapeutics that are effective for one patient may not work for every patient. However, past clinical experiences and scientific studies provide the foundation for therapeutic decision making. The concept of evidence-based medicine, or perhaps more appropriately called evidence-based practice, integrates clinicians' individual expertise with currently available external information sources in an attempt to improve patient outcomes.[2]

Evidence-based practice is not a new concept: it was used in part by clinicians in ancient Greece.[3] Recent interest in evidence-based practice has arisen in part because of justification of the rising costs of human health care. Aside from human health management decisions, evidence-based practice reinforces the need for due diligence when justifying therapeutic decisions.

A hierarchy ranking of the types of evidence is shown in **Fig. 1**.[4] The strongest evidence for therapeutic interventions is almost universally considered to be systematic review of randomized, triple-blind, controlled trials of a homogeneous population with excellent follow-up. These studies are rare in veterinary dentistry. Client testimonials and expert opinion are considered the weakest form of evidence. Some argue that expert opinion should be viewed as a separate type of knowledge that does not fit well into evidence hierarchies.[5] Expert opinion and client testimonial can be more likely influenced by bias. However, expert opinion is often the only available evidence for uncommon veterinary oral conditions. Even when other sources of empiric evidence are available, expert opinion is an integral part of the knowledge required for therapeutic decision making.[5]

ANAMNESIS

Anamnesis is the medical case history of a patient. The history is the first important step to making appropriate diagnostic and therapeutic decisions. Some simple approaches to obtaining a history will increase chances of gaining helpful information. Use of open-ended questions allows a client to tell his or her full story and provides

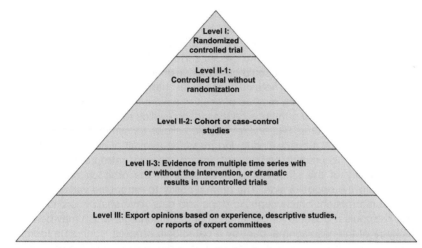

Fig. 1. An early proposed hierarchy of clinical evidence as stratified by the US Preventive Services Task Force. (*From* United States Prevention Services Task Force. Guide to clinical preventive services: report of the U.S. Preventive Services Task Force: United States Prevention Services Task Force; Washington, DC, 1989. p. 263; with permission.)

the clinician with a full understanding of the owner's perspective when coupled to attentive listening. Providing structure is necessary to redirect the conversation if open-ended questions result in tangential conversation. Pointed questions probe deeper in areas that seem important to explore. A good history taker allows the client to tell his or her story to obtain a complete understanding of what is occurring with the patient, and what is important to the client.

PHYSICAL EXAMINATION

The physical examination provides the foundation for decision making and brings the clinician one step closer to a therapeutic plan. A patient with the presenting complaint of halitosis leads us toward a diagnosis of periodontal disease even before we perform our physical examination, but it is important to thoroughly examine even the most straightforward of presenting complaints. Periodontal disease is the most common cause of halitosis, but any given case of halitosis may be caused by a necrotic tumor, endodontic disease, idiopathic osteomyelitis/osteonecrosis, stomatitis, lip fold dermatitis, uremic ulcers, or gastrointestinal disease. Ten to twenty percent of all cases of human halitosis are due to systemic causes, such as gastric, hepatic, pancreatic, and renal insufficiencies; trimethylaminuria; upper and lower respiratory tract infection; and medications.[6]

The physical examination provides information necessary to assess risk for elective procedures. Auscultation is performed in a quiet area to listen for cardiac murmurs or arrhythmias. The lungs are auscultated to listen for evidence of pulmonary pathology that may affect anesthetic plans. The trachea is palpated, especially in the proximal neck and thoracic inlet area of small-breed dogs, to check for a cough that may be indicative of collapsing trachea.

The head, neck, and oral examinations are done after the general examination, because the patient may be painful in these areas if presenting for an oral problem. The head and neck examination begins with extraoral observation of the head, face, eyes, ears, and neck using visual observation, palpation, and smell. Using gloved hands to avoid transmission of disease between patients and caregivers, palpate each side of the face, head, and neck for symmetric comparison. Assess the temporal and masseter muscles for the presence of atrophy, enlargement, or pain. Palpate the ventral, lateral, and medial surface of the left and right mandibles for the presence of swelling that could be evidence of neoplasia, infection, or fracture.

Visually inspect the ears and note evidence of discharge, odor, or pain on palpation. Pain upon opening the mouth may be a result of severe middle ear disease (**Fig. 2**). The eyes are palpated using thumbs on the closed eyelids to gently push (retropulse) both eyes at the same time. Bilateral retropulsion allows for symmetric comparison of depth and firmness. If a space-occupying mass (as a result of neoplasia, inflammation, or infection) is present behind or beneath the eye, retropulsion may find a decreased ability of the globe to move caudally in the orbit on one side when compared with the opposite side. The normal ability to retropulse varies depending on facial conformation: brachycephalic dogs and cats have shallow orbits and less ability to retropulse. Observe for evidence of ocular discharge, which may be caused by blockage of the nasolacrimal duct by a pathologic process, such as a tooth root abscess or neoplasia. Evaluation of the neck includes palpation of the right and left mandibular salivary glands beneath the skin of the ventral neck. The mandibular salivary gland is the only easily palpable major salivary gland in dogs and cats. The 3 other major salivary glands are either too diffuse to palpate easily (parotid, sublingual glands) or are not superficial enough to palpate (zygomatic gland). The mandibular gland is easily distinguished from the mandibular lymph nodes because it is softer, larger than, and caudomedial to the mandibular lymph nodes. Once the salivary glands are located, the mandibular lymph nodes can be identified by moving the finger tips cranially. The mandibular lymph nodes are palpated bilaterally for symmetry and firmness. In the cat, mandibular lymph nodes are difficult to palpate unless they are enlarged. In the dog, mandibular lymph nodes are generally always palpable, ranging in size from 0.5 to 1.5 cm in diameter depending on the size and age of the patient. Other nodes that drain the head (retropharyngeal, parotid) are not normally

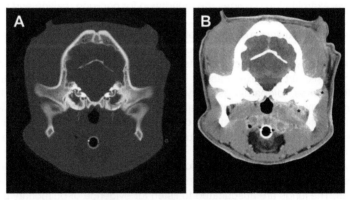

Fig. 2. A 2-year-old French bulldog with a history or prior ear infections was presented emergently for lethargy and pain on opening the mouth. (*A*) Computed tomography (CT) bone scan shows severe bilateral thickening of the cortices of the tympanic bullae (*arrows*) with a possible fissure through the ventral left bulla. (*B*) CT soft tissue scan after administration of intravenous contrast shows increased contrast uptake on each side of the left condylar process of the mandible, suggestive of peri-bullar cellulitis (*asterisks*). The close proximity of the temporomandibular joint to the bulla may result in pain on opening the mouth in patients with middle ear disease.

palpable. Nine percent of dogs have an additional lymph node that is palpable in the subcutaneous tissue dorsal to the maxillary third premolar tooth. This node is referred to as the facial or buccal lymph node and may be seen unilaterally or bilaterally.[7,8]

The occlusion should be evaluated before intubation by noting any teeth that are positioned incorrectly. Attention is paid to discrepancies of jaw length, the spatial relationship of the teeth as they erupt, and the relationship of the erupting teeth with the soft tissues and dental structures of the opposing jaw. Note any deciduous teeth that have not exfoliated by the time their permanent counterparts have erupted. Persistent deciduous teeth may create increased risk of periodontal disease (due to crowding and lack of normal gingival collar around the permanent tooth) and abnormal position of permanent tooth eruption.

The intraoral examination consists of evaluation of the soft tissues of the oral cavity, the dental structures, and the periodontium, a term that describes the supporting structures of the teeth. Some of this information can be obtained in the conscious patient, but assessment of the periodontium requires anesthesia. Begin by observing the skin and mucosa of the upper and lower lips. Some breeds are prone to lip fold dermatitis caudal to the mandibular canine tooth that can cause oral malodor unrelated to periodontal disease. Vestibular or labial mucosa refers to the mucosa that begins at the mucocutaneous junction and lines the cheeks and lips. Alveolar mucosa refers to the mucosa that lay against the bone of the upper or lower jaw, which meets with the gingiva at the mucogingival junction. The normal appearance of the mucosa may be pink or pigmented, and the mucosa should exhibit no lesions, ulcerations, or swellings. Mucosa that lay adjacent to periodontally diseased teeth may have painful mucosal ulcerations as a response to bacteria in the plaque, often referred to as contact stomatitis or mucositis. Observe the caudal cheek mucosa in the region of the carnassial and molar teeth. This mucosa frequently becomes pressed between the teeth during chewing, creating a condition known as "cheek-chewing lesions." Similarly, mucosa beneath the tongue may also show signs of chewing lesions referred to as "tongue-chewing lesions," which are usually bilateral (**Fig. 3**). These lesions usually do not require treatment unless the lesions are not bilaterally similar or if

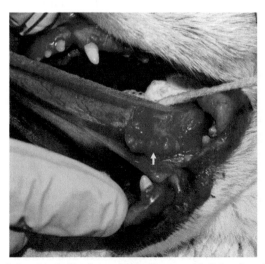

Fig. 3. A sublingual chewing lesion (*arrow*) in a 13-year-old Chihuahua. The lesion (*arrow*) was removed and histopathological evaluation showed hyperplasia and granulation tissue.

the lesions are ulcerated. In these cases, the affected mucosa may be removed and submitted for histopathological evaluation.

Two raised bumps are found on the alveolar mucosa dorsal to the maxillary fourth premolar and first molar teeth. Salivary secretions from the parotid and zygomatic salivary glands travel through ducts leading to these duct openings. Two similar raised bumps can be found beneath the tongue just caudal to the mandibular symphysis, which are the caruncles of the mandibular and sublingual glands. Care should be taken to avoid trauma to these structures when possible to avoid development of sialoceles (**Fig. 4**).

Small-breed dogs with advanced periodontal disease may be affected by bone loss and pathologic fracture of the mandible, which may be found as an incidental finding in the examination room. If severe periodontal disease is suspected in a small-breed dog, care should be taken to avoid creating a pathologic fracture when opening the mouth during the conscious examination or during intubation.

The roof of the mouth is composed of the hard and soft palates. The hard palate is covered by palatal mucosa arranged in prominent ridges, called rugae. These rugae range from 8 to 10 in number. In brachycephalic dogs, the rugae are closely positioned, and hair and debris can accumulate in these rugal folds. On the midline of the hard palate, just caudal to the incisor teeth, the incisive papilla is a round, slightly raised structure. Lateral to the incisive papilla, a small bilateral communication with the incisive duct and vomeronasal organ exists. The vomeronasal organ is a paired sensory organ involved in detection of pheromones and other volatile compounds. Palpation of the area lateral and caudal to the incisive papilla may normally feel as if there is air trapped beneath the mucosa as a result of the communication between the mouth and these nasal structures. The soft palate consists of mucosa and muscle that separate the oropharynx and nasopharynx. Two prominent bony structures can be palpated just lateral to the midline of the soft palate that are the hamular processes of the bilateral pterygoid bones. If one or both hamular processes are difficult to palpate, this may be due to the presence of a nasopharyngeal mass.

The pharynx should be evaluated for evidence of inflammation or neoplasia. When the patient's mouth is open, bilateral folds of pharyngeal mucosa will be evident lateral to the tongue. These are the palatoglossal folds, and this area and the mucosa lateral to these folds may be inflamed in cats with caudal stomatitis.

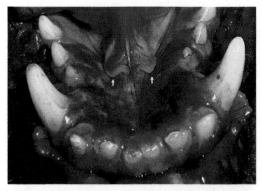

Fig. 4. The left and right sublingual caruncles are seen in the raised, redundant mucosa lateral to the lingual frenulum. The mandibular and sublingual salivary ducts empty into the oral cavity at this site (*arrows*).

Gently hold the tip of the tongue to enable visual examination of the dorsal, ventral, and lateral surfaces. The firm, tubular structure palpable on the midline of the rostral tongue is called the lyssa, which helps to provided structure and coordinated movement of the rostral tongue. Lift the tongue to observe the mucosa of the floor of the mouth and the base of the tongue. In the conscious patient, the examiner's thumb may be used extraorally to push the tongue dorsally for better visualization of the ventral surface of the tongue. The dorsal surface of the tongue is covered by thousands of papillae, some of which contain taste buds. The large, distinctive papillae located at the caudal third of the tongue are the vallate papillae, which are spaced in a curved line separating the body from the root of the tongue. Depress the tongue to visualize the tonsils, noting any enlargement or change in color or texture. The color of a normal tonsil is typically more hyperemic than the color of the adjacent mucosa. Normal tonsils may be fully contained within the tonsillar crypt and may be difficult to visualize.

The next step in the intraoral examination is evaluation of the teeth and their supporting structures. First, determine the presence or absence of teeth in each quadrant. Missing teeth can be documented on the dental chart by darkening or circling the missing tooth. Radiographic evaluation of areas of missing teeth is imperative because dentigerous cysts can develop as a result of an unerupted tooth. A periodontal probe and dental explorer are used to evaluate the tooth and its attachment structures. These dental instruments are important clinical tools for obtaining data about the health status of each tooth. Consider the adult canine mouth as containing 42 patients and the adult feline mouth containing 30 patients, each patient requiring a thorough evaluation and treatment planning. The periodontal probe has a round or flat working end, which is marked in millimeter increments, ending in a blunt tip. The probe is used like a miniature intraoral ruler to measure attachment levels, sulcus and pocket depths, loss of bone in furcation areas, and size of oral lesions. It is also used to assess the mobility of teeth and the presence of gingival bleeding. Periodontal probes are available in an assortment of styles, with variations in thickness of the diameter of the working end and variations in increments of millimeter markings.

The dental explorer has a slender, wirelike working end that tapers to a sharp point. It is used to explore the topography of the tooth surface. When the explorer is held with a light modified pen grasp (**Fig. 5**), the examiner acquires a tactile sense to locate tooth surface irregularities, including caries, tooth resorption, calculus deposits, and pulp

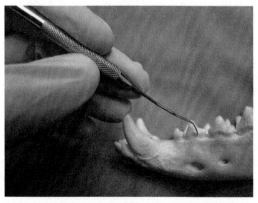

Fig. 5. The modified pen grasp is used to hold an explorer while feeling for defects at the cervical portion of the left mandibular second premolar tooth.

exposure. The explorer is also used to determine the completeness of treatment following calculus debridement and to ensure smooth transitions of dental restorations. Several designs of explorers are available. Varying degrees of flexibility contribute to the degrees of tactile sensitivity.

The assessment of the periodontium and teeth should begin at the midline of the mouth and systematically evaluate each tooth, one at a time, by using both visual observation and tactile use of the probe and explorer. Begin detecting excessive tooth mobility by placing the tip of the probe against the tip of the tooth and gently attempting to move the tooth in a buccolingual direction. Movement is estimated on a scale of 1, 2, or 3, based on the distance beyond normal physiologic mobility the tooth moves in one direction. A slight amount of movement is normal as a result of the periodontal ligament that connects the tooth to alveolar bone. The most severe mobility, a classification of 3, includes any tooth with vertical movement. As each tooth is approached to check for mobility, visually notice the characteristics of the gingiva for color, shape, texture, and consistency. Healthy gingival tissues are pink (except where normally pigmented), stippled (orange peel appearance), firm, tapered to a thin margin, and scalloped to follow the contour of the cementoenamel junction (CEJ) and underlying alveolar bone. Any area of the gingiva that deviates from these normal characteristics should be examined closer by use of the probe.

The probe is gently inserted into the sulcus (physiologic term) or pocket (pathologic term), ensuring that the probe is kept as close to parallel to the long axis of the root as possible, with the side of the probe tip in contact with the tooth. When physical resistance is felt at the base of the sulcus or pocket, note the marking level on the probe that is adjacent to the gingival margin. The probe is then "walked" around the tooth to assess the entire circumference of the tooth. Abnormal measurements (those greater than 3 mm in dogs, greater than 1 mm in cats) should be noted on the dental chart, along with the specific location of the pocket measurement (ie, MP for mesiopalatal). Probe measurements between millimeter markings are rounded up to the larger measurement. For accurate readings, it is essential to develop skills in consistent probing forces (between 10 to 20 g of pressure). This pressure amount can be practiced by pressing the probe tip into the pad of a thumb until the skin is depressed approximately 2 mm.

In areas where the height of the free gingival margin has migrated apically toward or beyond the CEJ, the probe is used to measure gingival recession. Recession is measured in millimeters from the CEJ to the level of the gingival margin. Attachment loss is a term that truly describes the periodontal state of a tooth because it accounts for both pocket depth and gingival recession. Gingival hyperplasia occurs when the free gingival margin migrates toward the crown of the tooth. An increased pocket depth may be due to hyperplasia or attachment loss, so clinical examination findings are necessary to determine if the increased probing depth is attributable to a true pocket or a pseudopocket.

When multirooted teeth are approached, the probe is used to assess loss of bone in the areas between and around the roots. A bifurcation is the furcation between 2-rooted teeth and should be assessed from the buccal and lingual-palatal surfaces. Trifurcations of 3-rooted teeth should be assessed between each of the 3 roots. The extent of bone loss determines the furcation classification.

During the periodontal evaluation of each tooth, also observe the hard structures of the tooth and use the dental explorer when noticing any chips, fractures, pulp exposure, or abnormal wear patterns of abrasion or attrition. Abrasion refers to tooth wear associated with aggressive chewing on external objects, such as toys, rocks, bones, and ice cubes. Attrition refers to 2 possible scenarios. Physiologic attrition refers to the normal wear associated with tooth-to-tooth contact of a patient over time with normal mastication. Pathologic attrition is caused by a malocclusion resulting in abnormal wear of teeth as a result of contact with teeth of the opposing jaw.

Dental caries (commonly referred to by the lay term of "cavities") result from demineralization of the enamel and dentin from acids produced by certain oral bacteria. These lesions occur most commonly on occlusal (flat) surfaces of the molar teeth. Gently explore for pits and fissures of the occlusal surfaces of the maxillary first and second molars and the distal half of the mandibular first molar, feeling for areas of demineralization. Use the explorer to check for clinical signs of tooth resorption by dragging the sharp point horizontally across the cervical portion of each tooth. Sometimes it is challenging to determine whether a concavity in the area of a furcation is a resorptive lesion or merely mild furcation exposure. If tooth resorption is present, the explorer tip will "catch" on the edge of the concavity, whereas the explorer will freely move out of the concave area as easily as it fell into it when encountering mild furcation exposure. When tooth fractures are present, gently drag the sharp point of the explorer across the tooth surface, feeling for any openings into the pulp. Teeth with significant abrasion may have a brown or black spot in the center of the worn tooth. This can be a sign of either chronic pulp exposure or a reparative material produced by the tooth in response to chronic wear (tertiary dentin). Pulp exposure can be distinguished from tertiary dentin by use of an explorer. If a tooth has pulp exposure, the tip of the explorer will "fall into a hole," whereas a discolored area caused by tertiary dentin will feel smooth as glass when the explorer is run over this area. This is an important clinical distinction because treatment of pulp-exposed teeth is necessary, but worn teeth without pulp exposure often require no treatment if radiographically normal.[9]

CAPTURING THE CLINICAL EXPERIENCE IN A RETRIEVABLE FASHION

Record keeping during the physical examination is important not only because it provides legal documentation, but also because well-documented cases provide us the opportunity to learn from our patients by reviewing and comparing these cases to future similar cases. During the soft tissue examination, any tissue variations from normal should be described by recording the size, shape, color, surface texture, and consistency (eg, soft, firm, hard, or fluctuant). A dedicated area of the dental record may be created to allow for documentation of any abnormalities of intraoral or extraoral structures (**Fig. 6**). Paperless dental charting systems are commercially available. Copies of digital dental radiographs and digital records may be saved automatically via online backup programs or external hard drives. Conventional dental radiographs are saved in the dental record and may be digitized by photographing with a digital camera. Preoperative and postoperative photos and videos of procedures can be archived and doubly saved on an external hard drive in both chronologic and categorical folders for ease of searching.

EXAMPLES OF COMMON PRESENTATIONS
Case 1: 13-Year-Old Yorkshire Terrier with Severe Periodontal Disease

Physical examination of Guinevere, a 13-year-old spayed female Yorkshire terrier, whose history was mentioned in the introduction, reveals a grade III/VI holosystolic murmur over the left and right chest. A repeatable cough is elicited on tracheal palpation in the thoracic inlet area. Mandibular lymph nodes are bilaterally enlarged. The patient is reluctant to have a thorough conscious oral examination, but as the dog pants, it is apparent that the mucous membranes are slightly pale except at the

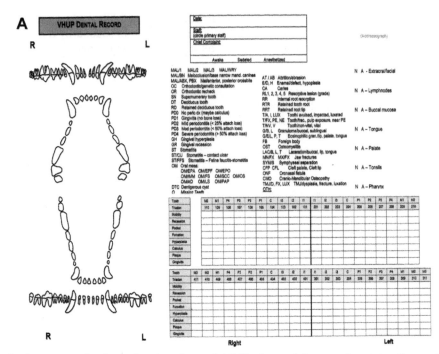

Fig. 6. An example of a canine dental record. (*A*) The front of the record contains diagnostic information.

gingival margin where gingivitis and gingival recession is seen around nearly all teeth. Severe calculus and plaque accumulation is present on the vestibular (buccal/labial) and palatal/lingual surfaces of all teeth. A gingival mass is seen arising from the gingiva of the left maxillary canine tooth (**Fig. 7**). A mild serous nasal discharge is present from the right nostril.

What did you prioritize as important information from the history and physical examination? Increased anesthetic risk is suggested by results of auscultation, tracheal palpation and mucus membrane color. Thoracic and cervical radiographs may be used to assess the trachea, heart, and lungs. Fluoroscopy may be used to assess dynamic changes of the trachea. Echocardiogram and electrocardiogram will provide further detail regarding cardiac abnormalities. Complete blood count and chemistry screen may elucidate a cause of mucus membrane pallor and will provide information on kidney and liver status.

The degree of overt periodontal disease in this patient and the lack of prior dental procedures suggest there are multiple hours of anesthesia necessary for this dog. Mortality rates associated with anesthetic procedures in veterinary patients have been documented to be between 0.17% and 5.00%, depending on the population studied and the study period.[10–12] Increasing American Society of Anesthesiologists (ASA) status was associated with an increased chance of anesthetic death in a recent study of 3546 dogs and cats.[11] ASA physical status classifications and examples are listed in **Table 1**.[13] **Fig. 8** shows an algorithm for potential decisions and outcomes regarding anesthetic risks in this patient.

If the decision is made to pursue treatment based on careful assessment of risk versus benefit, areas of the mouth causing the most morbidity should be prioritized,

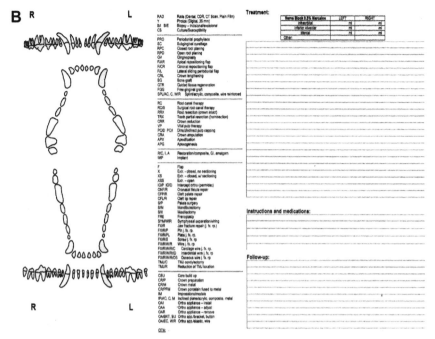

Fig. 6. (*B*) The back of the record contains treatment information.

as this procedure may require staging into more than one anesthetic episode. Assessment of how the patient eats may provide clues of which side is more painful. Plaque and calculus accumulation is often greater on the more painful side of the mouth, as less self-cleansing occurs because of less chewing on the painful side. **Fig. 9** shows

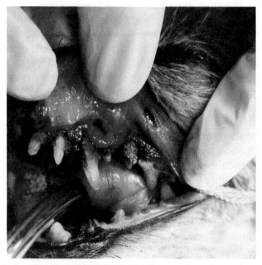

Fig. 7. Severe periodontal disease and gingival recession throughout the mouth of a 13-year-old Yorkshire terrier. Histopathology of the gingival mass over the left maxillary canine tooth revealed gingival hyperplasia and granulation tissue.

Table 1
American Society of Anesthesiologists physical status classification

Category	Physical Status	Example
I	Healthy patient	Removal of persistent deciduous teeth in a healthy young animal
II	Patient with mild systemic disease	Young healthy patient with a mandibular fracture due to dog fight
III	Patient with severe systemic disease	Cachexia, anorexia, and dehydration in a cat with severe stomatitis
IV	Patient with severe systemic disease that is a constant threat to life	Uremic, anorexic, anemic patient with bilateral pathologic mandibular fractures
V	A moribund patient not expected to survive 24 h with or without operation	Unresponsive patient with extreme shock, dehydration, active internal bleeding, pulmonary dysfunction, infection, and seizuring due to a terminal malignancy

Modified from Thurmon JC, Tranquilli WJ, Benson GJ, et al. Lumb & Jones' veterinary anesthesia. Baltimore (MD): Williams & Wilkins; 1996. p. 22.

an algorithm for treatment planning of periodontal disease in this patient. Decisions regarding how best to treat "borderline teeth" will depend on patient health status, the client's willingness to brush daily, and client interest level in saving teeth by performing regular professional dental cleanings in the future.

Case 2: 9-Month-Old Corgi Mixed Breed with a Fractured Tooth

A 9-month-old spayed female Corgi mixed breed is presented approximately 48 hours after fracturing its left maxillary canine tooth (tooth 204) while chewing on a deer antler (**Fig. 10**). The patient is otherwise healthy and was anesthetized 5 months earlier for ovariohysterectomy. Physical examination is nonremarkable except for a fractured cusp of tooth 204 with a red spot in the center of the cusp fracture indicative of pulp exposure. In this case, anesthetic risk, although always present at some level, is considered to be minimal and is outweighed by the benefit of treating the acutely fractured tooth. **Fig. 11** provides an algorithm regarding considerations for treatment of this patient. If the history was different, despite similar signalment (eg, motor vehicle trauma causing a fractured cusp of 204 in a 9-month-old dog), the anesthetic risk might be vastly different because of concerns for increased intracranial pressure, pulmonary contusions, blood loss, and internal bleeding.

Treatment options for a fractured tooth with pulp exposure include extraction, vital pulp therapy, or root canal therapy. An important consideration, when deciding if vital pulp therapy is appropriate, is elapsed time from onset of fracture until treatment. It has been shown that length of time of pulp exposure directly correlates with treatment outcome. A 36-month retrospective study compared the results of vital pulp therapy based on the duration of pulp exposure. Postoperative oral and radiographic examinations were performed at 3, 12, and 36 months following treatment. Based on the 36-month postoperative examinations 88.2%, 41.4%, and 23.5% of teeth were vital when treated within 48 hours, 1 week, and 3 weeks of pulp exposure, respectively. The conclusion from this study was that vital pulp therapy should be done as soon as possible after traumatic tooth fracture to improve outcome.[14] If vital pulp therapy does not provide the desired effect of keeping the tooth vital for the entire life of the

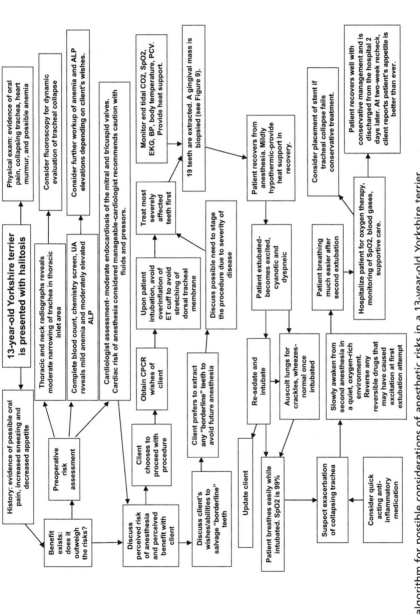

Fig. 8. An algorithm for possible considerations of anesthetic risks in a 13-year-old Yorkshire terrier.

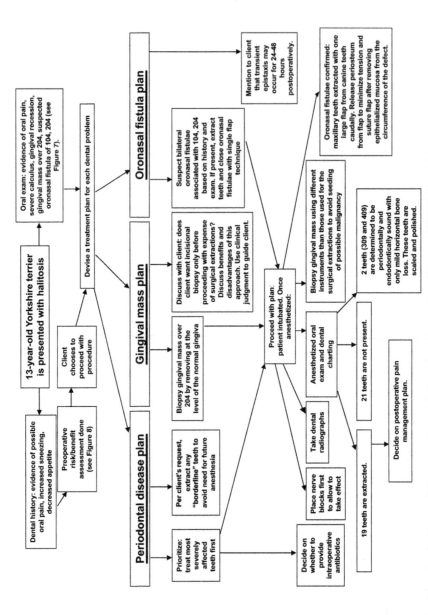

Fig. 9. An algorithm for decision making regarding periodontal treatment in a 13-year-old Yorkshire terrier.

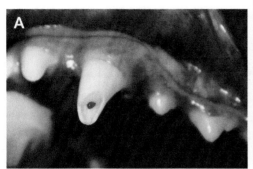
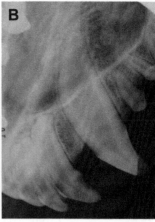

Fig. 10. A 9-month-old Corgi mix was presented with a fractured tooth approximately 48 hours after suspected trauma from chewing on a deer antler. (*A*) Photograph of tooth 204. (*B*) Dental radiograph of tooth 204.

patient, it may at least allow the tooth to mature enough that standard root canal therapy can be done once mature. Alternatively, if the pulp has been exposed for quite a while before treatment, root canal therapy may be considered if the root apex is developed enough to confine the root canal filling material, and if the maturing dentinal walls of the crown are thick enough to have a reasonable chance of avoiding future fracture.

FAILING TO PLAN = PLANNING TO FAIL

Planning of complicated dental or oral surgical procedures can be improved by using donated cadaveric material. The unwritten rule of the Dentistry and Oral Surgery residency program at the University of Pennsylvania is this: before performing a complex procedure on a living patient, this procedure is performed on a cadaver. Although no studies have evaluated the benefits of use of cadavers in veterinary dentistry and oral surgery, use of cadaveric material has been shown to improve outcomes and procedure times when teaching laparoscopy in human medicine.[15] Potential benefits for use of cadavers in veterinary dentistry and oral surgery include reaffirmation of anatomic knowledge, familiarity with instrumentation, and relief of operator stress during the actual procedure. For more involved maxillofacial procedures, computed tomography or magnetic resonance imaging may be performed and evaluated before the actual procedure date to allow for ample time to assess, plan, and perform cadaver procedures.

Another important planning aspect is review of instrumentation before anesthetizing the patient. Reviewing the surgical armamentarium before the procedure ensures all necessary equipment is ready for use and allows an opportunity to define roles when performing "4-handed dentistry" with an assistant. What is on my tray and what needs to be on my tray?

Planning for potential complications is also important. From our previous example, if our 13-year-old Yorkshire terrier awakes from anesthesia, and on extubation, becomes cyanotic and severely dyspneic, do we have the expertise, equipment, and staff to place a nitinol stent if indicated and if other treatment options fail? If not, what can we do as an alternative? Although no pet owner wants to think about what they would do if cardiac or respiratory arrest occurs, do we have a

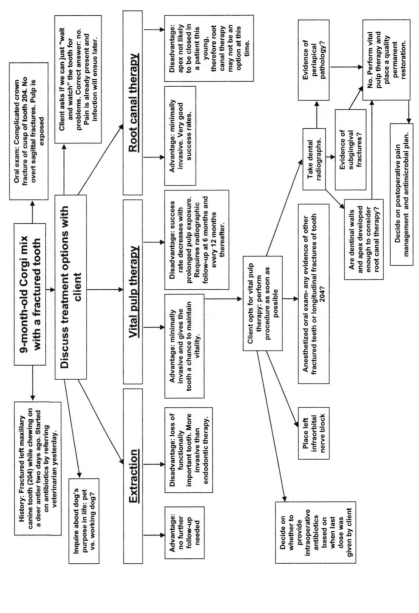

Fig. 11. An algorithm for decision making regarding treatment of a fractured tooth in a 9-month-old Corgi mix.

plan regarding whether the client would like cardiopulmonary cerebral resuscitation performed?

SUMMARY

Making successful therapeutic decisions involves an amalgamation of inputs, including history, physical examination, previous clinical experiences, and available literature. Although there is very little Level I evidence for veterinary dental conditions, the body of literature grows every day. If the details of the case are captured in memory or in dental records, even the most common case provides the opportunity to learn something new.

REFERENCES

1. Feinstein AR. Clinical judgment. Baltimore (MD): Williams & Wilkins; 1967.
2. Sackett DL, Rosenberg WM, Gray JA, et al. Evidence based medicine: what it is and what it isn't. BMJ 1996;312(7023):71–2.
3. Woolf SH, George JN. Evidence-based medicine. Interpreting studies and setting policy. Hematol Oncol Clin North Am 2000;14(4):761–84.
4. United States Prevention Services Task Force. Guide to clinical preventive services: report of the U.S. Preventive Services Task Force; Preface by Robert S. Lawrence. Washington, DC: United States Prevention Services Task Force; 1989. p. 263.
5. Tonelli MR. In defense of expert opinion. Acad Med 1999;74(11):1187–92.
6. Feller L, Blignaut E. Halitosis: a review. SADJ 2005;60(1):17–9.
7. Casteleyn CR, van der Steen M, Declercq J, et al. The buccal lymph node (lymphonodus buccalis) in dogs: occurrence, anatomical location, histological characteristics and clinical implications. Vet J 2008;175(3):379–83.
8. Shelton ME, Forsythe WB. Buccal lymph node in the dog. Am J Vet Res 1979; 40(11):1638–9.
9. Bassert JM, McCurnin DM, McCurnin DM. McCurnin's clinical textbook for veterinary technicians. St Louis (MO): Saunders Elsevier; 2010.
10. Brodbelt D. Feline anesthetic deaths in veterinary practice. Top Companion Anim Med 2010;25(4):189–94.
11. Bille C, Auvigne V, Libermann S, et al. Risk of anaesthetic mortality in dogs and cats: an observational cohort study of 3546 cases. Vet Anaesth Analg 2012;39(1): 59–68.
12. Hosgood G, Scholl DT. Evaluation of age and American Society of Anesthesiologists (ASA) physical status as risk factors for perianesthetic morbidity and mortality in the cat. J Vet Emerg Crit Care 2002;12(1):9–15.
13. Thurmon JC, Tranquilli WJ, Benson GJ, et al. Lumb & Jones' veterinary anesthesia. Baltimore (MD): Williams & Wilkins; 1996. p. 22.
14. Clarke DE. Vital pulp therapy for complicated crown fracture of permanent canine teeth in dogs: a three-year retrospective study. J Vet Dent 2001;18(3):117–21.
15. Levine RL, Kives S, Cathey G, et al. The use of lightly embalmed (fresh tissue) cadavers for resident laparoscopic training. J Minim Invasive Gynecol 2006; 13(5):451–6.

Oral and Dental Imaging Equipment and Techniques for Small Animals

Curt R. Coffman, DVM, FAVD*, Glenn M. Brigden, DVM

KEYWORDS

- Dental radiograph equipment • Veterinary dental radiography
- Digital dental radiographs

KEY POINTS

- Intraoral dental radiographs are necessary for the proper diagnosis and treatment of oral and dental diseases in dogs and cats.
- Equipment that is specifically manufactured for intraoral dental radiography should be used to obtain optimal oral and dental radiographic images.
- Digital intraoral radiography offers many advantages over the use of standard dental radiographic film, including rapid image generation, easier exposure correction, enhancement, and paperless storage.
- Digital image receptors can be divided in to 2 main types, direct digital systems using charged coupled devices and complementary metal oxide semiconductor sensors, and indirect digital systems using phosphor plates with a computerized scanner. Each system is paired with a computer software system to allow handling, visualization, enhancement, sharing, and archiving of the images.
- Proper positioning of the patient and digital sensor must be paired with angulation and exposure settings of the x-ray beam to produce diagnostic oral and dental images.

INTRODUCTION

In the past 2 decades, dentistry has evolved from an ancillary service offered by veterinarians into an integral part of the professional services provided by companion animal practices. With this evolution, dental radiography has become a key component in the proper diagnosis, treatment planning, follow-up evaluation, and medical record keeping for veterinary patients. The combination of proper clinical examination and dental radiography provides the veterinary clinician with the most objective

Arizona Veterinary Dental Specialists, PC, 7908 East Chaparral Road 108, Scottsdale, AZ 85250, USA
* Corresponding author.
E-mail address: curtcoffman@cox.net

Vet Clin Small Anim 43 (2013) 489–506
http://dx.doi.org/10.1016/j.cvsm.2013.02.007
0195-5616/13/$ – see front matter © 2013 Elsevier Inc. All rights reserved.

way to evaluate and diagnose dental and periodontal disease. A veterinarian who is forced to perform dental treatment without the aid of dental radiographs is at a great disadvantage, and may overlook or improperly diagnose dental and periodontal disease.

Intraoral radiography involves placing an image-capturing device such as film, digital sensor, or phosphor plate into the mouth to image a particular tooth or segment of the mandible or maxilla. The intraoral technique has the advantage of clarity and definition of the subject because of the absence of superimposition from the opposing dental arch. In this article, the terms dental radiography and dental imaging imply that the intraoral technique is used unless otherwise indicated. Historically, oral and dental diagnosis has been attempted using extraoral radiography, but the availability and advantages of intraoral radiography have made extraoral radiography using standard veterinary x-ray units obsolete. The rapid technological advancement of dental imaging has dramatically increased the number and complexity of imaging systems available for use by veterinarians. The purpose of this article is to inform veterinarians about the current concepts and latest radiographic imaging techniques in modern veterinary practice.

IMAGING EQUIPMENT AND TECHNOLOGY

There are 2 main equipment components of a dental imaging system, an x-ray generator and an intraoral receptor. Another important part of any digital imaging system is a computer imaging software program. Understanding and properly integrating each of these components will help ensure that high-quality diagnostic images are produced.

Dental X-Ray Generators

Although x-ray tube positioning is critical for adequate image quality, the generating machine itself will also affect image quality. Most dental x-ray generators marketed for veterinary use are machines that were developed for use in human dentistry. In some cases minor changes are made in the control panels or longer extension arms are added to adapt the machines for veterinary patients, but the inner workings of the machines are generally identical to those marketed for human dentists. A typical dental x-ray unit consists of a tube-head assembly that generates the x-rays and an accompanying control panel, which controls the exposure. The tube head has a hollow cylinder that is commonly called the cone or position indicating device (PID), which collimates and helps aim the x-ray beam. In veterinary practices the tube head is often mounted on an extension arm that is attached to wall or ceiling in the dental operating suite. The control panel is mounted behind a nearby wall or shielded area. Hand-held or cart-mounted x-ray generators are also available. Control panels and exposure trigger switches come in various configurations (**Figs. 1–3**). Exposure settings are indicated on the control panel with numerical values, anatomic images that represent pre-programmed settings, or both. Depending on the manufacturer, the exposure control panel may be located on the x-ray unit, may be remotely mounted, or may be configured as a removable faceplate that can be either mounted on the x-ray unit or remotely mounted. Most manufacturers offer a corded exposure trigger switch either as standard equipment or as an option.

The different properties of an x-ray generator can affect the radiographic image in several ways. Radiographic density relates to the degree of "darkness" or "blackness" of a radiograph. The mA (milliamperage) and exposure time are the primary variables used to control image density.[1] The mA and exposure time are both directly

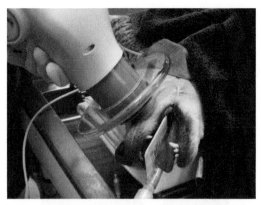

Fig. 1. A hand-held x-ray generator (Nomad Examiner; Aribex Inc, Orem, UT, USA).

related to the quantity of x-rays produced by the x-ray generator. Because most dental x-ray units have a fixed mA (7–15 mA) setting, the exposure time is used to control the quantity of x-rays produced and, thus, film density. Radiographic contrast relates to the number of "grays" visible on a radiograph. High contrast has few shades of gray, and low contrast has many shades of gray.[1] The kVp (kilovoltage peak) is the primary variable used to control film contrast. kVp controls the quality by controlling the wavelength and energy of the x-ray beam. Lower kVp settings produce higher contrast films. Most dental x-ray units have a fixed kVp setting between 60 and 90 kVp.[2] Low-contrast films with many grays (high kVp) are often preferred for visualizing osseous changes. High-contrast images with fewer grays (low kVp) are preferred for visualizing caries and for endodontic procedures. With the increased use of digital imaging systems, varying the kVp setting on an x-ray

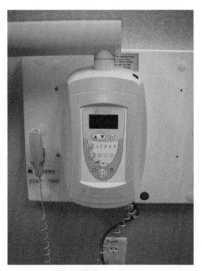

Fig. 2. A wall-mounted x-ray generator with veterinary control panel and wired trigger for remote exposure (Vet Vision DC, Progeny-Midmark, Lincolnshire, IL, USA).

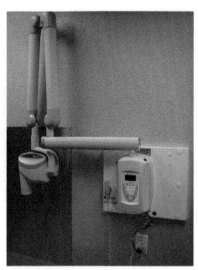

Fig. 3. An example of a wall-mounted veterinary dental x-ray generator with an extension arm for easy movement between operation tables (Vet Vision DC, Progeny-Midmark, Lincolnshire, IL, USA).

generator to control contrast is less important because the contrast of digital images can be manipulated with imaging software. Some older generators with preset exposure times cannot properly integrate with new digital receptors that require short exposure times.[3]

In the past, most dental x-ray generators applied alternating current (AC) to the tube when generating x-rays. However, some newer units apply a nearly constant potential to the tube. These units are referred to as direct current (DC) generators. DC generators produce a relatively constant stream of radiation and a greater percentage of higher-energy "useful" radiation. With an AC generator, voltage across the tube goes from zero up to the maximum kVp, then back to zero. This cycle produces x-ray photons of varying energies. The lowest-energy photons are filtered out, but the average photon energy produced by an AC tube for a given kVp is still lower than the average photon energy produced by a DC tube at that same kV. The patient more readily absorbs lower-energy photons,[1] so the more homogeneous beam of higher-energy photons produced by DC units may slightly reduce patient exposure. When using standard film, the lower average photon energy of an AC unit will produce films of higher contrast than will a DC unit (for a given kVp).[3]

Another consideration is the very low exposure times often used in digital radiography. AC units may not provide exposures as consistent as DC units at very short exposure times (ie, 0.04 seconds), because AC generators produce a sinusoidal waveform and x-rays are generated only in the "positive" portion of the waves. Depending on at what point in the waveform the exposure was initiated, less "usable" portions of the waves may be captured.[3] At very low exposure-time settings, this could result in variability in the overall x-rays generated for a given exposure. DC may reduce patient exposure slightly and may produce more consistent exposures at the very short exposure times associated with digital radiography. Overall, these differences are relatively minor, and AC and DC units are both capable of producing diagnostic images using either conventional film or digital radiography.

Types of Intraoral Receptors

- Standard dental x-ray film
- Direct radiography systems
- Computed radiography systems

Standard dental x-ray film is composed of a plastic/polyester base covered with a silver halide/gelatin emulsion. The silver halide crystals are affected by the x-rays and eventually form an image during film processing. During processing the film is exposed to a series of chemicals in a darkroom. This process can be time consuming, and incorrect exposures or mistakes in the development process require retakes, exposing the patient to additional radiation. The chemicals used for processing also require special handling and disposal. Because of these negative aspects and the availability of digital imaging, standard dental film is becoming less frequently used.

Digital receptors generally require less radiation and produce images much quicker than conventional radiographic films, often instantly viewable on a computer monitor. Digital receptors can be divided into direct and indirect receptor systems. Direct systems are often referred to as DR (direct radiography) systems, and indirect systems are termed CR (computed radiography) systems.

DR systems include charged coupled devices (CCD) and complementary metal oxide semiconductor (CMOS) sensors that contain silicon crystals, which convert photons to electrons. For CCD sensors, pixel charges are transferred to an output source for conversion, whereas for CMOS sensors the conversion takes place at each pixel.[4] Once digitized, the signals are converted by the system's software into images for viewing on a computer monitor. Each sensor type can be fabricated into typical intraoral sizes (except size 4 occlusal), but their active areas are somewhat smaller than on corresponding standard dental film. The nature of their components, along with cable connection and electrical supply, makes DR sensors thicker than standard film (**Fig. 4**). Wired and wireless DR sensors are available.

Because of their solid-state nature, DR sensors are more x-ray sensitive in comparison with conventional films or CR plates, allowing lower exposure times,[5–8] and they also offer almost instantaneous image generation. One reported drawback with direct sensor systems has been the occurrence of blooming artifacts.[4,6,7] Such an artifact may occur on areas of the sensor open to high x-ray exposure, causing the individual pixel capacity to be exceeded. If exceeded, the charge may subsequently leak into

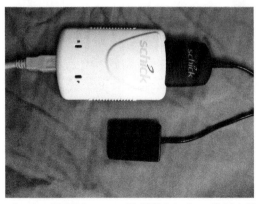

Fig. 4. An example of a size #2 DR Sensor with USB interface (Schick Vet, Schick Technologies, Inc, Long Island City, NY, USA).

neighboring pixels, leading to blooming. Blooming is usually seen as excessively dark areas where the charge overflow has occurred. As the technology of DR sensors and accompanying software has advanced, these limitations are being overcome.[4,9] Comparison of the image quality of the CMOS with CCD-based detectors showed minimal difference in diagnostic capabilities.[10] Another disadvantage is the thickness of DR sensors, which can make placement in smaller patients difficult.

CR systems use photostimulable storage phosphor plates (PSP) for dental imaging. The wireless photostimulable phosphor plate is also known as an imaging plate, storage phosphor imaging plate, or digital cassette. The CR imaging plates resemble standard intraoral films, and can be designed into similar-sized plates (including occlusal size 4). The thin nature of the plates may make them easier to place in the patient's mouth in comparison with DR sensors.

The photostimulable phosphors in the imaging plate have a property termed phosphorescence or photoluminescence, which allows them store x-ray energy and later free the energy as emitted light. To prepare the imaging plate for an x-ray exposure, the plate is exposed to intense light to erase any previous image. When exposed to x-rays, the phosphors are ionized and the number of trapped electrons is proportional to the amount of x-rays absorbed locally. These trapped electrons constitute a latent image. Owing to thermal motion, over time the electrons will slowly be liberated, so the latent image should be read without extended delay.[7]

After x-ray exposure the CR plate is inserted into a scanning unit and the plate is "read" with a laser light (**Fig. 5**). The laser scans the imaging plate while the plate is moved past the scanning beam. The laser stimulates the trapped electrons, leading to liberation of energy in the form of light emission. The emitted light is collected and digitized, and the image is stored in a computer as a digital matrix with each pixel having a gray-scale value determined by the amount of light emitted from the corresponding dot on the imaging plate. The system's computer software then transforms the matrix into a usable image. CR imaging plates have a wider dynamic range and exposure latitude than standard dental film and DR sensor systems. Although the required amount of radiation exposure needed for CR plates is similar to that of standard film systems, the uniform image density, even with overexposure and

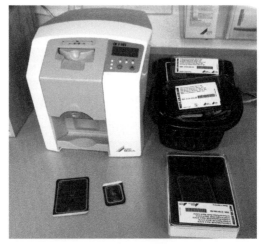

Fig. 5. An example of a CR system including digital image scanner and size #2 and #4 CR plates (CR7 Vet, IM3 Inc, Vancouver, WA, USA).

underexposure, is improved in comparison with standard film. This improvement may lead to fewer retakes following incorrect exposures. However, for most diagnostic tasks in dentistry, CR plates will provide images similar to those of CCD/CMOS sensors.[11]

Advanced 3-Dimensional Imaging

Medical-grade computed tomography (CT) scanners have become more widely available in veterinary medicine, and may provide additional information beyond the 2-dimensional images offered by intraoral dental radiographs. The 3-dimensional nature of the CT image may be helpful in certain challenging clinical situations. Cone-beam CT (CBCT), a relatively new diagnostic imaging modality, has been used in human dental imaging recently. CBCT uses a cone beam instead of the fan-shaped beam used in medical-grade CT to acquire images. In humans it offers relatively high-resolution, isotropic images when compared with medical-grade CT images.[11] Although promising, the current state of CBCT technology may be of limited clinical use in dogs and cats.[12]

DIAGNOSTIC IMAGING TECHNIQUES
Patient Preparation and Positioning for Dental Radiographs

All veterinary patients that require dental radiographs should be under general anesthesia, thus ensuring that movement will not affect detail of the radiographs and expensive digital sensors, and that plates will not be damaged. The authors recommend that standard anesthetic monitoring be used, including electrocardiography, blood pressure, pulse oximetry, and CO_2 monitoring with intravenous fluid administration.

The use of lead aprons and thyroid protectors is always recommended, along with dosimeters to protect staff against radiation exposure. Fortunately, the radiation produced by dental x-ray generators is minimal compared with standard medical x-ray machines. When using digital DR sensors, the radiation is further reduced in comparison with the level used with standard dental film.[13] General safety rules to observe when exposing dental radiographs include:

- Never stand directly facing the beam.
- Always stand behind or 90° to the side of the beam.
- Be at least 6 ft (1.8 m) away from the subject during exposure.
- Avoid using your hands to hold the generator or sensor in position.

If the x-ray generator tube head is drifting, adjusting the joints of the extension arm will prevent the drift. Sensor holders are available commercially through veterinary and dental distributors; however, the authors find that folded paper towels or gauze sponges are very convenient, readily available in the clinic, and inexpensive for positioning sensors or plates. Consider using beanbags placed on each side of the patient to assist in positioning during radiography.

Imaging Procedures

Full-mouth dental radiographs in most cats can be achieved with 7 radiographs. The number of exposures needed of full-mouth radiographs in a dog may vary from 8 to 20 exposures using a size-2 sensor depending on the size of the patient. The use of #4 size film or CR plate can reduce the amount of radiographs required. DR sensors are limited to size-2 sensors or smaller, whereas CR systems such as the CR7-Vet (IM3 Inc. Vancouver WA, USA) or the ScanX-Duo (Air Techniques Inc, Melville, NY) have sizes up to size-4 intraoral plates. These devices also have options for larger, custom plates that may be useful in exotic animal and avian practices.

When first learning to radiograph patients, use the preprogrammed exposure times on the x-ray generators as starting points for individual patients. If the radiographs are too light then additional exposure time is needed, and vice versa if the radiographs are too dark. These initial radiographs will determine proper exposure times for individual teeth and different sizes of patients, and can be used to develop a simple exposure technique chart. With time the clinician will become more familiar with the equipment and will build a working knowledge of the time of exposure needed to produce quality and consistent dental radiographs. Each individual x-ray generator may vary slightly in the exposures.

Imaging Techniques and Positioning

Patient positioning and angulation of the x-ray beam are very important in obtaining optimal dental radiographic images. A summary of techniques used to obtain dental radiographs is provided here. Individuals who are learning how to obtain dental radiographs should enroll in a hands-on laboratory to develop and refine proper techniques.

There are two main target areas commonly imaged by dental radiographs in dogs and cats, one of which is the alveolar bone in relation to the roots of the teeth. This area is important when evaluating the bone height and density for periodontal disease. The amount of bone loss visualized radiographically can help categorize the severity of periodontal disease, which is important for evaluating and assigning a prognosis to individual teeth. The second area is the apex of the root, which is important when endodontic disease is suspected. The target areas of the radiographs should be either centered in the image or at least 3 to 5 mm from the edge of the image to provide the most accurate assessment of the area. Ultimately, visualizing the entire tooth is best, but this is not always possible because of the size of the patient and teeth; this holds particularly true for canine teeth. In large dogs, when using size-2 sensors 2 radiographs may be required to visualize the entire tooth. When taking radiographs of a particular tooth, it is always helpful to radiograph the contralateral tooth for comparison. Often what appears to be apical abnormality on a tooth may actually be normal anatomy.

There are 2 basic methods for placing the sensor or plate when taking dental radiographs: intraoral and extraoral. Both techniques have advantages and disadvantages. Intraoral radiographic techniques are most frequently used to image individual teeth, and form the main point of discussion here. Specific instances for using extraoral techniques are mentioned later in the article.

When describing dental radiographic positioning, most people are familiar with the terms "parallel and bisecting-angle" techniques. Understanding these techniques is frequently a source of frustration for those who are learning dental radiographic techniques and those who cannot mentally visualize the root structure beneath the mucosa and bone. Having an anatomically correct clear dental model (**Fig. 6**) and skulls of the dog and the cat (**Fig. 7**) are a necessity when first learning intraoral techniques. The clear models allow the operator to visualize the relative position of the roots as they exist in a patient, and better understand the theory of the bisecting-angle technique. The skulls allow the operator to practice dental radiographic techniques without prolonging anesthetic procedures for the patient.

The parallel technique, the use of which is limited to the caudal mandibular premolars and molars, is the easiest understand and learn. This technique involves lining up the sensor or plate parallel to the desired tooth and then aiming the tube head and x-ray beam at a 90° angle to the sensor and tooth (**Fig. 8**). When placing the DR sensor

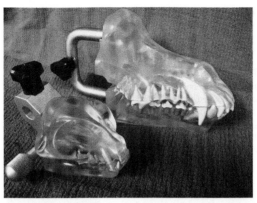

Fig. 6. Clear plastic dental models are an invaluable aid for learning dental anatomy as well as helping with client education (Columbia Dentoform Corporation, Long Island City, NY, USA).

in the mouth, the cord should always be toward the front of the mouth and the flat side of the sensor toward the cone. When using CR plates, the positioning guide (usually a white/silver or black dot in one corner of the plate) should be toward the front of the mouth to allow consistent orientation of the images (**Fig. 9**). In all radiographic techniques, the tube head should be placed as close to the subject and sensor as possible to give the most accurate and detailed image. The inverse square law governs the intensity of the radiation in relation to the distance between the x-ray generator and to the sensor. In general terms, if the distance between the x-ray tube head and the sensor is twice as far away; the intensity of the radiation received at the sensor is reduced by 4-fold,[1] thus requiring a significantly increased exposure time to account for the extra distance.

The bisecting-angle technique is required for imaging all other teeth in the mouth, because the normal anatomy of the mouth prevents the placement of the sensors or plates directly parallel to the other teeth. The bisecting technique is based on the line angle of the film in relation to the line angle of the tooth root of interest. The

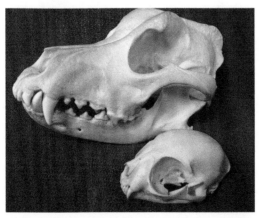

Fig. 7. The best way to learn the proper positioning needed to obtain quality dental radiographic images is to practice with canine and feline skulls. Only genuine skull specimens can be used to produce images (Skulls Unlimited International, Oklahoma City, OK, USA).

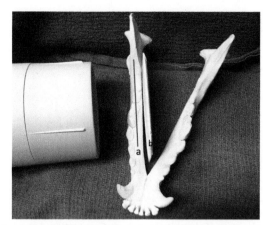

Fig. 8. The caudal mandibular premolars and molar are imaged using the parallel technique. With the parallel technique the film, plate, or sensor (b) is placed directly behind and parallel to the subject teeth (a). The cone and x-ray beam are directed perpendicular to the film and teeth.

midpoint or bisecting angle between the 2 previously determined angles (film, tooth root) is where the x-ray beam should be aimed. This technique is easier to illustrate than explain (**Fig. 10**).

For individuals who are averse to geometry, there are other ways to develop the skills needed to obtain quality dental radiographs consistently. The use of digital dental radiographs and models are key in either respect. Another useful training method involves using a clear anatomic model, a flashlight to represent the x-ray generator, and the blank side of a business card to represent the sensors. Using the flashlight, the images of the teeth in the clear model are projected on the business

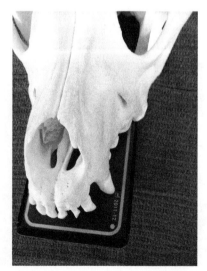

Fig. 9. A CR plate showing the white dot used for orientation of the plate. The dot should always be placed toward the rostral direction or the "front" of the mouth for proper communication with the scanning software.

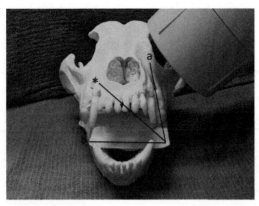

Fig. 10. The maxillary premolars are imaged using the bisecting-angle technique. With the bisecting-angle technique the film, plate, or sensor (b) is placed in a horizontal or "flat" position in the mouth, and the cone and x-ray beam are directed perpendicular to a line (*asterisk*) halfway between the film (b) and the long axis of the subject teeth (a).

card. This projection mimics what occurs with x-ray exposure of dental radiographs, but with the flashlight beam one can visualize the effect of the different angles used to produce the image immediately (**Fig. 11**). Some of the most common mistakes made during dental radiography are elongation, foreshortening (**Fig. 12**), and failure to image

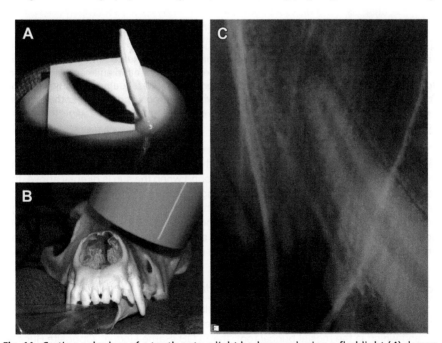

Fig. 11. Casting a shadow of a tooth onto a light background using a flashlight (*A*) demonstrates what occurs with x-ray exposure of dental radiographs using the bisecting-angle technique (*B*). A radiographic image produced using the bisecting technique (*C*) essentially "shadows" the image onto the film or sensor. Using the flashlight demonstration, simply changing the angle that the flashlight beam shines toward the tooth will mimic how different exposure angles will affect the image.

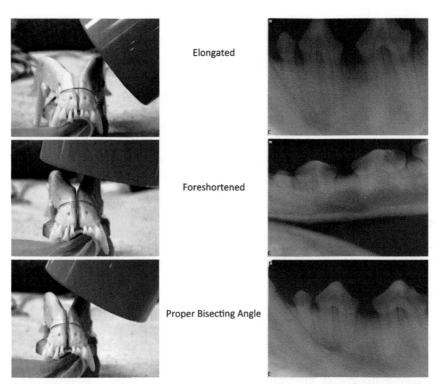

Fig. 12. When using the bisecting-angle technique, changing the aim or angulation of the x-ray beam will cause a specific corresponding change in the resulting image. In the examples shown, aiming the beam in a more vertical position will result in an image of roots that appear shorter than normal anatomy (foreshortening). Conversely, aiming the beam along a more horizontal angle will result in an image where the roots appear longer than normal anatomy (elongation). Using a proper bisecting angle will result in an image that reproduces normal anatomy.

the apex of the target tooth. This flashlight method helps illustrate how to correct these errors. Much like a person's shadow on the ground when the sun is directly above, the shadow is short and almost nonexistent. During the periods of sunrise and sunset, the shadow is elongated out to infinity. Somewhere between sunrise/sunset and high noon, the shadow length will equal the person's height. This concept can be easily applied to dental radiographs, matching the angle of the sun (x-ray generator), the person (the target tooth), and the ground (the sensor).

Techniques for Specific Areas of the Oral Cavity

Intraoral imaging of the maxillary fourth premolar roots frequently requires specialized technique. When determining which root of the maxillary fourth premolar is the palatal root and which is the mesial buccal root, the SLOB (Same Lingual, Opposite Buccal) rule, also known as the Tube-Shift rule or Clark rule, is used.[14,15] Two exposures of the tooth are often required. The first exposure is made using basic bisecting-angle positioning as a reference. The tube head is then shifted in either a rostral or caudal direction while still aiming toward the target tooth. The position change of the roots on this second radiographic image will determine which root is the palatal and which is the mesial buccal. If the tube head is shifted rostrally, the root that shifts the same way is the lingual (or in this case the palatal) root. The tooth shifting the opposite direction is the buccal (or mesial buccal) root.

In the case of the maxillary premolars in cats, the best intraoral technique by which to visualize the roots is intentional elongation, which allows one to radiograph the teeth "under" the zygomatic arch. A normal bisecting-angle technique will project the roots of these teeth with superimposition of the zygomatic arch, which may prevent an accurate evaluation and diagnosis. An alternative approach for the feline maxillary premolars is an extraoral technique, whereby the sensor or plate is placed outside the mouth parallel to the long axis of the premolars to be imaged. With the mouth open and the head in a lateral oblique position, the x-ray beam is directed through the oral cavity at the premolars in a slight oblique angulation. Extraoral techniques may also be useful in visualizing the caudal mandible, to avoid bending the plates or forcing sensors to fit into the oropharynx.

Using the parallel technique for visualizing the mandibular first/second premolars in dogs and third premolar in cats is not possible in most patients. In both dogs and cats, the mandibular symphyseal joint prevents placement of the sensor parallel to the tooth roots, so a bisecting-angle technique is commonly required to properly image these teeth. This positioning technique for the rostral mandibular premolars also provides perspective of the root apex of the mandibular canine tooth. In many cases, exposing multiple views (rostral and lateral projections) using the bisecting-angle technique for the mandibular canine teeth will allow a more complete assessment of the teeth (**Figs. 13** and **14**). Similarly, multiple views of the maxillary canines may provide a better assessment of the health of the palatal bone support of these teeth.

The presence of the mental foramen on the radiographic images can mimic apical abnormality, especially near the roots of the mandibular first or second premolars.

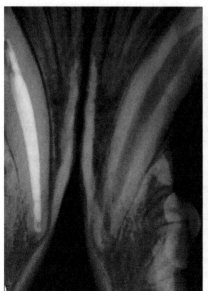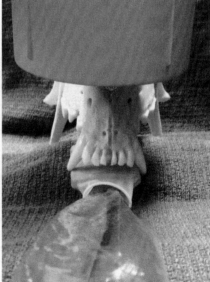

Fig. 13. In the rostral projection of the mandibular canines, the x-ray beam is aimed in a near-parallel angulation to obtain views of both the left and right mandibular canines. (Note: the right mandibular canine shows a partially obturated root canal.)

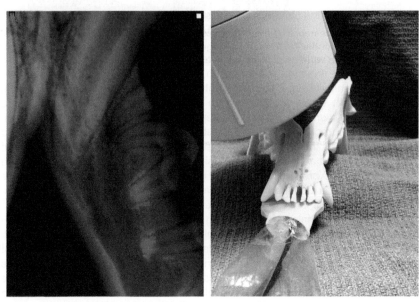

Fig. 14. To obtain a lateral projection of the mandibular canine, the cone is shifted in a slightly lateral direction to obtain a second view of the apex of the left mandibular canine and rostral premolar.

Obtaining a second radiograph of the area at a slightly different angle can help distinguish normal anatomy from pathologic appearance. Because DR sensors provide almost instantaneous results, it is easy to make small adjustments to the angle of the x-ray beam or exposure times to obtain a second image. Normal skeletal structures such as the mental foramen will appear to "move" from the tooth apex with the slight angle shift of the beam.

Imaging Errors and Artifacts

Elongation and foreshortening of the radiographs can cause to the clinician to miss a diagnosis. With elongation, the apex of the roots may be too close to the edge of the image or even off the edge. Accuracy and quality of the image increase toward the center of the image. The tooth or area of interest should always be centered on the sensor, plate, or film. Foreshortening may also disguise the lesions by making them appear smaller. Adjusting the angle of exposure, as already discussed, will provide more accurate images.

Cervical burnout occurs with overexposure of the radiograph. Overexposure can give the false impression of abnormality, and may mimic tooth resorption and the loss of tooth/crown structure. Retaking the radiograph at a lower time setting will allow accurate evaluation of the teeth and bone structures. In the opposite situation, a radiograph that is too light (underexposed) does not show enough detail to be diagnostic. This artifact can be seen as a very light or even bright pixelated distortion on the radiograph. Increasing the exposure time will remedy this problem.

Cone cut occurs when part of the sensor is not exposed owing to improper alignment of the cone of the x-ray tube in relation to the digital sensor or film. Not only does this make the radiographs look unprofessional, but critical information can be missed when evaluating the images. It appears as a rounded and well-defined margin of white, indicating that no exposure and no data were received on that part of the sensor. Readjusting and centering the cone and x-ray beam to cover the entire sensor will eliminate this problem with smaller-sized sensors. This problem occurs more commonly when using size-4 plates or film, owing to the size of the film being larger than the diameter of the collimated beam emitted from the tube head.

Bending of the plate during placement in the mouth can cause distortion of the image with both standard x-ray film and CR plates. The distorted image will appear like a reflection produced in a "wavy" carnival mirror. Using an appropriately sized plate in the mouth will prevent the need for bending during placement. Forceful placement of sensors may lead to injury of the sublingual mucosa when positioning a DR sensor using the parallel technique to radiograph the caudal premolars and molars in small dogs and cats. Gentle placement and lubrication of the sensor and mucosa can help prevent trauma to the mucosa.

Careful handling procedures when using digital sensors will prevent the sensors from being bitten by the patient under anesthesia. Having the patient in a stable plane of general anesthesia will prevent biting. The use of mouth gags will also help prevent both personal injuries to fingers and damage to the sensors, but prolonged episodes of mouth-gag use should be avoided. Always use provided plastic covers to protect the sensors and plates from scratching and other damage, and avoid allowing DR sensors to be dropped or the connection cords to be stretched. When touching or handling CR plates the phosphor surface should be avoided, so as to prevent finger-print defects and scratches. Using appropriate plastic protectors will help prevent image artifacts caused by scratching the phosphor surface. When feeding the plate into the scanner one must make sure that the plastic protector is free of debris to avoid contamination of the interior of the scanner.

Digital Image Handling and Manipulation

When interpreting images, it is important to take a consistent, systematic approach to assessing the entire radiographic image. A detailed discussion of interpretation is presented in articles "Radiographic Imaging – Dog Interpretation" by Kris Bannon and Radiographic Imaging – Cat Interpretation by Matt Lemmons elsewhere in this issue, so a brief description of handling digital images is offered here. An obvious benefit of DR is that computer manipulation and processing of DR images may facilitate extraction of items of diagnostic interest. Image processing has been shown to improve diagnostic quality, but certain processing parameters must be used for specific diagnostic tasks. Digital manipulation will be most effective if the original digital image is of optimal quality and is acquired using proper exposure parameters. Numerous image-processing algorithms exist for different diagnostic tasks, and articles are available that explain how imaging algorithms modify a dental radiograph.[16,17] Studies using contrast enhancement have found it to be useful for specific diagnostic tasks.[4] One study reported that images[18] that were contrast enhanced outperformed film for evaluation of the size of periapical lesions. It is also important to understand that inappropriate processing of images has been shown to degrade image quality and render the radiograph nondiagnostic.[19] Put simply, there is no single image-processing or manipulation method that will provide ideal enhancement for all diagnostic tasks.

Examples of common software manipulation options (CDR DICOM Ver. 4.5. Schick Technologies Inc, Long Island City, NY. www.schicktech.com)

- Equalization: Equalizes the image contrast, allowing evaluation of radiographs that are too light and making them more readable.

- Positive/negative manipulation: Reverses the shades of gray, which can help highlight some fine details in the image.
- Revealer: Maximizes the contrast of the image; which allows better visualization of the image.
- Flashlight: Similar to revealer but only highlights a chosen area of the radiograph. It can be moved to different locations on the radiograph using the mouse.
- Emboss: Used to view the radiographs in a simulated 3-dimensional format by raising the foreground layer of the radiograph.
- Reorient: Allows spatial manipulation of the images to ensure a consistent viewing of the teeth or image taken in the wrong view box.
- Importing/exporting: Moving images into and out of the patient examination in formats including, but not limited to, Digital Imaging and Communications in Medicine (DICOM), TIFF, Windows Bitmap, and JPEG.
- Detaching: Sorts and displays only the appropriate or diagnostic images for the examination. The software retains all detached images in searchable archives. Images can be restored to the original examination, as needed, using the software.

Different brands of DR and CR systems each have their own examination setup and layout options on the computer desktop. Most software programs allow users to customize examination layouts that best suit their needs, which helps the clinician to assess the images quickly, easily, and consistently. Each digital software package has multiple preset options for manipulation of digital images. These options use built-in algorithms to allow the clinician to manipulate the original image by selecting a button on the computer screen. The preset options aim to enhance a particular characteristic of the original image to increase the diagnostic value of the image. Computer hardware can also have a direct effect on the usability and diagnostic value of DR images. The ability to diagnose carious lesions with digital images in humans was found to be significantly better in a room with lower ambient light and on a monitor with well-adjusted brightness and contrast values than in a room with bright light and on an unadjusted monitor.[20]

Image Sharing and Compression

Images are ideally saved in tagged image file (.tif) format to avoid loss of information. Alternatively, they could be saved in DICOM format. DICOM is the universal standard for medical image encoding for transmission and archival purposes. It allows images generated by different units using different acquisition and processing software to be read without loss of diagnostic information. Saving and sending images electronically are integral components of digital radiology, and images can be reduced in size for storage or transmission purposes. However, some proprietary software formats for image viewing may limit electronic transfer and accessibility of the digital image.[21] However, evidence suggests that high compression ratios can have a negative impact on the diagnostic quality of digital radiographs.[22] Analysis of the effect of a reduction in size of digital images on diagnostic outcome of maxillary and mandibular premolars revealed that reduction in image size might lead to a loss of diagnostic information.[23]

SUMMARY

Dental radiography has become vital to delivery of state-of-the-art veterinary dental care today. Digital intraoral imaging has several advantages over standard dental film, and has facilitated more rapid diagnosis and delivery of treatment by veterinary dentists. Careful selection of an x-ray generator, digital image receptor system, and computer software system that integrate easily will help ensure the foundation for efficacious dental imaging in the veterinary office. The ability to view digital radiographs rapidly and then use software for image enhancement may aid diagnosis, but the clinician's ability to position and properly expose the radiograph is still of utmost importance. It is the combination of clinical aptitude combined with the proper use of contemporary equipment and technology that will ultimately provide the best diagnostic outcome.

REFERENCES

1. Thrall DE, Widmer WR. Radiation physics, radiation protection and darkroom theory. In: Thrall DE, editor. Textbook of veterinary radiology. Philadelphia: WB Saunders; 2002. p. 1–17.
2. Dupont GA, DeBowes LJ. Equipment. In: Atlas of dental radiography in dogs and cats. St Louis (MO): WB Saunders; 2009. p. 255.
3. Synopsis of Intra-Oral X-ray Units (Project 05-02) Air Force Medical Service USAF Dental Evaluation & Consultation Service. Available at: http://airforcemedicine. afms.mil/decs. Accessed April, 2005.
4. Litwiller D. CCD vs CMOS: maturing technologies. Photon Spectra 2005;1:154–8. Available at: www.photonics.com/. Accessed August 1, 2005.
5. Paurazas SB, Geist JR, Pink FE, et al. Comparison of diagnostic accuracy of digital imaging by using CCD and CMOS-APS sensors with E-speed film in the detection of periapical bony lesions. Oral Surg Oral Med Oral Pathol Oral Radiol Endod 2000;89(3):356–62.
6. Berkhout WE, Beuger DA, Sanderink GC, et al. The dynamic range of digital radiographic systems: dose reduction or risk of overexposure? Dentomaxillofac Radiol 2004;33(1):1–5.
7. Borg E. Some characteristics of solid-state and photo-stimulable phosphor detectors for intra-oral radiography. Swed Dent J Suppl 1999;139:1–67.
8. Pfeiffer P, Schmage P, Nergiz I, et al. Effects of different exposure values on diagnostic accuracy of digital images. Quintessence Int 2000;31(4):256–60.
9. Inglese JM, Farman TT, Farman AG. The sixth-generation: introduction of two new high fill factor complementary metal oxide semiconductor (or SuperCMOS) intraoral X-ray detectors. In: Computer assisted radiology and surgery. Proceedings of the 18th International Congress and Exhibition, Chicago, 2004. p. 1152–6. Accessed June, 2004.
10. Kitagawa H, Scheetz JP, Farman AG. Comparison of complementary metal oxide semiconductor and charge-coupled device intraoral X-ray detectors using subjective image quality. Dentomaxillofac Radiol 2003;32:408–41.
11. Nair MK, Nair UP. Digital and advanced imaging in endodontics: a review. J Endod 2007;33(1):1–6.
12. Van Thielen B, Siguenza F, Hassan B. Cone beam computed tomography in veterinary dentistry. J Vet Dent 2011;29(1):27–34.
13. Dupont GA, DeBowes LJ. Atlas of dental radiography in dogs and cats. St Louis (MO): Saunders; 2009. p. 259–60.
14. Mulligan TW, Aller MS, Williams CA. Atlas of canine and feline dental radiography. Trenton (NJ): Veterinary Learning Systems; 1998. p. 16–22.
15. Oakes A. Introduction radiology techniques. In: DeForge DH, Colmery BH, editors. An atlas of veterinary dental radiology. Ames: Iowa State University Press; 2000. p. XXI–XXII.

16. Analoui M. Radiographic image enhancement (part I: spatial domain techniques). Dentomaxillofac Radiol 2001;30:1–9.
17. Analoui M. Radiographic digital image enhancement (part II: transform domain techniques). Dentomaxillofac Radiol 2001;30:65–77.
18. Farman AG, Avant SL, Scarfe WC, et al. An in-vivo comparison of Visualix-2 and Ektaspeed Plus in the assessment of periapical lesion dimensions. Oral Surg Oral Med Oral Pathol Oral Radiol Endod 1998;85:203–9.
19. Tyndall DA, Ludlow JB, Platin E, et al. A comparison of Kodak Ektaspeed Plus film and the Siemens Sidexis digital imaging systems for caries detection using receiver operating characteristic analysis. Oral Surg Oral Med Oral Pathol Oral Radiol Endod 1998;85:1131–8.
20. Hellén-Halme K. Quality aspects of digital radiography in general dental practice. Swed Dent J Suppl 2007;184:9–60.
21. ADA Council of Scientific Affairs. The use of dental radiographs: update and recommendations. J Am Dent Assoc 2006;137:1304–12.
22. Eraso FE, Analoui M, Watson AB, et al. Impact of lossy compression on diagnostic accuracy of radiographs for periapical lesions. Oral Surg Oral Med Oral Pathol Oral Radiol Endod 2002;93:621–5.
23. Versteeg CH, Sanderink GC, Lobach SR, et al. Reduction in size of digital images: does it lead to less detectability or loss of diagnostic information? Dentomaxillofac Radiol 1998;27:93–6.

Clinical Canine Dental Radiography

Kristin M. Bannon, DVM, FAVD, DAVDC

KEYWORDS

- Canine intraoral radiographs • Periodontal disease • Endodontic disease
- Dental anatomy • Intraoral radiograph orientation • Developmental anomalies

KEY POINTS

- Intraoral radiographs should be performed with every canine dental procedure.
- More pathology is identified with intraoral radiographs than with clinical examination alone.
- Understanding of proper anatomy, radiograph orientation, and normal variations is essential to identifying pathology.
- Performing intraoral radiographs when appropriate allows for better patient care, which also improves practices.

INTRODUCTION

Dental and oral diseases are a common problem in companion animals. Dental radiography is an important piece of the puzzle that helps practitioners with diagnosis and treatment. In one study of dental radiograph diagnostic value, radiographs identified clinically relevant problems in visibly normal teeth in 27.8% of dogs and incidental findings in clinically normal teeth in 41.7% of dogs, and, in teeth clinically diagnosed with disease, 50% more information was obtained with radiographs than without.[1]

Because of this important diagnostic value, every dental procedure should include intraoral radiographs – taking intraoral radiographs is a black and white issue. Interpretation of those radiographs, however, brings in the shades of gray that make life complicated. The purpose of this article is to introduce practitioners to dental radiographic interpretation and make some sense out of the chaos that can be canine intraoral radiography.

DENTAL RADIOGRAPHS: WHEN AND WHY?

As stated previously, full mouth radiographs in clinically normal patients identify clinically relevant disease that would not have been identified in any other way. The

Veterinary Dentistry and Oral Surgery of New Mexico, LLC, 2001 Vivigen Way, Santa Fe, NM 87505, USA
E-mail address: aggiekris@aol.com

Vet Clin Small Anim 43 (2013) 507–532
http://dx.doi.org/10.1016/j.cvsm.2013.02.011   vetsmall.theclinics.com
0195-5616/13/$ – see front matter © 2013 Elsevier Inc. All rights reserved.

American Animal Hospital Association recommends full mouth intraoral radiographs as a baseline, then as needed thereafter.[2] The teeth should be cleaned before the exposure of the radiographs. Calculus is radio-opaque, is visible on radiographs, and may obscure correct interpretation of the radiographs (**Box 1**).

NOMENCLATURE
Tooth Identification

The current standard for identifying teeth in companion animal medicine is the Triadan system.[3] In the Triadan system, the teeth are organized into 4 quadrants and each quadrant is assigned a group number. The individual teeth within the quadrant also have a number, so that each unique tooth has a 3-digit number that identifies it by quadrant and type of tooth. The 4 quadrants are the right maxillary quadrant (100s), the left maxillary quadrant (200s), the left mandibular quadrant (300s), and the right mandibular quadrant (400s).

Within each quadrant are 4 types of teeth: incisors, canines, premolars, and molars. The teeth are numbered consecutively from the midline moving toward the back of the mouth, starting with the central incisors. The incisors are 01 through 03. The canine is 04. The premolars are 05 through 08 and the molars are 09 through 11.

Therefore, a right maxillary canine tooth is designated as 104, and a left mandibular third premolar is identified as 307. This system allows for easy and rapid identification of a tooth for record keeping as well as discussion with colleagues and specialists.

Box 1
Indications for intraoral radiographs

- Missing teeth
- Fractured teeth
- Discolored teeth
- Resorptive lesions
- Pre-extraction
- Post-extraction
- Periodontal pockets
- Worn/abraded teeth
- Gingival enlargements, masses, and tumors
- Painful or sensitive teeth
- Draining tracts
- Nasal discharge
- History of oral pain, drooling, or pawing at mouth
- Client education
- Decreased interest in chew toys or bones
- Epistaxis
- Evaluation of prior treatment
- Evaluation of disease progression
- Medical-legal record keeping
- And many more!

In the oral cavity, each tooth is examined and identified as a separate entity. This allows for proper record keeping and identification of abnormalities in association with certain parts of the tooth. For example, if a periodontal pocket is identified on only one aspect of a particular tooth, this is documented in the medical record so that it is evaluated at the next dental procedure and accurate comparisons are made over time.

Directional Terminology

The most common directional terms used in association with oral and dental structures are *mesial, distal, buccal, lingual, palatal, interproximal, coronal,* and *apical.*[3]

- Mesial—toward the midline of the maxilla or mandible
- Distal—away from the midline
- Buccal—toward the buccal mucosa
- Lingual—toward the tongue
- Palatal—toward the palate
- Interproximal—the space in between the teeth
- Coronal—toward the tip of the crown of the tooth
- Apical—toward the root apex

The nomenclature of the tooth names and directions are important when discussing radiographs so that practitioners can understand, document, and relay to colleagues and clients the correct location of pathology in relation to normal structures.

PATIENT POSITIONING

To obtain diagnostic radiographs of the canine dentition, patients must be under general anesthesia. Patients are positioned in any recumbency that is convenient for the veterinarian. In the author's practice, patients are positioned in dorsal recumbency and then the head can be tilted from side to side as needed for access to a specific area of the dentition without disturbing the anesthetic monitors. The primary goal for obtaining intraoral radiographs is to visualize the structures of the tooth that cannot be seen clinically. The most important part of the tooth to examine radiographically is the root structure. A common mistake made when obtaining radiographs is to center the film on the visible portion of the tooth. Unfortunately, in most situations, this does not allow visualization of the structures of the tooth that are below the gingival margin and within the bone. There are 2 commonly used methods of obtaining dental radiographs. One is the parallel technique, and the other uses a bisecting angle.

Parallel Technique

The parallel technique for obtaining intraoral radiographs is similar to taking a radiograph of an abdomen or thorax. The film, or digital sensor, is placed on the opposite side of the target structure (tooth) from the x-ray generator. The film is generally centered on the gingival margin of the tooth and angled so that it is parallel to the tooth structure. The x-ray generator is activated and the image is obtained. Because the film has to be directly parallel to the entire tooth structure, this technique is limited to use for the mandibular molars and caudal mandibular premolars, where the film can be placed next to the mandible. Use of the parallel technique is the preferred radiographic technique when it is possible because it minimizes distortion.[4]

Bisecting Angle Technique

The bisecting angle is typically used for imaging all other teeth. The specific details of using this technique are discussed elsewhere in this issue by Coffman. With practice, this technique is useful to image any tooth in the mouth, no matter the location or orientation.

RADIOGRAPH ORIENTATION

Intraoral radiographs can be obtained using standard intraoral film, a direct digital sensor, or indirect phosphor plates (described elsewhere in this issue by Coffman). However an image is obtained, there are guidelines for orienting the image correctly. Just as thoracic and abdominal radiographs have a standard orientation for review, so do intraoral radiographs. This allows for easy and consistent evaluation of images between reviewers, ease of recognizing pathology, and discussion with colleagues.

If film is used, then the raised dot on the film should be positioned toward the reviewer. If the intraoral image is obtained digitally, this orientation is already set. All intraoral radiographs should be reviewed as if a patient were standing in front of the reviewer. This means that radiographs of maxillary teeth should be positioned so that the crowns are pointing down and the roots are pointing up (**Fig. 1**A). Radiographs of mandibular teeth should have their crowns pointing up and the roots pointing down (see **Fig. 1**B). Keep in mind that the raised dot on the film should always be toward the reviewer, so the images should be rotated to be positioned correctly rather than flipped over. This keeps the image consistent with proper viewing orientation.

Once an image is oriented with the raised dot toward the reviewer and the crowns and roots positioned correctly for a maxillary or mandibular image, then the reviewer can easily identify if the image is of a right or left quadrant. If oriented correctly, dental radiographs of the left maxillary and mandibular quadrants are positioned so that the most mesial aspect of the radiograph is to the reviewer's left (**Fig. 2**A), and radiographs of the right maxillary and mandibular quadrants have the mesial aspect to the right (see **Fig. 2**B). This mimics the view expected as if a patient were standing in front of the evaluator. This consistent positioning allows for easy determination if an image is a right side or left side without the traditional radiographic markers that are used for other parts of the body.

Some intraoral radiographs do not have mesial and distal sides clearly delineated, such as views of the rostral maxilla and mandible (**Fig. 3**). For these images, the right and left sides are determined by recognizing if an image was obtained in a ventrodorsal or dorsoventral manner. This means that, just like for a dorsoventral thoracic radiograph, the right side of a patient is on the left side of the image.

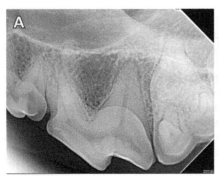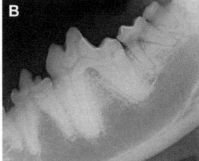

Fig. 1. Normal left maxillary (*A*) and mandibular (*B*) caudal teeth showing the correct orientation for viewing intraoral radiographs as if the patient were standing in front of the reviewer.

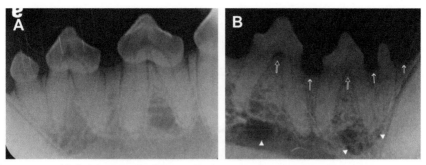

Fig. 2. Normal left (*A*) and right (*B*) mandibular premolars showing the correct orientation for positioning intraoral radiographs. The mental foramina (*arrowheads*) are normal structures that can mimic endodontic lesions. The interdental alveolar bone (*arrows*) should be 1 mm to 2 mm apical to the cementoenamel junction. Furcational bone (*open arrow*) should fill the space between the roots.

NORMAL ANATOMY

To most effectively recognize pathology in intraoral radiographs, it is important to understand the normal anatomy. There are many normal structures identified in all intraoral radiographs, and there are some that are specific to certain locations in the mouth.

Radiographic Anatomy of a Tooth

The normal canine tooth has a clinically visible crown structure, which is above the alveolar bone margin, and a root structure that is only visible radiographically. All parts of the tooth are visible radiographically, (**Fig. 4**). The crown of the tooth is composed of 3 layers: the inside is the pulp chamber, which is radiographically radiolucent; the

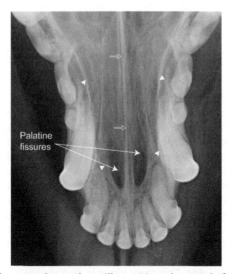

Fig. 3. Radiograph of a normal rostral maxilla positioned correctly for review. The left side of the patient is on the right side of the image. Nasal sinuses (*arrowheads*), palatine fissures (*arrows*), and the vomer bone, which forms the midline (*open arrow*), are normal structures visualized in the rostral maxilla.

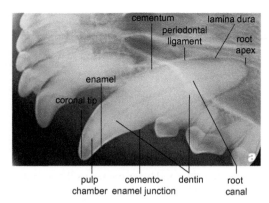

Fig. 4. A normal left maxillary canine tooth showing the parts of the tooth and adjacent bone.

middle layer is a moderately radiodense layer—dentin; and the outer coating on the tooth is a thin but extremely radiodense layer—the enamel (see **Fig. 4**).

The pulp chamber in the crown is continuous with the root canal, which is the radiolucent center extending through the length of the root. The dentin layer of the crown is continuous with the dentin layer in the root. There is a thin layer of cementum on the surface of the root, which is normally not clinically visible. The cementoenamel junction is the location on the tooth where the cementum of the root meets the enamel of the crown. On the outside surface of the root is a thin radiolucent line, which typically closely follows the shape of the root. This is the periodontal ligament. Next to the periodontal ligament is a radiodense layer of the alveolar bone, the lamina dura (see **Fig. 4**).

The alveolar bone margin is the margin of the maxillary or mandibular bone to which the gingiva is attached. In a normal healthy mouth, this bone is radiographically 1 mm to 2 mm apical to the cementoenamel junction (see **Fig. 2**B).[5] The bone between the roots of a multirooted tooth is the interradicular bone. The area of the tooth where the roots join the crown is the furcation. The furcation area is normally covered by bone and gingiva but can become exposed in teeth affected by pathology (discussed later).

Maxillary Teeth

The maxilla has several normal anatomic features, which consistently superimpose over the maxillary tooth roots (see **Fig. 4**).[6] Without a clear understanding of the normal structures, interpretation of radiographs of the maxillary teeth can be difficult.

Radiographs of the maxillary incisors and canines often include the palatine fissures, which appear as large symmetric radiolucent areas in the rostral maxilla near the apical area of the incisors (see **Fig. 3**). The conchal crest is visible as a radiodense line that extends from the root of the canine tooth to the third premolar (**Fig. 5**A). There is a normal radiodense line that extends from the palatine fissures to the caudal maxilla, and it is typically visible along the apical third of the roots of the maxillary canines, premolars, and molars. This is the line created by the joining of the vertical body of the maxilla to the palatine process, which creates the lateral border of the floor of the nasal cavity (see **Fig. 5**A). The nasal sinus is also visible in many radiographs of the maxilla (see **Figs. 4** and **5**A).

The normal maxillary incisors vary in size and shape but all have a single root (see **Fig. 3**). The central maxillary incisors (also known as the first maxillary incisors:

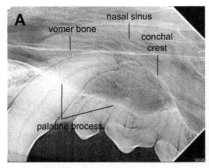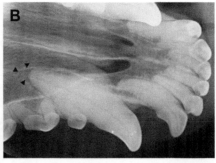

Fig. 5. Normal rostral maxillary structures on a lateral view: (*A*) canine tooth and premolars showing the normal maxillary structures, which can overlap the area of interest, and (*B*) canine tooth demonstrating the chevron effect, which is a normal variation on some teeth (*arrowheads*).

101/201) are the smallest of the incisors and have straight roots. The second maxillary incisors (102/202) are slightly longer and thicker than the first incisors. The lateral maxillary incisors (also known as the third maxillary incisors: 103/203) are longer and typically wider than the second incisors. They also have a slight banana-shaped curve to the root. This curve is normal, and it can create difficulty when attempting to extract this tooth.

The maxillary canine tooth (104/204) is the largest and longest tooth in the maxilla. It also has a single banana-shaped root, with the widest part of the tooth below the alveolar margin (see **Fig. 5**B). The normal maxillary canine tooth often has an approximately triangular-shaped radiolucent area at the apex of the tooth. This has been called a *chevron effect* (see **Fig. 5**B).[5] The effect is created by the radiolucent periapical trabecular bone and vascular structures, which are next to the denser alveolar bone. This effect is also commonly noted on the maxillary incisors and the mandibular first molar.

The maxillary premolars vary in size, shape, and number of roots. The first maxillary premolar (105/205), is a small, single-rooted tooth (see **Fig. 5**A). The second and third maxillary premolars (106/206, 107/207 respectively) are typically 2-rooted teeth. The roots of each tooth are of equal length, and the second premolar is usually slightly smaller than the third premolar. The maxillary fourth premolar (108/208) is a 3-rooted tooth, and is the largest of the 4 premolars (see **Fig. 1**A). This tooth is also known as the carnassial tooth.[3] The 3 roots of the maxillary fourth premolar are the large distal root, and the 2 smaller mesiobuccal and mesiopalatal roots. All 3 roots are approximately the same length, but the distal root is wider than the 2 mesial roots (see **Fig. 1**A).

Identification of the roots of the maxillary fourth premolar is a common place for difficulty. There are many ways to radiographically identify the individual roots. If a radiograph is obtained directly perpendicular to the tooth, the mesial roots overlap and may appear to be 1 root (**Fig. 6**A). To distinguish the individual mesial roots of the fourth premolar, the image must be obtained at an angle to the tooth.

One of the most commonly used techniques for identifying individual roots is the same lingual, opposite buccal (SLOB) rule.[7] The angle that generates the radiograph is used to determine the identity of the mesial roots of the maxillary fourth premolar. The root that is closest to where the x-ray machine is positioned is the more lingual (or palatal) root, and the one that is further away from the angle of the radiograph is the buccal root.

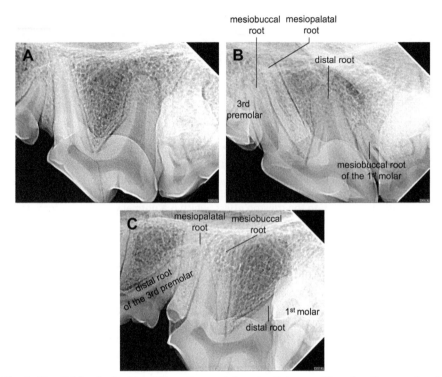

Fig. 6. The SLOB rule for identifying the mesial roots of the maxillary fourth premolar. A straight lateral radiograph (*A*) often overlaps the mesial roots and makes them difficult to evaluate. When viewed in a distobuccal to mesiopalatal direction (*B*), the mesial roots may be split and evaluated but may overlap the third premolar. The angle can also be changed to a mesiobuccal to distopalatal direction (*C*), which can allow better detail of the mesial roots but the distal root may overlap the first molar. All 3 views are needed for review in some situations.

If a radiograph is obtained from the distobuccal aspect of the tooth aiming toward the mesiopalatal aspect, all 3 roots are visible although they may be overlapping the distal root of the maxillary third premolar (see **Fig. 6**B). If a radiograph is obtained from the mesiobuccal aspect and aimed toward the distopalatal aspect, the mesial roots are typically easy to distinguish but the distal root is often overlapping the roots of the first molar (see **Fig. 6**C). In situations where the health or integrity of the maxillary fourth premolar is in question, many practitioners take views from all 3 directions of the tooth before making a determination and a treatment plan.

There are 2 maxillary molars in each quadrant. The first molar (109/209) is the larger molar, which is distal to the carnassial tooth (**Fig. 7**). The first molar has 3 roots, the mesiobuccal, distobuccal, and palatal. The palatal root is large, wide, and short compared with the 2 longer but thinner buccal roots. These roots are difficult to isolate radiographically and typically have to be evaluated with the crown overlapping. The maxillary second molar (110/210) is a small molar, which also has 3 roots. In many patients, however, 1 or more of the roots are fused together to form fewer, but larger roots. The roots of the maxillary second molar are typically short and are prone to rapid bone loss and subsequent periodontal disease.

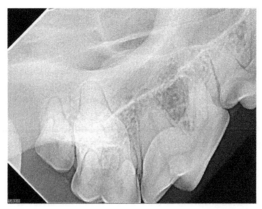

Fig. 7. Normal maxillary right fourth premolar and molars. The smaller second molar is on the left of the image.

Mandibular Teeth

In the mandible, there are no naturally occurring 3-rooted teeth. There are 3 incisors in each quadrant, 1 canine tooth, 4 premolars, and 3 molars. The incisors are single-rooted teeth that are all similar in size and shape, unlike the maxillary incisors. The mandibular canines are single rooted and similar in size and shape to the maxillary canines. These teeth of the rostral mandible (the 6 incisors and 2 canines) are typically imaged in 1 radiograph (**Fig. 8**).

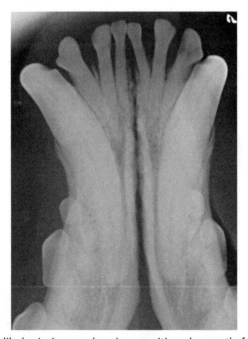

Fig. 8. Normal mandibular incisors and canines, positioned correctly for review. Similar to the maxillary incisors, the left side of the patient is on the right side of the image. The normal mandibular symphysis is cartilage. Therefore, as shown here, the left and right mandibles have a slight radiographic gap where they join, which is normal.

There are 4 premolars in the normal canine mandible. The first premolar is a small, single-rooted tooth distal to the canine tooth. The second, third, and fourth premolars are 2-rooted teeth and gradually increase in size (see **Fig. 2**A). The first molar is the largest of the 3 molars in the mandible. It has 2 roots. The mesial root is typically larger than the distal root, both in width and length. The second molar is a small, 2-rooted tooth with roots that normally diverge with the distal root oriented in a distal direction. The third molar is a small, short, single-rooted tooth that tapers at the root tip (see **Fig. 1**B).

There are fewer normal anatomic structures to overlap the radiographic interpretation in the mandible compared with the maxilla. The middle and caudal mental foramens are visible, in some radiographs of the rostral mandible premolars (see **Fig. 2**B). The location of the foramen can sometimes overlap the root tips and can appear to be lesions of endodontic origin. The most common way to determine if the anomaly on the radiograph is a true endodontic lesion or a foramen is to take another radiograph from a different angle. If the anomaly moves with the change of the angle with respect to the tooth, then it is most likely to be the foramen. Conversely, if the anomaly remains near the root in question, then a lesion of endodontic origin is more likely.

In some mandibular intraoral radiographs, the ventral mandibular cortex is visible (**Fig. 9**). Dorsal to the mandibular cortex is the mandibular canal. The mandibular canal is radiographically a radiolucent line that extends along the length of the mandible, which extends from the inferior alveolar foramen in the distal mandible to the mental foramen in the rostral mandible (see **Fig. 9**). The dorsoventral width of the canal can vary, and in some situations the roots of the first molar radiographically overlaps the mandibular canal. This can also mimic a lesion of endodontic origin, due to the decreased radiodensity in the periapical area (see **Fig. 9**).

Radiographic Changes with Age

Dogs are diphyodonts, meaning they have 2 sets of teeth during their life. The deciduous teeth and the first permanent molar have radiographically visible calcification at birth.[4] The formation of the deciduous teeth is almost complete by day 55, and they

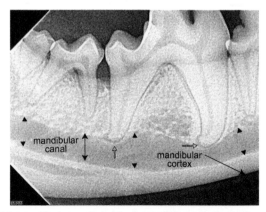

Fig. 9. Normal right mandibular molars. The large first molar is on the right of the image. The mandibular cortex (*arrow*) and mandibular canal (*arrowheads*) are seen. Where the mandibular canal overlaps the root tips of the molar, a more radiolucent area is seen (*open arrow*). This is a normal chevron effect on a mandibular first molar.

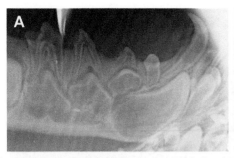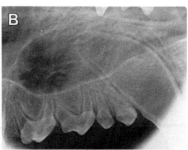

Fig. 10. Intraoral radiographs during tooth development. (*A*) A 14-week-old dog with normal mandibular deciduous dentition erupted and developing permanent tooth buds. A white processing artifact is noted dorsal to the deciduous fourth premolar. (*B*) A 6-month-old dog with normal maxillary permanent canine and premolar development. The apex of the canine is open, which is normal at this age. A supernumerary first premolar is seen.

begin to erupt at 3 to 4 weeks of age.[4] All the deciduous teeth should be erupted by 12 weeks of age. By that time, the permanent tooth buds are developing lingual and palatal to the deciduous teeth and show radiographic evidence of calcification (**Fig. 10**A). All the deciduous teeth should naturally exfoliate and the permanent teeth should erupt by 6 to 7 months of age (see **Fig. 10**B). Development and maturation of the root structure follows eruption and can last up to 18 months in some larger dogs.[4] Maturation of the tooth continues through a dog's life, as evidenced by an increasing thickness of the dentin wall and a decrease in the width of the pulp chamber and root canal with increasing age (**Fig. 11**). This maturation of the teeth is used to estimate a patient's age.

PATHOLOGY
Periodontal Disease

Periodontal disease is the most common disease of small animal medicine.[8] In some situations, the extent of the disease is obvious on clinical evaluation. Even though it may appear clinically obvious, radiographs should always be obtained in situations of known or suspected periodontal disease. Intraoral radiographs identify the extent of the periodontal disease, both in the number of teeth that are involved and the extent of involvement of an individual tooth. These radiographs can then be used to determine treatment options and evaluate the progression of healing or continued destruction over time.

Radiographic evidence of periodontal disease is characterized by widening of the periodontal ligament space (vertical bone loss) and loss of alveolar bone height (horizontal bone loss).[9] In most situations, horizontal bone loss is more difficult to manage and results in a poorer prognosis for the tooth. Vertical bone loss can be severe, but if an owner wishes, it can be managed in some situations with in-clinic periodontal therapy and ongoing home care.

An example of horizontal bone loss is seen in **Fig. 12**. The alveolar bone height is affected over several teeth, indicating chronic inflammation and attachment loss. Horizontal bone loss can be mild, moderate, or severe, depending on the extent and chronicity of the disease process. Horizontal bone loss is clinically visible by gingival recession, loss of alveolar bone height, and root exposure.

Vertical bone loss is often less clinically evident. Generally, vertical bone loss is isolated to 1 tooth or 1 interdental space (**Fig. 13**). Radiographically, vertical bone loss is

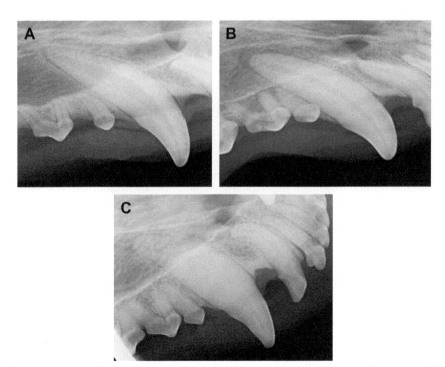

Fig. 11. Right maxillary canine teeth in dogs of varying ages. The root canal narrows with time as odontoblasts create a thicker wall of dentin. This process stops if the tooth becomes nonvital. The canal width is used to approximately estimate a dog's age and evaluate a tooth in comparison to others to determine vitality: (*A*) 1 year old, (*B*) 3 years old, and (*C*) 9 years old.

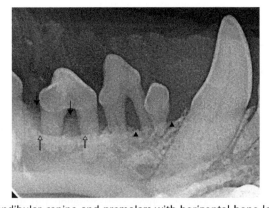

Fig. 12. Right mandibular canine and premolars with horizontal bone loss. The degree of periodontal disease is severe based on the apical location of the alveolar bone margin (*arrowheads*) and the exposure of the furcation area of the 2-rooted teeth. Due to the loss of the periodontal support, the second premolar is extruding and shifting distally. The third premolar has more significant bone loss on the lingual side (*open arrow*) than the buccal side (*closed arrow*).

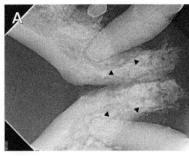 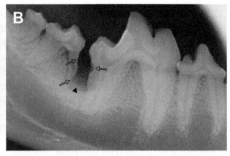

Fig. 13. Vertical bone loss caused by (A) periodontal disease. The periodontal ligament space (*arrowheads*) is wider than normal. (B) Interdental wedging of a foreign body. The alveolar bone margin is apical shifted (*arrowhead*). External root resorption is seen from pressure necrosis and chronic root exposure (*open arrows*).

identified by a widening of the periodontal ligament space and a clinically evident separation of the tooth and bone partially or completely down the length of the root. This may be from chronic periodontal disease (see **Fig. 13**A) or from interdental wedging of a foreign body (see **Fig. 13**B).

Patients with periodontal disease typically have combinations of horizontal and vertical bone loss throughout the mouth, sometimes even on the same tooth (**Fig. 14**). This is clinically important because the treatment of teeth affected by horizontal and vertical bone loss is different. Because horizontal bone loss has changed the alveolar bone height over the entire tooth, it is difficult to treat or reverse. Vertical bone loss creates a periodontal pocket, which can be cleaned, débrided, and treated. With the right circumstances, patient care, and owner home care, vertical bone loss can be halted or reversed and the tooth affected by vertical bone loss saved.

Radiographs have limitations when evaluating the extent of periodontal disease. Radiographic evidence of periodontal disease is characterized by bone demineralization and loss. Because bone loss does not become radiographically visible until approximately 40% of the bone is demineralized, radiographic findings may underestimate the extent of periodontal disease.[4] Also, superimposition of tooth or bone over vertical bony pockets may mask radiographic abnormalities. Combining radiographic findings with a detailed oral examination allows for the best interpretation of the extent and character of periodontal disease.

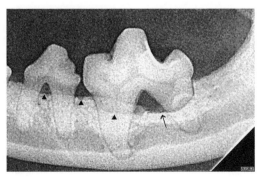

Fig. 14. Left mandibular fourth premolar and first molar with a combination of horizontal (*arrowheads*) and vertical (*arrow*) bone loss.

Endodontic Disease

Clinically, endodontic disease should be suspected when a tooth is fractured or discolored or if a draining fistula is present in the area of a tooth root. Radiographs are needed, however, to evaluate the extent of the disease, determine treatment options that are available, and monitor the progression of healing over time. Radiographic evidence of endodontic disease is caused by inflammation around the apex of the tooth. The alveolar bone surrounding the tooth root is very vascular, which makes it particularly susceptible to damage from inflammation and inflammatory mediators.[5]

Radiographic evidence of endodontic disease includes

- Resorption of the root tip (**Figs. 15** and **16A**)
- Loss of the lamina dura (the radiodense white line around the root) (see **Fig. 16**)
- Approximately circular lesions, which can have either distinct or indistinct borders (see **Fig. 16**)
- Changes in the width of the pulp and root canal in comparison with a contralateral tooth (either a wider root canal indicating pulp necrosis or a narrowed canal, indicating irritation of the pulp) (**Fig. 17**)
- Increased width of the periodontal ligament space (**Fig. 18A**)

As discussed previously, some teeth have a normal increased radiolucency at the apex—the chevron effect. The most common teeth for this effect are the maxillary incisors, the maxillary canines, and the mandibular first molars. The chevron effect is distinguished from a true endodontic lesion by evaluating the shape and the size of the lesion. In most situations, the chevron effect is a triangular-shaped area of relative radiolucency with a normal periodontal ligament and lamina dura around the margin (see **Fig. 5B**).

Combined Periodontal-Endodontic Disease

In some situations, periodontal disease and endodontic disease can affect the same tooth. If a tooth develops endodontic disease from a fracture, pulpal trauma, or other cause, this can progress to periodontal disease. As the inflammation progresses around the apex of the tooth, the inflammatory mediators can create a draining tract that follows the periodontal ligament of the tooth (see **Fig. 18A**). This can mimic the

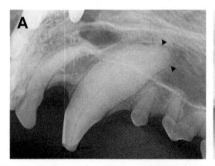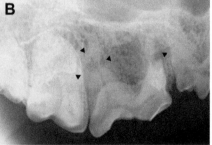

Fig. 15. Radiograph evidence of endodontic disease: root resorption. (*A*) This left maxillary canine tooth has a small enamel and dentin fracture (*arrows*), which did not expose the pulp but has compromised the integrity of the crown. Endodontic disease is seen by blunting of the apex (*arrowheads*). (*B*) The right maxillary fourth premolar has a coronal fracture, which exposed the main pulp horn (*arrow*). This has led to chronic endodontic disease, which caused external resorption of the roots (*arrowheads*).

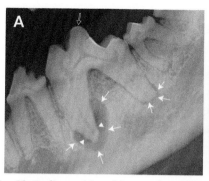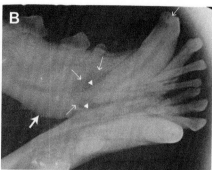

Fig. 16. Radiographic evidence of endodontic disease: loss of lamina dura. (*A*) The left mandibular first molar has abrasion (*open arrow*), which was clinically minimal. But radiographic changes include severe apical root resorption (*arrowheads*), periapical rarefaction (*thin arrows*), and loss of the normal lamina dura. (*B*) Pulp exposure from a fracture (*arrow*) on the right mandibular canine tooth caused apical root resorption (*arrowheads*), periapical rarefaction (*thin arrows*), loss of the lamina dura, and reactive thickening of the nearby mandibular cortex (*thick arrow*).

vertical bone loss associated with periodontal disease and is known as an endo-perio lesion.

   If a tooth develops periodontal disease that progresses down the length of the root to the apex, bacteria and inflammatory mediators can enter the root canal, causing pulpal necrosis. This is a perio-endo lesion (see **Fig. 18**B).

   In some cases, it is difficult to determine which process was the initiator of disease. If a patient has widespread periodontal disease and significant horizontal bone loss in the area of the affected tooth, periodontal disease is the likely initial insult to the tooth.

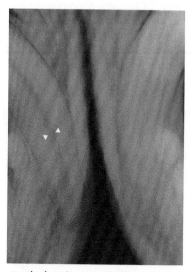

Fig. 17. Mandibular canine teeth showing comparative changes in root canal width. Endodontic disease was confirmed in the right mandibular canine with the wider root canal chamber (*arrowheads*) due to cessation of development with pulp necrosis and odontoblast death.

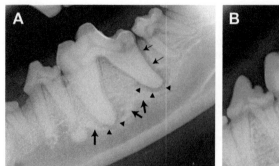
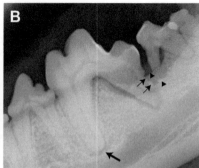

Fig. 18. Combined endodontic and periodontal disease. (*A*) The left mandibular first molar has a slight coronal compromise, which caused endodontic infection, as evidenced by periapical rarefaction (*arrowheads*) and reactive thickening of the mandibular bone (*thick arrows*). The endodontic disease progressed coronally on the distal root (*thin arrows*) creating a periodontal pocket. An incidental finding of condensing osteitis is noted near the distal root of the 4th premolar. (*B*) Periodontal disease between the left mandibular first molar and second molar caused vertical bone loss (*arrowheads*), root resorption (*thin arrows*), and endodontic disease as evidenced by the periapical rarefaction on the mesial root (*thick arrow*).

If evaluation of the crown of the tooth elucidates injuries or evidence of trauma or fractures, however, the origin of the problem is likely endodontic disease.

Tooth Resorption

Although often thought of as primarily a feline problem, idiopathic tooth resorption also occurs in dogs. In 1 study of 224 dogs presented to a university for a dental procedure, tooth resorption was identified in 53.6% of canine patients, with older and large breed dogs affected more commonly.[10] Clinically, a tooth with resorption can vary in appearance from completely normal, to a small pink area on the crown of the tooth, to a large defect in the tooth with sharp edges. To evaluate the extent of tooth resorption, intraoral radiographs are needed. Radiographically, a tooth with idiopathic resorption often appears ghostly, with more extensive involvement than is generally visible by clinical evaluation (**Fig. 19**).

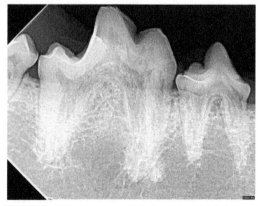

Fig. 19. Right mandibular fourth premolar and first molar with idiopathic tooth resorption.

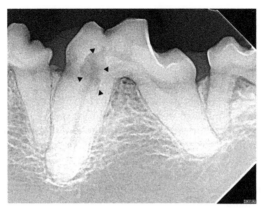

Fig. 20. Left mandibular first molar with internal root resorption (*arrowheads*), likely from inflammation within the pulp chamber.

Dogs can also be affected by internal and external root resorption. Internal root resorption occurs from inflammation within the pulp chamber or root canal (**Fig. 20**). External resorption can occur from chronic periodontal or endodontic disease (see **Figs. 16**B and **18**B). In some cases it is difficult to determine the cause of the resorption. Most teeth affected by idiopathic tooth resorption appear to be clinically normal except for the resorption, whereas a tooth affected by internal or external resorption generally has clinical evidence of the causative agent.

Caries

Carious lesions, otherwise known as cavities, are not nearly as common in dogs as they are in people.[11] They do occur, however, with some frequency. Caries result from bacterial destruction of the normal tooth structures, typically occurring in dogs in the occlusal pits, fissures, and grooves of the molars. They can occur, however, on any surface of a tooth. Radiographically, caries appear as an approximately spherical radiolucent defect with diffuse margins (**Fig. 21**). Because more than 40% of a

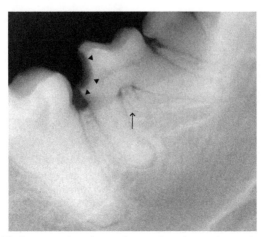

Fig. 21. Left mandibular second molar with a carious lesion (*arrowheads*) on the mesial aspect of the crown. The tooth also has a supernumerary root (*arrow*).

tooth must be demineralized before the lesion is visible radiographically, the extent of the carious lesion may be more severe than radiographs suggest.[4] Treatment usually involves a cavity preparation and a restoration. If the caries is large or deeply affecting the pulp chamber, then root canal therapy or extraction may be required.

Neoplasia

Benign and malignant neoplasia of the oral cavity combined account for 6% of all canine neoplasia.[12] Radiographic evidence of oral neoplasia varies greatly, but the characteristics of the neoplastic process tend to account for the radiographic characteristics visible. In general, aggressive or malignant neoplasms tend to have bone lysis, whereas benign oral neoplasms typically have bone proliferation or calcification of the soft tissues.[13] Many oral neoplasms cause swelling or distortion of the soft tissues. Neoplasia can also present in canine patients as an area of teeth that are mobile or a nonhealing extraction site.

Malignant melanoma is the most common oral neoplasia in dogs.[12] Radiographically, melanoma frequently invades the bone aggressively and extensively, causing a diffuse area of irregular bone loss, often without disturbing the teeth. This can lead to the appearance of the teeth floating in soft tissue (**Fig. 22**).

Acanthomatous ameloblastoma is a locally aggressive but benign oral neoplasm in dogs.[12] Like malignant melanoma, patients with acanthomatous ameloblastoma often have bone destruction, but the teeth are usually moved aside by the enlargement of the tumor (**Fig. 23**). Radiographs of acanthomatous ameloblastoma may show varying degrees of soft tissue calcification or osteolysis, or combinations of both.

Acanthomatous ameloblastoma is only one of several odontogenic tumors. These tumors are generally benign and have histologic characteristics that resemble periodontal ligament, suggesting that they are derived from periodontal structures.[13] Fibromatous epulis, preferentially referred to as a peripheral odontogenic tumor, is a common finding in canine patients. The ossifying epulis is a histiologic variant of the peripheral odontogenic tumor.[13] The peripheral odontogenic tumor (fibromatous epulis) is characterized by a supragingival soft tissue swelling which appears to

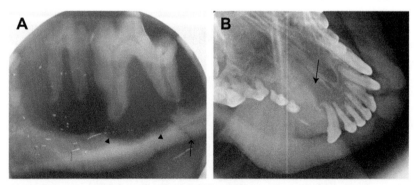

Fig. 22. Malignant melanoma. (*A*) Left mandible of a dog with severe bone lysis (*arrowheads*) and a pathologic fracture of the mandible (*thin arrow*) from melanoma. The teeth also have pulpitis as evidenced by irregularity in the root canal width. Film handling artifacts are seen as small white marks on the image. (*B*) Melanoma of the right maxilla in a small dog. The palatine fissure and normal nasal structures are destroyed (*arrow*). The canine tooth naturally exfoliated and the premolars are severely mobile from the bone destruction. A film processing artifact is seen as a white line down the image.

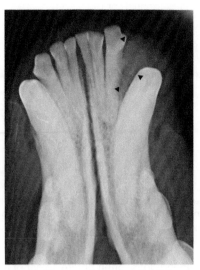

Fig. 23. An acanthomatous ameloblastoma between the left mandibular canine tooth and the third incisor (*arrowheads*), which has displaced the incisors mesially.

originate from around a tooth. It is generally minimally ossified to nonossified, does not change the periodontal ligament space or the tooth structure, and does not cause lysis of the alveolar bone margin (**Fig. 24**A). The ossifying epulis variant is similar in clinical characteristics to the peripheral odontogenic tumor, but radiographically osseous proliferation is seen within the soft tissue enlargement (see **Fig. 24**B).

Odontomas are gingival enlargements consisting of normal dental tissues in an abnormal location or arrangement (hamaratoma).[5] Odontomas are benign but can cause clinical discomfort. They can become large and cause tissue and bony destruction with expansion. Complex odontomas have enamel, dentin, and cementum within the swelling in a mixture that radiographically appears as a disorganized radio-opaque mass. Compound odontomas have distinct, normal arrangements of enamel, dentin, and cementum in small, tooth-like structures, called *denticles* (**Fig. 25**). Odontomas

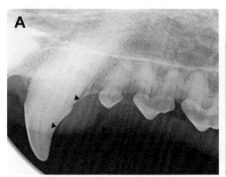 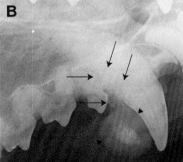

Fig. 24. Peripheral odontogenic tumors: (A) Left maxillary canine tooth with a peripheral odontogenic tumor (*arrowheads*). (B) Ossifying epulis variant on a right maxillary canine tooth (*arrowheads*). Ossification is seen within the primary mass and extending down the distal aspect of the canine tooth (*arrows*), but no bone lysis or tooth displacement is noted.

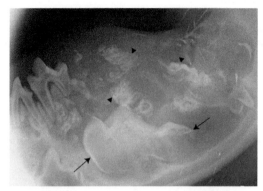

Fig. 25. Compound odontoma in the left mandible of a 14-week-old dog. Multiple denticles are seen, composed of normal enamel, dentin, and cementum in small tooth-like but abnormal structures (*arrowheads*). The normal mandibular first molar is seen at the ventral aspect of the tumor (*arrows*).

are typically identified in young dogs, often before 1 year of age, and require surgical removal of the abnormally located dental tissues.

DEVELOPMENTAL ANOMALIES
Supernumerary Tooth

A supernumerary tooth is an extra tooth within the arcade caused by a twinning of the tooth bud during development. The most common supernumerary tooth is the maxillary first premolar (see **Fig. 10**B; **Fig. 26**A). The presence of a supernumerary tooth in a

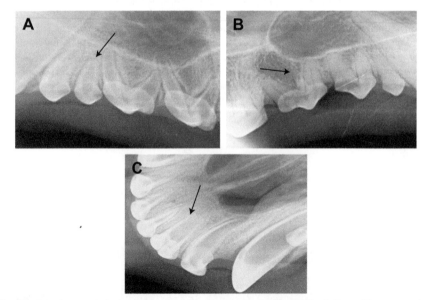

Fig. 26. Developmental anomalies: supernumerary structures. (*A*) The left maxillary premolars with a supernumerary first premolar (*arrow*), which is slightly smaller than the normal first premolar tooth. (*B*) The right maxillary premolars with a supernumerary root in the furcation area of the third premolar (*arrow*). (*C*) The left maxillary second incisor is a gemini tooth (*arrow*), which has 2 crowns and 1 root, caused by an incompletely split supernumerary tooth.

full arcade can cause crowding, which can precipitate early onset periodontal disease. If there is no clinical crowding of the teeth and radiographs confirm that the supernumerary tooth developed normally, generally no treatment is required. Supernumerary teeth are often bilateral.

Supernumerary Root

A supernumerary root is an extra root within a tooth, generally originating from the furcation area of a 2-rooted tooth (see **Figs. 21** and **26B**). This occurs during early development of the tooth. In most cases, the supernumerary root does not cause any clinical abnormalities. The presence of an additional root, however, which is not standard for the tooth, should be noted before extraction or endodontic therapy. Radiographs should be used before and after extraction to identify the location of the abnormal root and to confirm its complete removal.

Gemini Tooth

A gemini tooth is a tooth that has 2 crowns and 1 root. It is typically a supernumerary tooth that incompletely split (see **Fig. 26C**). A gemini tooth is distinguished from a fused tooth based on the number of normal teeth in the arcade. If the number of teeth in the arcade is correct, the abnormal tooth is a gemini tooth. If the number of teeth in the arcade is less than expected, however, the abnormal tooth is likely 2 tooth buds that fused together, instead of 1 tooth bud that incompletely split. This is typically an incidental finding and no treatment is required. Clinically, there is no significant difference between a gemini tooth or a fused tooth. Some breed show standards, however, may not be met if a dog has a fused tooth.

Radicular Groove

A radicular groove is a concave surface on an otherwise approximately circular root, which creates a double radiographic shadow down the length of the root (**Fig. 27**). This makes the root appear C-shaped when viewed coronal to apical. A deep radicular groove creates a lock-and-key effect of the root within the bone and prevent rotation during extraction.

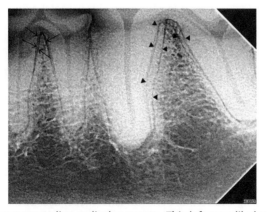

Fig. 27. Development anomalies: radicular groove. This left mandibular first molar has a double radiographic shadow (*arrowheads*) down the length of the distal aspect of the mesial root, in the furcation area, and on the mesial aspect of the distal root for approximately one-third of the length. A smaller groove can also be seen in the furcation area of the fourth premolar (*arrows*).

Persistent Deciduous Tooth

By the time most dogs are 7 months old, all permanent teeth should be erupted and all deciduous teeth exfoliated. As the permanent tooth erupts, the deciduous tooth should have a natural resorption of the root and exfoliation. In some situations, the deciduous tooth does not exfoliate. This can cause crowding and rapid onset of periodontal disease if the permanent tooth erupts next to the persistent deciduous tooth (**Fig. 28**). This is common in small breed dogs.

If the permanent tooth did not develop, the deciduous tooth may not naturally exfoliate at the appropriate time. A persistent deciduous tooth is distinguished from its permanent counterpart by the size and shape of the roots and the crown. A deciduous tooth has smaller, thinner roots and the crown of the tooth is smaller and less radiodense than a permanent tooth (see **Fig. 28**).

Dentin Dysplasia

Radicular dentin dysplasia manifests radiographically as a generalized lack of normal root structure (**Fig. 29**). Dentin dysplasia can occur when the body receives an insult at a young age, such as a systemic illness. The stage of development of the affected teeth generally indicates the age at which the insult occurred. Teeth with radicular dentin dysplasia can clinically appear normal if the timing of the insult was during the development of the root rather than the crown. In most cases, teeth with dentin dysplasia should be extracted due to the lack of normal healthy tooth structure.

Dilacerated Roots

A dilacerated root is a root that is misshapen from the normal. In most cases, the root tip is curved or angled in a way that is not expected for the normal shape of the tooth (**Fig. 30**A). If the dilaceration is at the root tip, this is not clinically a problem for patients until extraction of the tooth is attempted. Once the dilaceration is identified on a pre-extraction radiograph, steps should be taken during the extraction to minimize root tip breakage or trauma to the surrounding bone.

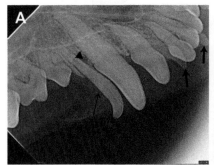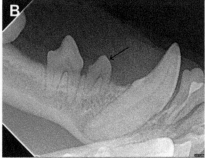

Fig. 28. (*A*) A persistent deciduous right maxillary canine tooth (*thin arrow*) in a young adult dog is causing crowding and vertical bone loss (*arrowhead*) against the permanent tooth. Persistent deciduous incisors (*thick arrows*) are visible, and the first premolar is absent. (*B*) Right mandibular premolars in a young adult dog. The first, second and fourth premolars are missing. The deciduous second premolar is persistent (*arrow*). The deciduous premolar is distinguished from its absent permanent counterpart because it is a smaller, thinner tooth with a blunt crown.

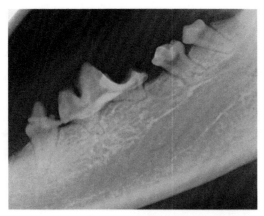

Fig. 29. Developmental anomalies: dentin dysplasia. Left mandibular fourth premolar and molars demonstrating radicular dentin dysplasia. The root structure of the first molar is severely blunted and irregularly shaped with no visible root canal. The fourth premolar and second molar have roots that are near normal length but fused together. The third molar developed at a different time and was unaffected by the dysplasia.

Convergent Roots

A more severe form of dilacerated roots is called *convergent roots*. Although dilacerated roots can be on any tooth, convergent roots are found only on a multirooted tooth. In most canine patients, the roots of multirooted teeth diverge, which allows for greater stability of the tooth within the bone during mastication. In some dogs, however, primarily small breeds, the roots of a multirooted tooth converge (see **Fig. 30**B). This forces the coronal tissues to crinkle together and can expose an opening into the root canal through which a bacterial infection can enter. Teeth with convergent roots should be extracted to prevent or treat future pain and infection. Great care must be taken, however, during the extraction because the roots are angled differently

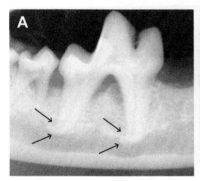
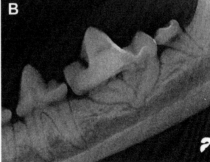

Fig. 30. Developmental anomalies: dilacerated roots. (*A*) The root tips of the right mandibular first molar are angled distally, or dilacerated (*arrows*). The interdental bone between the first and second molar is affected by horizontal bone loss and the furcational bone of the first molar has resorbed from periodontal disease. Extraction of this tooth is recommended due to the severe periodontal disease but is complicated by the hook at the end of each root. (*B*) A severe form is convergent roots. The roots appear to be fused at the tip, but this is a 2-D view of a 3-D structure so they may only be overlapping. The second molar is absent.

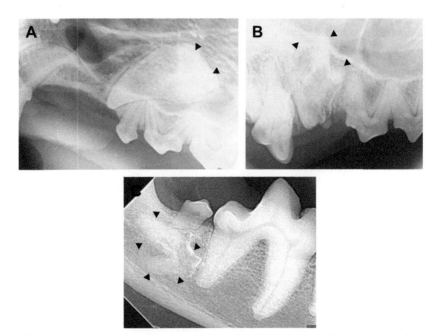

Fig. 31. Developmental anomalies: impacted teeth. (*A*) The left maxillary canine tooth root was damaged during development. This caused blunting of the root (*arrowheads*) and the normal eruption process ceased. (*B*) The right maxillary premolars and molars in a mature dog. The fourth premolar is misshapen, rotated, and impacted although it appeared to develop roots of average length (*arrowheads*). (*C*) The right mandibular second molar in this geriatric dog was found correctly formed but rotated so eruption did not occur (*arrowheads*). The tooth is naturally resorbing. The root development of the third molar was stunted by the presence of the impacted second molar.

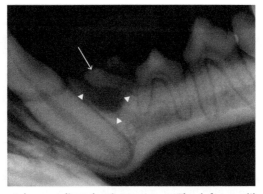

Fig. 32. Developmental anomalies: dentigerous cyst. The left mandibular first premolar (*arrow*) in this 14-month-old dog developed at an angle, which prevented normal eruption into the oral cavity. A cystic lesion is developing around it, which is causing bone lysis with expansion (*arrowheads*). The second premolar is absent and the crown of the persistent deciduous second premolar is visible dorsal to the cyst. Left untreated, this expansile lesion compromises the health and integrity of the surrounding teeth, including the canine and spontaneous mandibular fracture could occur.

than a normal tooth. The pre-extraction radiographs should be used to plan the extraction and bone removal if necessary.

Impacted Teeth

All clinically missing teeth should be radiographed. If there is a traumatic insult to an isolated tooth during development, the tooth can become malformed, and this can affect eruption (**Fig. 31**). Impacted teeth can be developed normally and simply not erupt; they can be misshapen and unable to erupt; or they can be angled incorrectly and unable to erupt into the oral cavity. When found at a young age, impacted teeth should be extracted. A dentigerous cyst can form around an impacted tooth, which causes bone destruction on expansion (discussed in next section). When identified in older patients, evaluation of the clinical situation around an impacted tooth should be considered to determine if extraction is appropriate.

Dentigerous Cyst

A dentigerous cyst is an epithelium-lined, fluid-filled sac that surrounds an unerupted tooth crown (**Fig. 32**). This most commonly occurs in unerupted mandibular first premolars but can occur with any tooth crown that remains embedded in bone. Once formed, without surgical removal and débridement of the cyst lining, the cyst continues to enlarge and can cause severe bone and tooth damage. Because of the destructive nature of these cysts, all clinically missing teeth should be radiographed and removed if impacted.

SUMMARY

Dental radiographs are invaluable when performing canine dental procedures. They are an important part of the medical-legal record and provide essential information when treatment planning. Readers are encouraged to take radiographs of every dental patient. The more a practitioner sees normal anatomy, the easier it is be to identify pathology. And the more radiographs that are obtained, the more pathology is identified and treated. This is better medical care for patients and better for the bottom line of a practice. This article provides only a brief introduction to the amazing world of canine intraoral radiology. There are many wonderful and informative books that have been written on this topic. As with all radiographs, interpretation is an art form that requires practice, patience, and repetition.

REFERENCES

1. Verstraete FJ, Kass P, Terpak C. Diagnostic value of full-mouth radiography in dogs. Am J Vet Res 1998;59(6):686–91.
2. Holmstrom SE, Bellows J, Colmery B, et al. AAHA dental care guidelines for dogs and cats. J Am Anim Hosp Assoc 2005;41(5):277–83.
3. Wiggs R, Lobprise H. Veterinary dentistry: principles & practice. Philadelphia: Lippincott-Raven; 1997.
4. Mulligan T, Aller M, Williams C. Atlas of canine & feline dental radiography. Yardley (PA): Veterinary Learning Systems; 1998.
5. DuPont G, DeBowes L. Atlas of dental radiography in dogs and cats. St Louis (MO): Saunders; 2009.
6. Gracis M, Harvey C. Radiographic study of the maxillary canine tooth in mesaticephalic dogs. J Vet Dent 1998;15(2):73–8.
7. Bellows J. Small animal dental equipment, materials and techniques: a primer. Ames (IA): Blackwell Publishing; 2004.

8. Niemiec BA. Periodontal disease. Top Companion Anim Med 2008;23(2):72–80.
9. Tsugawa AJ, Verstraete FJ. How to obtain and interpret periodontal radiographs in dogs. Clin Tech Small Anim Pract 2000;15(4):204–10.
10. Peralta S, Verstraete FJ, Kass P. Radiographic evaluation of the types of tooth resorption in dogs. Am J Vet Res 2010;71(7):784–93.
11. Hale FA. Dental caries in the dog. Can Vet J 2009;50(12):1301–4.
12. Withrow S, Vail D. Withrow and MacEwen's small animal clinical oncology. St Louis (MO): Saunders; 2007.
13. DeForge D, Colmery B. An atlas of veterinary dental radiology. Ames (IA): Iowa State University Press; 2000.

Clinical Feline Dental Radiography

Matthew Lemmons, DVM

KEYWORDS

- Dental radiography • Tooth resorption • Periodontal disease • Endodontic disease
- Feline

KEY POINTS

- Dental disorders cannot be fully assessed and diagnosed without good-quality intraoral radiographs.
- Dental radiographs make early detection of tooth resorption more likely and aid in surgical planning of extractions; they are necessary if crown amputation is to be performed.
- Dental radiographs are important in determining patterns of bone loss when assessing periodontal disease and ensuring that clinical findings are not caused by another pathologic process such as tooth resorption or neoplasia.
- Dental radiography provides good medical data that benefit patients and provide an economic benefit to the practice.

Even before the foundation of the American Veterinary Dental College in 1988, the value of dental radiographs in small animal veterinary practice was known. As early as 1971, dental film was reportedly used in small animal practice not only for assessment of the teeth but also of the nasal cavity and to evaluate extremities.[1] As the practice of veterinary medicine has continued to advance, the need and acceptance of dental radiography as a vital diagnostic tool has increased. It is invaluable when assessing periodontal disease, fractured teeth, tooth resorption, neoplasia, and maxillofacial injuries.

According to the American Animal Hospital Association's Dental Care Guidelines for Dogs and Cats, radiographs are necessary for accurate evaluation and diagnosis and standard views of the skull are inadequate when evaluating dental disorders.[2]

This is not to say that skull radiographs are not a valuable and necessary diagnostic modality. Skull radiographs are beneficial when assessing maxillofacial injuries, neoplastic processes, and tympanic bulla disorders.

When clinical examination findings were compared with dental radiograph findings in cats undergoing dental treatment, radiographs revealed clinically important information in 41.7% of cats that were not detected on examination only. In addition,

Circle City Veterinary Specialty and Emergency Hospital, Carmel, IN, USA
E-mail address: mlemmons@circlecityvets.com

Vet Clin Small Anim 43 (2013) 533–554
http://dx.doi.org/10.1016/j.cvsm.2013.02.003
0195-5616/13/$ – see front matter © 2013 Elsevier Inc. All rights reserved.

clinically essential information was revealed in 32.2% of teeth with lesions detected on examination. For example, in 8.7% of cats, tooth resorption was detected on radiographs when lesions were not detected clinically. Perhaps more importantly, in 98.4% of cats with clinically diagnosed tooth resorption, dental radiographs revealed additional information.[3,4] This additional information is necessary when treating tooth resorption if crown amputation with intentional root retention is to be used.

NORMAL ANATOMY

The adult cat has 30 teeth normally present. Each maxillary quadrant holds 3 incisors, 1 canine, 3 premolars, and a molar. The maxillary first molars are normally absent. Each mandibular quadrant holds 3 incisors, a canine, 2 premolars, and a molar. The mandibular first and second premolars are normally absent.

The incisors and canine teeth are always single rooted (maxilla and mandible). The maxillary second premolar may have 1 root or 2 fused roots or 2 independent roots.[4] The maxillary third premolar normally has 2 roots and the fourth premolar 3 roots. The maxillary molar may have 1 root, 2 fused roots, or 2 independent roots.[4]

The following describes the radiographic appearance of normal anatomy for the typical views for full-mouth radiographs of the cat. More specific details regarding positioning can be found in the article "Oral and Dental Imaging Equipment and Techniques for Small Animals" in this issue.

Occlusal radiographs of the maxillary incisors (**Fig. 1**) and the oblique projection of the maxillary canine tooth (**Fig. 2**) show the corresponding teeth and alveolar bone, incisive bone, rostral extent of the maxillae, palatine fissures, conchal crest, junction of the palatal process of the maxilla to the lateral portion, vomer bone, and possibly

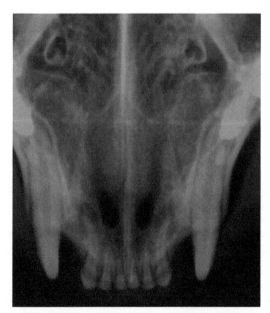

Fig. 1. Occlusal radiograph of the maxillary incisors clearly shows the crown, root, and alveolar bone of each incisor. The relative radiolucent line outlining the roots is the periodontal ligament space. When viewing this radiograph, the maxillary right of the patient is to the viewer's left and vice versa. The teardrop-shaped radiolucent structures apical to the first and second incisors are the palatine fissures.

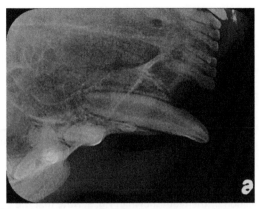

Fig. 2. On this oblique view of a right maxillary canine tooth, the conchal crest has been outlined in red. This structure can mimic the lamina dura and interfere with interpretation of the apical structures.

the nasal bone. Of particular interest are the conchal crest and junction palatal process of the maxilla, because these structures may interfere with assessing the canine tooth.[5] This structure may be mistaken for the lamina dura and thus affect how the apical health of the tooth is interpreted.

On lateral projections of the maxillary premolars and molar, the ventral border is the corresponding crowns and alveolar crest. The dorsal aspect of the radiograph is the nasal cavity. The zygomatic bone is superimposed over the third and fourth premolars and molar when the radiograph is exposed using strict bisecting angle technique (**Fig. 3**). When using intentional elongation or an extraoral image, the zygomatic bone is dorsal to the teeth (**Fig. 4**).

Cats have 2 paired mandibles that connect rostrally through a fibrocartilaginous symphysis. The symphysis is represented radiographically as a radiolucent border between the two mandibles (**Fig. 5**). The portions of the mandibles associated with the symphysis are roughly parallel.

The mandibular premolars and molar have 2 roots. The roots of the premolar are typically nearly equal in size. The mesial root of the molar is 2 to 3 times the width of the distal root.

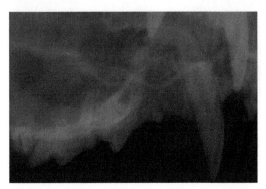

Fig. 3. Lateral projection of the right maxillary premolars and molar. Note the zygomatic arch is superimposed over the third and fourth premolars and molar.

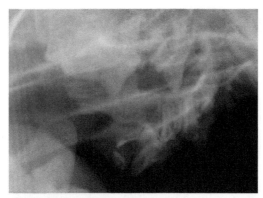

Fig. 4. Extraoral projection of the teeth shown in **Fig. 3**. Note that the zygomatic arch is no longer masking the third and fourth premolars and molar.

The lateral projection of the feline mandible is bordered by the ventral cortex ventrally and the cusps of the premolars and molar dorsally (**Figs. 6** and **7**). A radiolucent area is visible directly dorsal to the ventral cortex and ventral to the tooth roots. This area is the location of the mandibular canal, which contains the inferior alveolar artery vein and nerve.

When evaluating any tooth, the following are evaluated: crown (and enamel) and pulp chamber, root and root canal, periodontal ligament space, and alveolar bone. The crown is located coronal to the alveolar bone. It is covered by a more radiodense margin, which is the enamel, and the bulk is dentin, which is not as radiodense as enamel, but is radiodense compared with bone. At the center of the crown is the

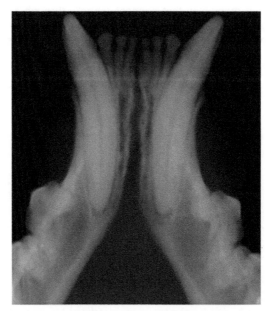

Fig. 5. Occlusal view of the mandibular canines and incisors. The radiolucent line between the mandibles is the location of the fibrocartilaginous symphysis.

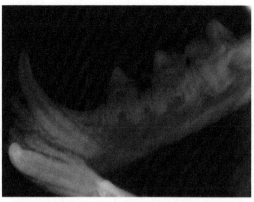

Fig. 6. The bisecting angle of the left mandibular premolars. The apex of the distal root of the molar is not completely within the field.

radiolucent pulp chamber, which contains the coronal portion of the pulp. Because the bulk of the root is made of dentin, it is of the same radiodensity as the crown. Because the cementum has nearly the same radiodensity as bone, it is not obvious radiographically. The center of the root is the radiolucent root canal, which houses the radicular portion of the pulp. The root canal and pulp chamber are widest where the tooth first erupts and the dentinal walls are thinnest. As the tooth matures, secondary dentin is produced, making the root canal smaller in diameter and the dentinal walls thicker.

A radiolucent line surrounds the root, which is the periodontal ligament space (the ligament cannot be visualized), known as the lamina lucida. It is wider early in age and is typically widest at the coronal and apical one-third of the root. If this space is absent, it may be because of dentoalveolar ankylosis or because the resolution of the radiograph does not allow it to be visualized.

Adjacent to the periodontal ligament space is a radiodense line that is congruent with the ligament space. This line is the cortical bone of the alveolus and is known as the lamina dura. Adjacent to it is the trabecular bone of the alveolus. In multirooted teeth, bone should be present up to the apex of the furcation. The alveolar crest is seen as a peak of bone adjacent to the tooth both distally and mesially and between teeth with proximal contacts.

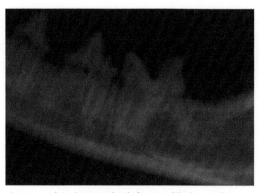

Fig. 7. Parallel technique used to image the left mandibular molar.

RADIOGRAPHIC FINDINGS WITH COMMON DENTAL DISORDERS
Tooth Resorption

Tooth resorption in cats is a progressive resorption of dental hard tissue from odonto-clasts. The exact cause is unknown. Vitamin D levels in the food, renal function, and peculiarities in the anatomy of the feline dentin and periodontal ligament are all thought to play a role. As tooth resorption progresses, it becomes painful for the patient, thus early detection and treatment are important.

When a trained veterinary dentist examined the mandibular teeth of cats and assessed radiographs of the same teeth, 1.4 times more tooth resorption of the crown and 2.4 times more tooth resorption of the roots were found using radiographs versus examination alone.[6] Radiographs are also necessary before crown amputation for treatment of tooth resorption, because not all resorbing teeth are candidates. Given that tooth resorption affects from 20% to 67% of cats, tooth resorption alone justifies the use of dental radiography in small animal practice.[7]

Tooth resorption is classified into 3 types. This classification signifies whether the tooth root is being replaced by new bone.

With all types of tooth resorption, radiolucent foci may be seen on or within the crown of the tooth. These foci are often congruous with grossly visible defects in the crown.

When type 1 tooth resorption is present, there is no evidence that the dental hard tissue is being replaced by bone. The periodontal ligament space is visible and the lamina dura is seen at the periphery of the periodontal ligament space. The roots are easily distinguished from the surrounding bone. An artist's rendering is shown in **Fig. 8**.

Often what is observed on radiographs is a focal or multifocal radiolucency present on the crown of the tooth. Typically this corresponds with a defect that is visible on examination. In this defect, the enamel of the crown is missing and the dentin is exposed. In later stages, the pulp of the tooth is exposed and often appears inflamed. A proliferation of soft tissue from the gingiva that covers or fills the crown defect is often observed. This soft tissue is not typically observed on radiographs.

A focal radiolucency on the root may not necessarily show external resorption. It may indicate internal resorption or resorption within the root canal. If the radiograph tube is shifted to slightly oblique, the radiograph external lesions will appear to move away from the pulp and internal lesions will remain contiguous with the pulp.

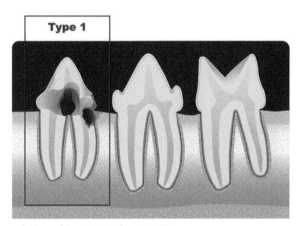

Fig. 8. Artist's rendering of type 1 tooth resorption.

In type 2 tooth resorption, the periodontal ligament is thin to absent in areas and the alveolar bone contacts the cementum and begins replacing the dental hard tissue with osteoid, and ankylosis of the tooth root to the alveolar bone (dentoalveolar ankylosis) occurs. When type 2 tooth resorption is present, the periodontal ligament space and lamina dura are not identifiable on the radiograph. The radiographic border of the root is indistinguishable from the radiographic border of the alveolar bone. An artist's rendering is shown in **Fig. 9**.

The radiodensity of the root is not homogenous when type 2 resorption is present. With type 1 resorption, the root is uniformly radiodense compared with the surrounding bone. With type 2 resorption, the overall radiodensity of the root is similar to that of the surrounding bone. However, there may be radiodense threads visible (**Fig. 10**).

With type 2 resorption, part of the root may be easily detectable with radiographs but the original borders of the root have been replaced by bone. There is still a radiolucent margin between the existing root and bone, and root may have a conical appearance. In these cases it is advisable to extract the visible and radiographically evident portion of the root while leaving the portion replaced by bone.

Type 2 resorption may be radiographically present without gross evidence of tooth resorption. It is generally thought that if there is no resorption coronal to the alveolar bone and no evidence of internal resorption, there is no associated pain. However it is impossible to predict how quickly this lesion will progress. It may be prudent to treat these teeth proactively.

When type 1 resorption is present, the roots may still display external resorption, which is seen as a focal radiolucency on the root or a scalloped appearance of the root. It is common to find that the associated alveolar bone is reduced in height or infrabony pockets are present. There is evidence that type I resorption is more common than type 2 resorption in the presence of concurrent periodontitis.[5] Periodontal bone loss is not a common finding in teeth with type 2 resorption. The alveolar bone height is often normal.

The periodontal ligament space is not always obvious in normal teeth. Inability to identify it on a radiograph does not necessarily indicate that the tooth is undergoing type 2 resorption. If the density of the root is uniformly more radiodense than the surrounding bone but the periodontal ligament space is not easily seen, it is possible that the periodontal ligament is too thin or the resolution of the radiograph not high

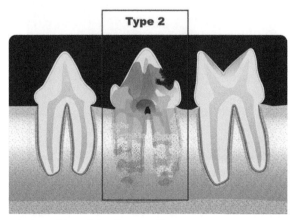

Fig. 9. Artist's rendering of type 2 tooth resorption.

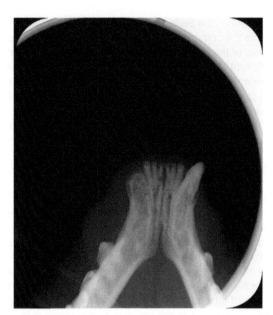

Fig. 10. Type 2 resorption of the right (stage 5) and left (stage 2) mandibular canine teeth.

enough to image the periodontal ligament space. In this case it cannot be assumed that type 2 resorption is present (**Fig. 11**).

Type 3 tooth resorption means that, in a multirooted tooth, one root is undergoing type 1 resorption and another is undergoing type 2 resorption (**Fig. 12**).

Tooth resorption is also staged on a 1 to 5 scale that signifies the degree of resorption.[8] This classification indicates how much dental hard tissue has been resorbed.

Stage 1 resorption indicates that only the cementum has been resorbed without the dentin being affected, which may be difficult to detect clinically. This stage could

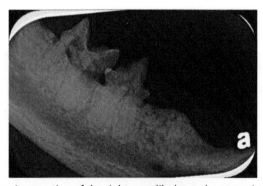

Fig. 11. Stage 3 type 1 resorption of the right mandibular molar, stage 1 type 1 resorption of the fourth premolar, and stage 5 type 2 resorption of the third premolar. The mesial root of the fourth premolar is losing the distinct border of the periodontal ligament space. However, the lamina dura and the roots are still visible. At this point, this tooth should be treated as type 1 resorption.

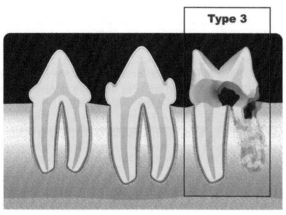

Fig. 12. Artist's rendering of type 3 tooth resorption.

indicate that only enamel is missing. However, for enamel to be lost, underlying dentin must first be resorbed.

Stage 2 indicates that there is some dentin loss; however, the lesion has not extended into the pulp. These lesions appear radiographically as focal or multifocal lucency on the crown and/or root.

Stage 3 resorption involves the pulp of the tooth. This may be seen grossly as a pink/red soft tissue bleb present within a defect in the crown. On radiographs, the lucency is contiguous with the root canal or pulp chamber.

Stage 4 indicates that a significant portion of the root is missing.

In teeth with stage 5 tooth resorption, the crown of the tooth is absent, but a spur of bone may be seen rising from the occlusal ridge of the jaw. These structures occasionally contain spicules of bone or osteoid that may protrude through the gingiva.

Again, it is only appropriate to perform crown amputation with intentional root resorption on roots undergoing type 2 resorption. Roots undergoing type 1 root resorption may not resorb and can remain as a nidus for inflammation (**Fig. 13**).

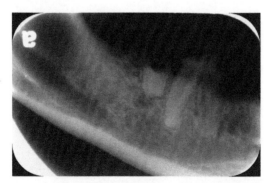

Fig. 13. Teeth with type 1 tooth resorption should not be treated with crown amputation. The roots do not resorb and may be a nidus for infection and inflammation, as shown by the periapical lucency and extrusion of the mesial root of the right molar. Note the U-shaped defect in the root, which may indicate that a previous clinician attempted to drill out the root.

Periodontal Disease

When assessing periodontitis radiographically, alveolar bone loss and expansion are assessed. Two patterns of bone loss are described: horizontal and vertical. Horizontal bone loss involves 2 or more adjacent teeth. The coronal crest of the alveolar bone recedes from the teeth uniformly and the new plane of the alveolar bone is parallel to the original plane (**Fig. 14**). It is possible to see loss of furcational alveolar bone (stage 3 furcation loss) with horizontal bone loss (**Fig. 15**).

Vertical bone loss describes bone loss of a single root. This pattern creates an infrabony periodontal pocket and resembles a triangular pattern of bone loss adjacent to a root. The most apical portion of the bony defect is apical to the adjacent bone (**Figs. 16** and **17**).

Most periodontal bone loss is a combination of horizontal and vertical bone loss.

In a study of periodontal bone loss in cats, only 28% had normal periodontal bone height, 55% had generalized horizontal bone loss, and 33% had focal vertical bone loss.[9]

When examining the canine teeth of the cat, the cementum may be visible. Conventional thought is that there is periodontal attachment loss caused by gingival and alveolar bone recession. When examining the gingiva closely, the normal architecture is often still present. When assessed radiographically, the crestal bone is still present and there is no evidence of periodontal bone loss. In these cases there is no periodontal attachment loss. Instead, there is either increased cementum production at the apex, increased apical bone deposition, or a combination of the two.[10] This condition is known as supereruption and is not necessarily pathologic. However, there may be a correlation between supereruption and tooth resorption.[11]

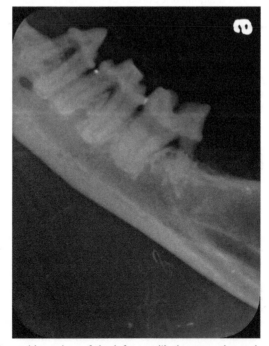

Fig. 14. Mild horizontal bone loss of the left mandibular premolar and molar characterized by crestal bone loss.

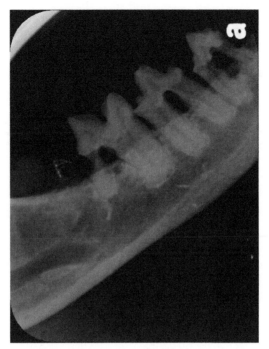

Fig. 15. Marked to severe horizontal bone loss of the right mandibular premolars and molar with type 1 tooth resorption of the third premolar and molar.

Chronic alveolar osteitis of the canine tooth may lead to a specific pattern of periodontitis called buccal bone expansion. This presents radiographically as a thickening of the buccal bone width of 1 or more canine teeth (**Fig. 18**). The buccal bone width of the canine teeth is normally less than 2 mm.[9] This pattern was shown to affect 53% of cats.[9] In severe cases, this may be associated with severe vertical bone loss and a spherical appearance to the alveolar bone (**Fig. 19**).[9] The author's experience is that supereruption is generally present when buccal bone expansion is present.

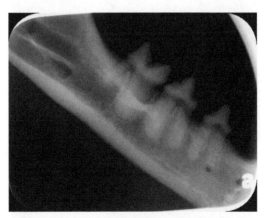

Fig. 16. Vertical bone loss of the mesial root of the right mandibular molar. The defect is single walled and located buccally. The location makes it difficult to visualize because the root disguises the bone loss.

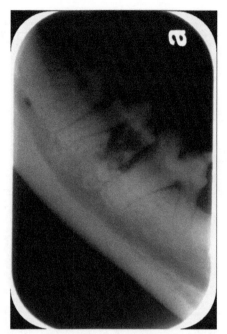

Fig. 17. Severe vertical bone loss of the right mandibular fourth premolar with concurrent type 1 tooth resorption.

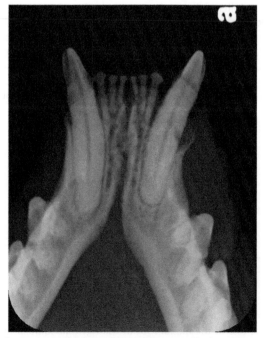

Fig. 18. Mild alveolar bone expansion of the right mandibular canine tooth and marked alveolar bone expansion of the left mandibular canine tooth with vertical bone loss.

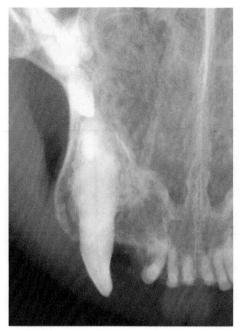

Fig. 19. Severe alveolar bone expansion of the right maxillary canine. Note concurrent vertical bone loss.

The exact relationship between tooth resorption and periodontal bone loss is unknown. It has been shown that the presence of tooth resorption increases the risk of decreased alveolar bone height.[9] This may be because inflammation associated with tooth resorption causes inflammatory resorption of the surrounding alveolar bone (**Figs. 20** and **21**).

Endodontic Disease

Death or infection of the dental pulp can lead to localized osteitis of the periapical bone, which is likely to be painful. Possible sequelae include secondary periodontitis, rhinitis, and, in rare cases, dacryocystitis.

If gross exposure of the pulp is noted, regardless of the radiographic findings, the tooth requires treatment. Radiographic findings of endodontic death include periapical rarefaction, focal widening of periodontal ligament space, widened root canal, external root resorption, internal root resorption, and supereruption.

Periapical rarefaction is a lucency of the periapical bone (**Fig. 22**) caused by loss of mineral of the alveolar bone. For periapical inflammation to be evident on radiographs, a certain portion of mineral needs to be resorbed from the bone or the buccal cortical bone plate needs to be perforated by the lesion. The percentage most commonly quoted is 30% to 50%. One study showed that as little as 7.5% mineral bone loss was apparent to observers.[12] The higher quoted number relates to observing osteoporotic bone and the second entails mechanically removing bone with a burr. Regardless of the number, not all cases with periapical inflammation have obvious radiographic lesions, and clinical examination is necessary.

Periapical rarefaction may be as subtle as widening of the periodontal ligament space. The periodontal ligament is widest at the apex and at the most coronal aspect

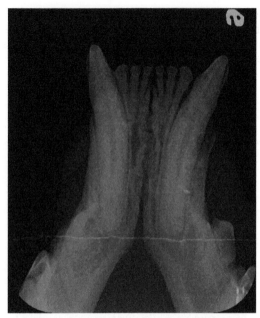

Fig. 20. Alveolar bone expansion of the left mandibular canine tooth with vertical bone loss. Note the radiolucent foci present on the root at the cervical region. This tooth is undergoing type 1 root resorption.

and thinnest at the middle of the root. Thus widening of the periodontal ligament space should not be overinterpreted. Periapical lucency has also been noted with severe vertical periodontal bone loss but has not been associated with tooth resorption,[13] which may strengthen the argument for treating type 2 resorption with crown amputation.

The root canal widths of contralateral teeth should also be compared. As vital teeth age, more secondary dentin is produced, thickening the dentin layer and, in turn, narrowing the root canal. A tooth with a root canal wider than its counterpart may have stopped maturing because of pulp death (**Figs. 23** and **24**).

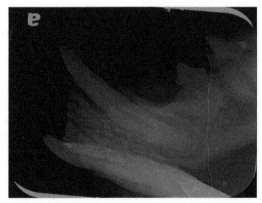

Fig. 21. The same tooth as in **Fig. 20** viewed from an oblique angle. Note that the radiolucent area on the root has stayed in the same location, confirming that the lesion is on the root.

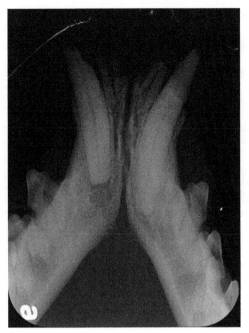

Fig. 22. Periapical lucency and extrusion of the right mandibular canine tooth with a complicated crown fracture.

Inflammation (the apices of feline teeth are less round than canine teeth). However, inflammation may cause external resorption of the apex and lead to a blunted appearance of the apex. External odontoclastic resorption may be sufficiently extensive for significant portions of the root to be missing (**Figs. 25** and **26**). Although odontoclasts are involved, this process is not likely related to idiopathic tooth resorption.

In cases of chronic pulp inflammation, internal resorption may be observed (**Fig. 27**), which does not necessarily indicate that the tooth is undergoing typical feline

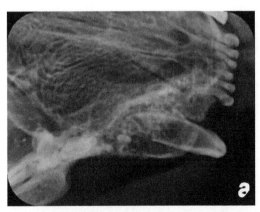

Fig. 23. Widened root canal of the right maxillary canine tooth. The width of the root canal with little secondary dentin production indicates that the tooth was injured soon after it erupted.

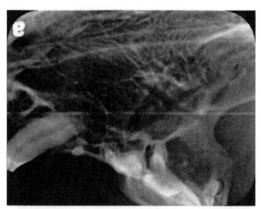

Fig. 24. The left maxillary canine tooth of the patient shown in **Fig. 23**. Note that the root canal is more narrow.

idiopathic tooth resorption. However, it may decrease the prognosis for successful root canal therapy.

The author has observed that some teeth with chronic apical periodontitis secondary to pulp inflammation may cause supereruption of the tooth.

Teeth with uncomplicated crown fractures (dentin is exposed but pulp is not directly exposed) should always be assessed radiographically. In the case of an uncomplicated crown fracture, pulp contamination is possible via bacterial ingress through exposed dentinal tubules, which can lead to a septic pulpitis. Cats may be at a higher risk than dogs of septic pulpitis because of uncomplicated fractures.

Neoplasia

Squamous cell carcinoma

Squamous cell carcinoma is the most common oral malignancy of the cat.[14] This carcinoma is a highly aggressive lesion with poor prognosis. In the mandible, a mixed pattern of sclerosis and lysis is often seen.[15] It may appear as an expansile lesion with periosteal new bone formation.[16] The alveolar bone may be radiolucent and, if in the

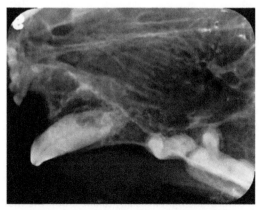

Fig. 25. External root resorption of a left maxillary canine tooth that has been chronically fractured. The patient presented for chronic sneezing and left-sided nasal discharge.

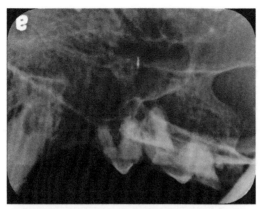

Fig. 26. Lateral view of the same lesion seen in **Fig. 25**.

mandible, the ventral cortex may appear to be absent (**Fig. 28**). The initial clinical findings may be a mobile tooth or a small tumor associated with a tooth. In a study of 24 cats with oral swellings, 12 were histologically confirmed to be malignant lesions.[16] Biopsy is recommended whenever an unexplained growth or radiographic bone lysis is noted.

Osteoma
An aggressive variant of osteoma of the mandible has been described in the cat.[17] The radiographic findings might be expected to show a well-defined lesion resembling

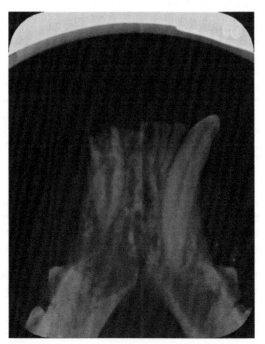

Fig. 27. Severe periapical lucency, extrusion, and widened root canal with internal resorption of a right mandibular canine tooth with a chronic complicated crown fracture.

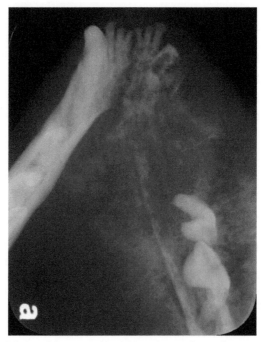

Fig. 28. The typical lysis of bone with periosteal new bone formation associated with squamous cell carcinoma.

new, compact bone formation without destruction (**Fig. 29**).[15,16] However, bone loss associated with osteoma has been reported,[17] which may be secondary to periodontal disease and shows the importance of relying not only on clinical and radiographic findings but also on histologic samples.

Other oral tumors have been reported in cats, but are less common and rarely reported. The author has diagnosed 2 calcifying odontogenic epithelial tumors and 1 ossifying odontogenic fibroma. In addition, an osteoma diagnosed by the author radiographically resembled squamous cell carcinoma. The lesion responded to surgical debulking. Radiographic findings of oral tumors can vary and histologic confirmation is always recommended.

Orthopedic injury

Traumatic symphyseal separation has been noted to be the most common orthopedic injury to the feline oral cavity.[18] These injuries often occur secondary to falls or vehicular trauma. Palpable instability of the symphysis is not pathognomonic for traumatic symphyseal separation. Instability may result from periodontal disease, laxity of the ligamentous attachment, neoplasia, or fracture of the mandible.[19] There may be fractured tooth roots. The symphysis often appears wider than normal and, if malaligned, the occlusal planes of the incisors and alveolar bone may be unequal when comparing left with right (**Fig. 30**).

Fractures of the rostral portion of the mandibular body may present similarly to symphyseal separation. A fracture may travel through the alveolus of the ipsilateral canine tooth (**Figs. 31** and **32**). Although rostral mandibular fracture and symphyseal separation may resemble each other clinically, radiographic assessment is crucial. A

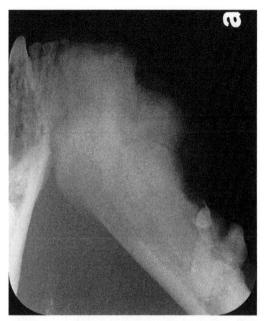

Fig. 29. Osteoma of the left mandible. These lesions are typically osteoproductive without lysis.

cerclage wire often suffices to treat a symphyseal separation. However, this same treatment does not immobilize a rostral mandibular fracture.

Fractures of the mandibular body, caudal to the canine tooth, are uncommon in the cat. When assessing the mandibular body for fractures, the direction of the fracture and the location of the fracture in relation to tooth roots should be evaluated. Oblique fractures of the mandible may be described as favorable or unfavorable according to the difficulty of immobilization. A fracture that travels caudodorsally is considered favorable, whereas a fracture that travels caudoventrally is considered unfavorable. This distinction results from the forces that the muscles of mastication place on the mandible.

Fractures that travel through the alveolus of a tooth ending at the apex have the potential to cause the endodontic death of the tooth.[20] In addition, any fracture

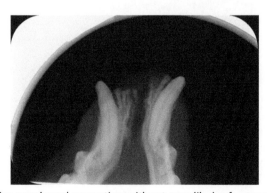

Fig. 30. Mandibular symphyseal separation without mandibular fracture.

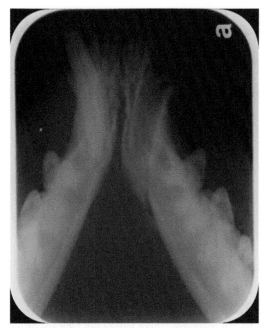

Fig. 31. A fracture of the rostral portion of the left mandible from traumatic luxation of the canine tooth. Although clinically it resembles a symphyseal separation, a rostral cerclage wire, as is used to stabilize separations, will not stabilize this fracture.

through the alveolus, regardless of whether it travels through the apex, has the potential to cause periodontal ligament death and subsequent root ankylosis and tooth resorption. There are differing opinions on how and when these teeth should treated, and this is beyond the scope of this article; however, there is the potential for future complications and follow-up with dental radiographs is prudent.

Maxillofacial trauma may lead to separation of sutures between the palatal process of the paired maxillae. A concurrent separation in the hard palate mucoperiosteum may also be present. Small lesions have been reported to heal spontaneously.[21]

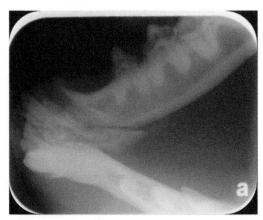

Fig. 32. The same fracture as in **Fig. 31**, shown from an oblique angle.

However, if the void does not heal, an oronasal fistula will be present and can lead to rhinitis. On a dorsoventral projection of the nasal cavity with a size 2 or 4 dental film placed in the mouth, this may be seen as a radiolucent gap between the left and right palatal process of corresponding maxilla, and this can be paired with a fracture of one or both maxilla, therefore additional radiographic views should be made.

Because of masking of lesions by superimposition of surrounding osseous structures, some fractures of the maxilla, palatine bone, and temporal bone may not be visible with standard or dental radiography. In these cases, computed tomography (CT) may be a superior diagnostic method. It has been shown that twice as many maxillofacial fractures are diagnosed using CT versus standard skull radiographs in dogs and cats with maxillofacial trauma.[22] If a patient has an abnormal or unstable dental occlusion after trauma and radiographs do not show a fracture or luxation, CT should be considered.

In addition to being necessary for complete diagnosis and assessment of dental and maxillofacial disease, radiographs are vital to ensuring the success of treatment. A common complication to extractions in veterinary dental practice is incomplete extraction and subsequent root retention.

When roots are retained (except in the case of type II tooth resorption), most veterinary dentists agree that the patient is often in pain. It is the experience of the author that there is often a marked focal gingivitis associated with root retention in cats (see **Fig. 13**). This gingivitis usually resolves after complete extraction of the root. A published case report also suggested that retained tooth roots and the associated infection and inflammation may have resulted in ketoacidosis in a cat.[23] It is unknown whether this cat was diabetic before treatment, but, after stabilization and removal of the retained roots, the patient showed marked clinical improvement. Radiographs are also necessary to evaluate successful endodontic treatment. Failure or success of root canal therapy cannot be determined by visual inspection alone.

SUMMARY

Dental radiography is an invaluable diagnostic modality not only in feline practice but in all small animal practice. Dental disorders cannot be fully assessed and diagnosed without good-quality intraoral radiographs. Dental radiographs make early detection of tooth resorption more likely and aid in surgical planning of extractions. They are necessary if crown amputation is to be performed. Dental radiographs are important in determining patterns of bone loss when assessing periodontal disease and ensuring that clinical findings are not caused by another pathologic process such as tooth resorption or neoplasia. Once the concepts are understood, dental radiography provides good medical data that benefit patients and provide an economic benefit to the practice.

REFERENCES

1. Use of dental film in small animal practice. J Am Vet Med Assoc 1971;159(7): 877–9.
2. Holmstrom SE, Bellows J, Colmery B, et al. AAHA dental care guidelines for dogs and cats. J Am Anim Hosp Assoc 2005;41(5):277–83.
3. Verstraete FJ, Kass PH, Terpak CH. Diagnostic value of full mouth rads. Am J Vet Res 1998;59(6):692–5.
4. Verstraete FJ, Terpak CH. Anatomical variations in the dentition of the domestic cat. J Vet Dent 1997;14(4):137–40.

5. Gracis M. Radiographic study of the maxillary canine tooth of four mesaticephalic cats. J Vet Dent 1999;16(3):115–28.
6. Gengler W, Dubielzig R, Ramer J. Physical examination and radiographic analysis to detect dental and mandibular bone resorption in cats: a study of 81 cases from necropsy. J Vet Dent 1995;12(3):97–100.
7. DuPont GA, DeBowes LJ. Comparison of periodontitis and root replacement in cat teeth with resorptive lesions. J Vet Dent 2002;19(2):71–5.
8. AVDC nomenclature. In: AVDC Web site. 2012. Available at: http://avdc.org/nomenclature.html#resorption. Accessed August 27, 2012.
9. Lommer MJ, Verstraete FJ. Radiographic patterns of periodontitis in cats: 147 cases (1998-1999). J Am Vet Med Assoc 2001;218(2):230–4.
10. Reiter AM, Lewis JR, Okuda A. Update on the etiology of tooth resorption in domestic cats. Vet Clin North Am Small Anim Pract 2005;35(4):913–42.
11. Lewis JR, Okuda A, Shofer FS, et al. Significant association between tooth extrusion and tooth resorption in domestic cats. J Vet Dent 2008;25(2):86–95.
12. Bender IB. Factors influencing the radiographic appearance of bony lesions. J Endod 1982;107(3):413–9.
13. Lommer MJ, Verstraete FJ. Prevalence of odontoclastic resorption lesions and periapical radiographic lucencies in cats: 265 cases (1995-1998). J Am Vet Med Assoc 2000;217(12):1866–9.
14. Liptak JM, Withrow SJ. Cancer of the gastrointestinal tract. In: Withrow SJ, Vail DM, editors. Withrow and MacEwen's small animal clinical oncology. Philadelphia: Saunders Elsevier; 2007. p. 455–75.
15. Forrest LJ. Cranial and nasal cavities: canine and feline. In: Thrall DE, editor. Textbook of veterinary diagnostic radiology. 5th edition. Philadelphia: Saunders Elsevier; 2007. p. 119–41.
16. Kapatkin AS, Manfra Marretta S. Mandibular swellings in cats: prospective study of 24 cats. J Am Anim Hosp Assoc 1991;27(6):575–80.
17. Fiani N, Arzi B, Johnson EG, et al. Osteoma of the oral and maxillofacial regions in cats: 7 cases (1999-2009). J Am Vet Med Assoc 2011;238(11):1470–5.
18. Wiggs RB, Lobprise HB. Domestic feline oral and dental disease. In: Veterinary dentistry, principles and practice. Philadelphia: Lippincott-Raven; 1997. p. 482–517.
19. Reiter AM. Symphysiotomy, symphysiectomy, and intermandibular arthrodesis in a cat with open-mouth jaw locking–case report and literature review. J Vet Dent 2004;21(3):147–58.
20. Schloss AJ, Manfra Marretta S. Prognostic factors affecting teeth in the line of mandibular fractures. J Vet Dent 1990;7(4):7–9.
21. Verstraete FJ. Maxillofacial fractures. In: Slatter D, editor. Textbook of small animal surgery, vol. 2, 3rd edition. Philadelphia: Saunders Elsevier; 2003. p. 2190–207.
22. Bar-Am Y, Pollard RE, Kass PH, et al. The diagnostic yield of conventional radiographs and computed tomography in dogs and cats with maxillofacial trauma. Vet Surg 2008;37(3):294–9.
23. Reiter AM, Brady CA, Harvey CE. Local and systemic complications in a cat after poorly performed dental extractions. J Vet Dent 2004;21(4):215–21.

Oral Inflammation in Small Animals

Milinda J. Lommer, DVM[a,b,*]

KEYWORDS

- Oral inflammation • Small mammals • Oral cavity

KEY POINTS

- In mammalian tissue, inflammation is a highly integrated, elaborate response to insult or injury.
- Its primary purpose is to contain and remove offending microorganisms and necrotic tissue, preventing infection and facilitating tissue healing.
- An aberrant or accentuated inflammatory process can itself cause tissue injury and dysfunction.
- As ongoing research yields an increasing understanding of the cellular and molecular mechanisms that modulate inflammation, efforts to treat and prevent oral inflammatory diseases can become more specific, targeting the precise cells and molecules responsible.

INTRODUCTION

The oral cavity can be affected by a wide variety of disorders characterized by recurrent or chronic, generalized or localized inflammation of the oral mucosa and gingiva. Based on their appearance, oral inflammatory lesions may be classified as ulcerative conditions, vesiculobullous diseases, or proliferative lesions (**Table 1**). Because the oral mucosa has a limited repertoire of responses, however, many different diseases may produce similar manifestations.[1] In particular, vesicles and bullae of canine and feline oral mucosa rarely persist long enough to be observed, due to constant trauma from chewing, playing, and grooming. Therefore, immune-mediated conditions normally producing vesiculobullous lesions may present as ulcerative lesions in the oral cavity.

Therefore, the various inflammatory conditions are discussed according to their underlying causes: inflammation associated with dental disease, infectious conditions,

Conflict of Interest: None.

[a] Aggie Animal Dental Center, 487 Miller Avenue, Mill Valley, CA 94941, USA; [b] Department of Surgical and Radiological Sciences, School of Veterinary Medicine, University of California, Davis, Davis, CA 95616, USA

* Aggie Animal Dental Center, 487 Miller Avenue, Mill Valley, CA 94941, USA.

E-mail address: mlommer@aggieanimaldentalservice.com

Table 1
Oral mucosal diseases categorized according to appearance

Ulcerative Conditions	Vesiculobullous Diseases	Inflamed Proliferative Lesions
Plaque-reactive mucositis	Mucous membrane pemphigus	Eosinophilic granuloma complex
Feline gingivostomatitis	Pemphigus vulgaris	Feline gingivostomatitis
Eosinophilic granuloma complex	Pemphigus foliaceous	Viral papillomas
Periodontal abscess	Bullous pemphigoid	Endodontic abscess with parulis
Feline calicivirus	Systemic lupus erythematosus	Foreign body reaction
Erythema multiforme	Erythema multiforme	Sublingual mucosal hyperplasia
Pemphigoid disorders		Extramedullary plasmacytoma
Systemic lupus erythematosus		Squamous cell carcinoma
Epidermolysis bullosa		Epitheliotrophic lymphoma
Uremia		Acanthomatous ameloblastoma
Chemical exposure		Benign buccal exostoses
Electrical injury		

idiopathic inflammatory responses, mucosal and cutaneous immune-mediated disorders, reactive lesions, and neoplastic conditions.

INFLAMMATION ASSOCIATED WITH DENTAL DISEASE

Localized ulceration or swelling limited to the gingiva and alveolar mucosa may be associated with a periodontal or endodontic abscess. Periodontal abscesses are typically associated with swelling and redness of the gingiva surrounding a single tooth, contiguous to a periodontal pocket (**Fig. 1**A).[2] Gentle pressure on the swollen tissue generally results in expression of purulent exudate. If a draining tract is present, it is coronal to the mucogingival junction. Periodontal abscesses may be associated with regional lymph node enlargement, fever, and acute discomfort.[2] Periodontal

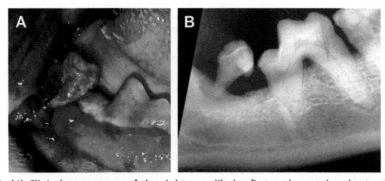

Fig. 1. (A) Clinical appearance of the right mandibular first and second molar teeth in a 7-year-old spayed female French bulldog. Significant ulceration of the gingiva and alveolar mucosa are evident at the second molar tooth. (B) Radiograph of the same teeth, showing combined horizontal and vertical bone loss with near total loss of attachment of the second molar tooth.

probing and intraoral radiographs confirm the presence of periodontal pockets and alveolar bone loss (see **Fig. 1**B).[2]

Microscopically, a periodontal abscess is a localized accumulation of neutrophils within the periodontal pocket wall.[3] Within the overlying epithelium, intracellular and extracellular edema and leukocyte invasion are evident.[3] Gram-negative anaerobic rods are the primary bacterial colonizers.[3]

By contrast, an endodontic abscess (more properly termed, *apical periodontitis*) is typically associated with swelling and mucosal inflammation apical to the mucogingival junction, and there may be a draining tract through the mucosa, apical to the mucogingival junction (**Fig. 2**A). Periodontal probing usually does not reveal the presence of pockets.[2] In dogs and cats, apical periodontitis is most commonly associated with dental fractures,[4] but abrasion[5] and pulp necrosis secondary to concussive trauma[6] are also common causes of apical periodontitis. Although rare, caries may also lead to pulp necrosis and apical periodontitis in dogs.[7]

Radiographically, a diagnosis of apical periodontitis is supported by the presence of any of the following: increased width of the periodontal ligament space in the region of the apex, changes in the trabecular bone pattern around the apex, a diffuse or well-defined periapical radiolucency (see **Fig. 2**B), arrested deposition of secondary dentin (indicated by a pulp cavity that is wider than that of the contralateral tooth or adjacent teeth), or inflammatory resorption of dental tissue at the apex.[8]

Although periodontal abscesses and apical periodontitis may be diagnosed based on periodontal probing and radiographs, biopsy may be indicated for lesions with slightly atypical features. In some cases, tumors occurring at or near the site of a fractured tooth may go undiagnosed if the tissue swelling and ulceration are assumed inflammatory (**Fig. 3**).

INFECTIOUS CONDITIONS

Acute ulceration of the oral mucosa and/or tongue has been associated with feline calicivirus,[9–13] feline herpesvirus,[14,15] feline panleukopenia,[16] feline leukemia virus,[14] feline immunodeficiency virus,[17–19] and canine parvovirus.[20,21] (There are also 2 reports from India of fungal-related stomatitis in dogs.[22,23]) Affected animals almost always display many other symptoms suggestive of systemic illness, such as lethargy, fever, and hematological and serum biochemical abnormalities, so diagnosis is not

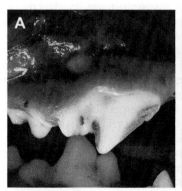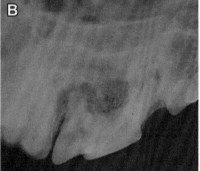

Fig. 2. (*A*) Clinical appearance of the right maxillary fourth premolar tooth in a 6-year-old neutered male labradoodle. (*B*) Intraoral radiograph of the same tooth, revealing large periapical lucencies and a wide pulp cavity relative to the adjacent teeth.

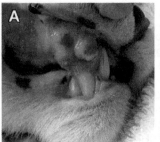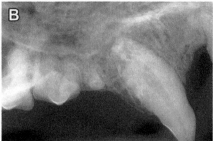

Fig. 3. (A) Clinical appearance of swollen alveolar mucosa at the buccal aspect of the right maxillary canine tooth in a 10-year-old neutered male domestic shorthair cat. The tooth had a complicated crown fracture of unknown duration. The swelling had not responded to oral administration of clindamycin, and the cat was referred for radiographs and biopsy. (B) Intraoral radiograph of the right maxillary canine tooth confirms a wide pulp cavity and moth-eaten bone loss around the root, but no distinct periapical lucency. The tooth was extracted and the surrounding mucosa was submitted for histopathologic analysis, which revealed round cell neoplasia consistent with lymphoma. Immunohistochemistry was supportive of a diagnosis of B-cell lymphoma, and the cat was treated with chemotherapy.

based on oral findings, and biopsy is rarely indicated. Treatment is primarily supportive, including appropriate analgesia and parenteral nutrition when oral ulceration is severe. Supplementation with L-lysine has been shown to reduce replication of herpesvirus[24] and reduce the severity of herpesvirus-related conjunctivitis,[25] although its effects on oral symptoms have not been specifically investigated. Recent investigations using feline recombinant interferon,[26,27] immune plasma,[28] and antiviral agents, such as famcyclovir[29,30] and plerixafor,[31] have shown promise as more-specific therapeutic options. In the future, targeted gene therapy, such as the use of small interfering RNA, may also be useful in inhibiting viral replication[32] and expediting resolution of acute viral infections.

IDIOPATHIC INFLAMMATORY CONDITIONS
Feline Chronic Gingivostomatitis

Of the oral inflammatory diseases commonly seen in veterinary practice, feline chronic gingivostomatitis (FCGS) has been the most researched, yet its etiology remains largely undetermined. Although several studies have found a higher prevalence of feline calicivirus in cats with FCGS than in nonaffected cats,[11,33–35] and transient oral ulceration has been observed in cats with acute calicivirus infection,[9,36–38] chronic oral inflammation has not been a sequela in either naturally occurring or experimentally induced acute calicivirus infection. Other microorganisms have been investigated as possible contributing factors to the development of FCGS, including feline immunodeficiency virus, feline leukemia virus, feline herpesvirus, *Bartonella henselae*,[17,33,35,39–42] and *Pasteurella multocida*,[43] but causal relationships have not been established. The presence of plaque bacteria is thought to be a major contributing factor.[44] It is likely that the development of chronic gingivostomatitis is related to an underlying immune abnormality, specifically with regards to the inflammatory mediators produced by lymphocytes and plasma cells in response to bacterial and/or viral infection. Initial histopathologic studies of FCGS revealed that the infiltrates into affected tissue are composed of plasma cells, with varying numbers of lymphocytes, neutrophils, and macrophages present.[45,46] Abnormalities of neutrophil function were not detected in affected cats.[47] Mast cells, although present in higher numbers in the gingiva of affected cats,[48,49] seem to play only a minor role, because there seems to be no significant difference in the numbers of mast cells in the gingiva of cats with FCGS, tooth resorption, or periodontitis.[50]

Serum biochemical changes in affected cats are typically limited to high serum globulin concentrations, composed of a polyclonal hypergammaglobulinemia,[46] which was further classified as composed of high serum IgG, IgM, and IgA.[51] Salivary immunoglobulin concentrations were also evaluated, with the result that cats with FCGS were found to have much higher salivary IgG, moderately higher salivary IgM, and lower salivary IgA than unaffected cats.[51] These findings coincide with recent findings that the majority of plasma cells in the oral mucosa of cats with FCGS were of the IgG isotype.[49] In that same investigation, severity of inflammation was positively correlated with the number of CD97a$^+$ cells (mostly plasma cells), CD3$^+$ T cells, and L1$^+$ cells (primarily neutrophils) and expression of MHC class II proteins in affected tissue.[49] Investigation of the cytokine profiles of cats with FCGS revealed a mixed helper T cells type 1 and type 2 cytokine profile compared with primarily a type 1 profile in cats with healthy mucosa.[52] All these studies suggest an underlying aberration in the immune response. The investigators also noted, however, that CD8$^+$ T cells (cytotoxic T cells) greatly outnumbered CD4$^+$ (helper T) cells, suggesting that intracellular pathogens, such as viruses, play a role in the pathogenesis of FCGS.[49]

Clinically, FCGS may appear as generalized or localized areas of ulceration (**Fig. 4**A) or proliferation (see **Fig. 4**B) within the oral cavity. Because periodontitis and tooth

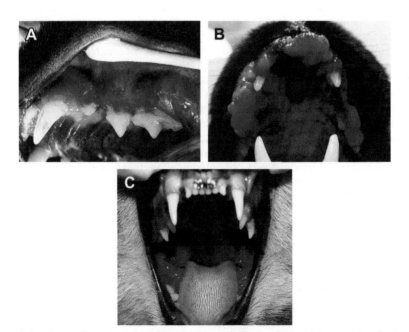

Fig. 4. (*A*) Left maxillary gingiva and buccal mucosa of a 3.5-year-old neutered male domestic shorthair cat who was presented for evaluation of ulcerative stomatitis. (*B*) Maxillary gingiva and buccal mucosa of a 10-year-old neutered male domestic medium-hair cat who was presented for evaluation of severe proliferative stomatitis. (*C*) Caudal oral mucosa of a 2.5-year-old spayed female domestic shorthair cat presented for treatment of severe, generalized stomatitis.

resorption may also be associated with generalized or localized inflammation, full-mouth radiographs and dental charting are important to distinguish between these 3 conditions. The presence of inflammation in the caudal oral cavity (ie, the areas lateral to the palatoglossal folds, sometimes incorrectly referred to as the fauces) and/or the oropharynx is one of the distinguishing characteristics of FCGS (see **Fig. 4**C).

Patients with periodontitis and/or tooth resorption alone do not have inflammation in these caudal areas. All 3 diseases, however, can be present concomitantly (**Fig. 5**).

Successful treatment of FCGS requires minimizing oral bacteria. Because daily plaque removal by mechanical means (eg, toothbrushing) is difficult in these painful patients, reduction of plaque-retentive surfaces by extracting teeth has proved the most effective way to minimize plaque and reduce oral inflammation. It has been demonstrated that 60% to 80% of cats with lymphocytic-plasmacytic gingivitis stomatitis significantly improve after extraction of all premolar and molar teeth, and surgical treatment is, therefore, the current standard of care for cats with FCGS.[53,54] Those cats that do not respond to premolar/molar or full-mouth extractions, however, present a therapeutic challenge. Because glucocorticoids have immunosuppressive effects (which include decreasing neutrophil diapedesis, redistributing lymphocytes to extravascular compartments, and down-regulating maturation of antigen-presenting cells)[55] and are easily accessible and inexpensive, they remain the most commonly prescribed medication for management of refractory stomatitis. The beneficial effects of steroid administration are inconsistent, however, and may be accompanied by deleterious effects, such as behavior changes, thinning of the skin, polyuria, polydipsea, and potential for development of diabetes mellitus.[55–57] Therefore, alternative treatments are sought. One option is cyclosporine, which has recently been Food and Drug Administration–approved for use in cats and is available in a liquid suspension (Atopica for Cats, Novartis Animal Health, Greensboro, North Carolina) which allows more precise dosing and is easier to administer than the capsule form commonly prescribed for dogs (Atopica for Dogs, Novartis Animal Health, Greensboro, North Carolina). In one retrospective analysis featuring 8 cats with FCGS who received oral cyclosporine (Sandimmune solution, Novartis Pharmaceutical Corporation, East Hanover, New Jersey) at 30 mg to 50 mg daily, 50% achieved remission of inflammation after 90 days, and the remaining 50% showed fair to good improvement of 40% to 70%.[58] Although it was reported that all cats in this study had previously received injectable steroids, it was not noted whether these cats had previously undergone periodontal treatment or dental extractions. In a prospective, placebo-controlled study of 16 cats with refractory FCGS (ie, those who had not completely responded to premolar/molar or full-mouth extractions), approximately 78%

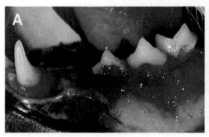
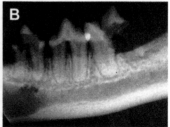

Fig. 5. (*A*) Photograph and (*B*) radiograph of a 10-year-old neutered male domestic short-hair cat with generalized stomatitis, severe localized periodontitis, and semigeneralized tooth resorption.

demonstrated improvement of 40% or more after 6 weeks of treatment compared with 14% of control cats; mean improvement in the cyclosporine group was 52.7% after 6 weeks.[59] Side effects are usually mild and consist primarily of transient vomiting or diarrhea.[60] Cyclosporine administration is not without risk, however, particularly for outdoor cats, because disseminated toxoplasmosis has been reported.[61–63]

In 2011, a multicenter, controlled, double-masked European investigation revealed that recombinant feline interferon omega delivered transmucosally was as effective as prednisolone in decreasing clinical lesions and pain scores.[26] With no significant deleterious side effects reported, this product is expected to be widely used once it becomes commercially available in the United States.

Contact Mucositis (Plaque-reactive Stomatitis)

Although cats are more frequently affected by stomatitis, an increasing number of dogs is being presented with symptoms, such as ptyalism, halitosis, decreased ability to prehend hard food, and reluctance to play with chew toys. General physical examination may reveal atrophy of the masticatory muscles and weight loss. Patients may be extremely reluctant to allow oral examination without sedation or anesthesia. Oral examination typically reveals ulceration of the vestibular (buccal) mucosa in areas that contact the tooth surfaces, particularly at the carnassial and canine teeth. Although histopathologic analysis of the lesions may reveal lymphocytes and plasma cells in the epithelium and lamina propria similar to that found in cats with FCGS, this syndrome (previously referred to as chronic ulcerative paradental stomatitis) differs from feline gingivostomatitis in that the lesions are almost exclusively localized to the areas in contact with the teeth and do not typically involve the caudal oral mucosa or the oropharyngeal mucosa.[64,65] In some cases, severe ulceration occurs in the absence of significant periodontitis (**Fig. 6**). In other cases, periodontitis may be evident based on clinical findings of severe gingival recession and/or radiographic findings of bone loss (**Fig. 7**).

As with cats, treatment of contact mucositis in dogs relies on effective plaque control. Although many dogs are amenable to daily toothbrushing, the discomfort associated with contact mucositis may make these patients uncooperative for home care. Professional periodontal treatment is essential, including extraction of any teeth demonstrating significant bone loss. This should be followed by administration of analgesic and anti-inflammatory medications, which may provide enough relief to enable

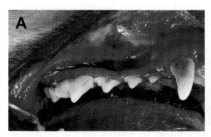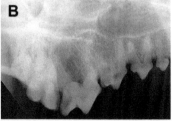

Fig. 6. (*A*) Ulcerative stomatitis featuring gingivitis, buccal mucositis, and glossitis in a 7-year-old spayed female shepherd mix. The lateral margins of the tongue were affected in the regions that contacted the lingual surfaces of the mandibular teeth. (*B*) Intraoral radiograph of the right maxillary premolar and molar teeth of the same dog. Replacement resorption is evident at the first premolar tooth, and there is evidence of inflammatory resorption at the third and fourth premolar teeth, but periodontal bone levels are near normal, with approximately 1 mm of horizontal bone loss apparent.

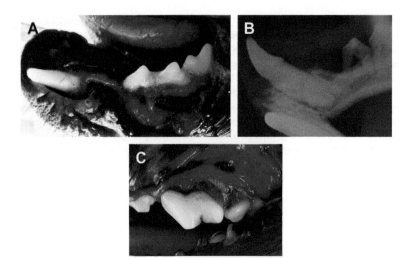

Fig. 7. (*A*) Severe gingivitis and buccal mucositis affecting the left mandible of a 9-year-old spayed female pug. (*B*) Intraoral radiograph of the left mandibular canine and third premolar teeth (the first 2 premolar teeth are missing); moderate horizontal bone loss is noted at the canine tooth, with severe horizontal bone loss affecting the mesial root of the third premolar tooth. (*C*) Severe localized gingivitis, gingival recession, and buccal mucositis at the left maxillary fourth premolar and first molar teeth in a 10-year-old neutered male golden retriever. Although intraoral radiographs should be performed as part of a complete examination when the dog is anesthetized, a diagnosis of stage 3–4 periodontitis can be made at the time of the initial examination based on these findings alone.

initial attempts to remove plaque using wet gauze on a finger. Chlorhexidine-based rinses and gels or drinking water additives that have demonstrated efficacy in reducing plaque (eg, products that have received the Seal of Acceptance by the Veterinary Oral Health Council) may be helpful adjuncts to toothbrushing. If these measures fail to resolve the areas of inflammation, medical management (as discussed previously, cyclosporine has fewer side effects than glucocorticoids and is, therefore, preferred) and/or surgical treatment by removing all teeth in the affected areas may be required. In the author's experience, a combination of selective extractions, professional dental cleaning at 3-month to 6-month intervals, and diligent home care is usually sufficient to prevent recurrence of contact ulcers. In several canine patients for whom home care was not feasible and long-term immunosuppressive medication was undesirable, however, extraction of all premolar and molar teeth was performed, resulting in resolution of the inflammation (**Fig. 8**).

MUCOSAL AND CUTANEOUS DISEASES
Eosinophilic Granuloma Complex

Eosinophilic granuloma complex is a common disorder in cats, affecting the skin (eosinophilic plaque), upper lip (indolent ulcer) (**Fig. 9**), palate, and/or tongue (eosinophilic granuloma). Although rare, eosinophilic lesions have been described in the oral cavity of dogs as well,[66–69] who may be presented with symptoms of clearing the throat, difficulty swallowing, coughing during and after eating, or difficulty eating.[68] Rather than a disease, eosinophilic dermatoses should be thought of as a reaction pattern to a variety of different stimuli.[70] Histologic findings are typical, with an eosinophilic infiltrate and a variable number of mast cells, histiocytes, and lymphocytes.[70]

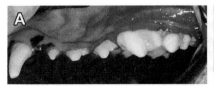
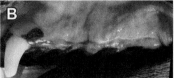

Fig. 8. (*A*) The left maxillary quadrant of a 4-year-old neutered male Australian cattle dog mix who was presented due to severe oral pain, which manifested in symptoms including halitosis, ptyalism, hiding, and refusal to play. Oral examination revealed severe gingivitis and contact mucositis associated with the caudal premolar and molar teeth in all 4 quadrants, with moderate contact mucositis adjacent to the canine and rostral premolar teeth. (*B*) Daily plaque control at the caudal teeth was not possible, so extraction of all premolar and molar teeth was performed, which resolved the inflammation. This photograph was taken 10 months after extraction of all premolar and molar teeth; the patient was allowing daily toothbrushing of the remaining canine and incisor teeth.

Feline herpesvirus-1 may occasionally result in skin or oral lesions resembling eosinophilic plaques or ulcers.[40,71]

The most common underlying cause is a hypersensitivity reaction to environmental antigens, foods, or parasites, and it is important to attempt to identify and address the underlying cause before administering immunosuppressive medications, such as glucocorticoids or cyclosporine.[58] In some cases, treatment with amoxicillin trihydrate–potassium clavulanate alone may result in near-resolution of eosinophilic plaques or indolent ulcers.[72]

Erythema Multiforme

Erythema multiforme (EM) is a rare disorder, leading to vesicular and ulcerative lesions on skin and mucus membranes, with some histologic findings typical of pleocellular inflammation but featuring characteristic keratinocyte apoptosis and lymphocyte satellitosis.[73] It is hypothesized that EM results from a host-specific cytotoxic T-lymphocyte attack on keratinocytes expressing nonself antigens, typically microbes and drugs.[73] In many cases, EM is initiated by administration of medications.[73,74] In some cases, viral infection of skin and mucosal epithelial cells results in activation of cytotoxic T lymphocytes, which then induces keratinocyte apoptosis.[20,21] In dogs, the oral cavity is involved in approximately one-third of cases with EM,[75] and dysphagia and/or ptyalism secondary to oral ulceration may be the primary complaint

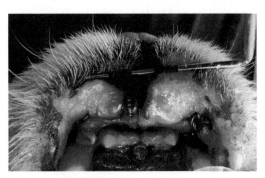

Fig. 9. Eosinophilic ulcers on the maxillary lip of a 4.5-year-old spayed female domestic shorthair cat.

at presentation.[76] In some cases, it may be difficult to distinguish EM from epitheliotrophic lymphoma, and immunohistochemistry may be required to identify neoplastic intraepithelial CD3+ T cells within a focus of pleocellular inflammation.[76] Proper diagnosis is crucial, because the prognosis for epitheliotrophic lymphoma is poor, whereas EM may resolve once the triggering factor is removed.[76] In the future, administration of intravenous immunoglobulins may comprise part of the treatment plan for EM patients.[74]

Pemphigus Foliaceous

Pemphigus foliaceous is most common antibody-mediated, autoimmune skin disease of dogs,[77] but mucosal lesions are rare, reported in approximately 2% of dogs with pemphigus foliaceous.[78] A major antigen responsible was recently identified as desmocollin-1, a calcium-dependent transmembrane glycoprotein involved in intercellular adhesion.[79] Clinical features include facial and footpad lesions consisting of vesicles and pustules (which evolve rapidly to erosions covered with crusts).[77] Histopathology reveals acantholytic keratinocytes accompanied by neutrophilic infiltration and a variable number of eosinophils. The prognosis is generally good, because patients usually respond to immunosuppressive doses of corticosteroids (2 mg/kg/d).[77]

Pemphigus Vulgaris

Although rare, lesions of pemphigus vulgaris may first develop in the oral cavity or at mucocutaneous junctions and then spread to haired skin.[80,81] German shepherd dogs and collies may be predisposed, and male dogs predominate.[81] Vesicles evolve rapidly into irregular erosions and areas of sloughing.[80] The prognosis is guarded and referral should be made to an internist or dermatologist to discuss appropriate treatment options.

Mucous Membrane Pemphigoid

Vesicles, erosions, and ulcers are seen primarily in or around the oral cavity, nasal planum, eyes, ear canals, anus, and genitals[82,83] German shepherd dogs may be predisposed to mucous membrane pemphigoid. IgG autoantibodies directed against basement membrane proteins result in subepidermal and submucosal vesiculation, with few inflammatory cells.[83]

Epidermolysis Bullosa Acquisita

Epidermolysis bullosa acquisita is characterized by severe clinical signs, including sloughing of the oral epithelium and footpads, and carries a poor prognosis.[82] Great Danes are overrepresented. Autoantibodies target collagen VII, resulting in subepidermal and submucosal vesicles without inflammation or with subepidermal alignment of neutrophils.[82] Immunohistochemistry is required to differentiate epidermolysis bullosa acquisita from mucous membrane pemphigoid or bullous pemphigoid (which does not usually present with oral mucosal ulceration).[82]

Systemic Lupus Erythematosus

It is unusual for patients with systemic lupus erythematosus to present with primarily oral signs, because joint pain and stiffness (attributable to polyarthritis), together with dermatitis, are more common presenting complaints. Erythematous, crusty skin lesions on the face, and ulceration of the lip margins may be apparent (**Fig. 10**). Affected animals test positive for circulating antinuclear antibody.[81]

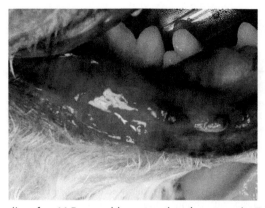

Fig. 10. Left lower lip of a 14.5-year-old neutered male coton de Tulear suspected of having immune-mediated disease. However histopathologic analysis of the ulcerated region at the mucocutaneous junction resulted in a diagnosis of lymphocytic-plasmacytic cheilitis, and the ulcer resolved after periodontal treatment and topical application of antibiotic ointment.

REACTIVE LESIONS

In addition to the intrinsic immune disturbances (described previously), many external stimuli can result in oral inflammation. When attempting to determine the underlying cause of an oral inflammatory lesion, whether the lesion is localized or generalized within the oral cavity and whether it is ulcerative or proliferative should be considered.

Generalized ulcerative lesions may result from viral infections (in particular, feline calicivirus, as discussed previously), chemical exposure,[84,85] administration of pancreatic enzyme supplements,[86] or uremia. Obtaining a thorough history, which includes travel history, exposure to toxins, known traumatic incidents, and administration of any dietary supplements as well as prescription medications, is important whenever patients present with evidence of oral ulceration. In most patients with generalized oral ulceration caused by viral infection, chemical exposure, or uremia, the oral signs are not the primary complaint, and patients display other significant symptoms that direct the path of diagnostic testing.

Generalized proliferative lesions may include viral papillomatosis, drug-induced gingival enlargement, and familial gingival hyperplasia.

A localized ulcer may result from a penetrating wound, an electrical injury (**Fig. 11**), or eosinophilic indolent ulcer.

Conditions presenting with localized proliferation of oral mucosa include focal fibrous hyperplasia, foreign body reaction, and sublingual mucosal hyperplasia (**Fig. 12**). Sublingual mucosal hyperplasia may be both proliferative and ulcerated, depending on whether there is masticatory trauma, and is usually bilaterally symmetric, although one side may be larger than the other. Excisional biopsy not only yields a diagnosis but also in most cases is curative.[87]

Treatment depends on the underlying cause. Localized ulcerative lesions may respond well to débridement and supportive care. In the future, stem cell therapy may play a role in the treatment of oral inflammation, because local injection of mesenchymal stem cells derived from bone marrow was found to accelerate the healing of chemically induced oral ulcers in an experimental model using dogs.[88]

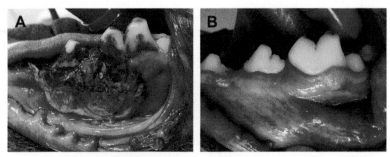

Fig. 11. (*A*) Ulcerative, necrotic gingival, and mucosal lesion affecting the left mandibular fourth premolar and first molar teeth of a 10-year-old neutered male Weimaraner. Radiographs were unremarkable. The lesion was biopsied and débrided. Histopathology revealed no evidence of neoplasia, with changes suggestive of electrical cord injury. (*B*) Despite complete loss of the attached gingiva and alveolar mucosa at the buccal aspect of the fourth premolar and first molar teeth, 6 weeks later the area had healed completely and appeared almost normal.

NEOPLASTIC LESIONS

Although many oral neoplasms appear as masses, several may first present as ulcerations or even simply as erythematous areas on the gingiva or oral mucosa. Squamous cell carcinoma (**Fig. 13**) in cats and epitheliotrophic lymphoma in dogs are 2 malignant neoplasms that commonly have an ulcerative rather than exophytic appearance. Biopsy and histopathologic analysis is recommended for any abnormal-appearing tissue in the oral cavity, in particular, nonhealing extraction sites; early diagnosis and appropriate intervention may mean the difference between a satisfactory and unsatisfactory outcome.

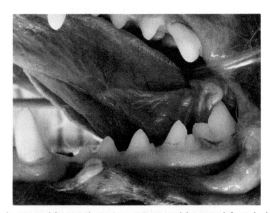

Fig. 12. Sublingual mucosal hyperplasia in a 10-year-old spayed female bichon frise. These lesions are usually bilateral and tend to occur in small breed dogs. Surgical excision is usually only performed if they are inflamed and/or are traumatized during mastication.[88]

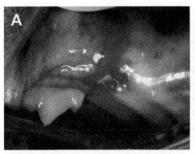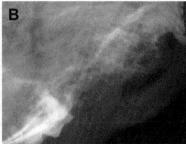

Fig. 13. (*A*) Clinical and (*B*) radiographic appearance of an ulcerative lesion at the site of a recent tooth extraction (the right maxillary third premolar tooth, P3). The radiograph reveals subtle permeative and subtle moth-eaten osteolysis in the region extending from the region of the missing P3 to the (also missing) canine tooth site. Histopathologic analysis of bone and soft tissue collected from the P3 site confirmed a diagnosis of squamous cell carcinoma.

SUMMARY

In mammalian tissue, inflammation is a highly integrated, elaborate response to insult or injury. Its primary purpose is to contain and remove offending microorganisms and necrotic tissue, preventing infection and facilitating tissue healing.[89] An aberrant or accentuated inflammatory process, however, itself can cause tissue injury and dysfunction. As ongoing research yields an increasing understanding of the cellular and molecular mechanisms that modulate inflammation, efforts to treat and prevent oral inflammatory diseases can become more specific, targeting the precise cells and molecules responsible.

REFERENCES

1. Bradley G. Diseases of the oral mucosa. Can Fam Physician 1988;34:1443–51.
2. Melnick PR, Takei HH. Treatment of a periodontal abscess. In: Newman MG, Takei HH, Klokkevold PR, et al, editors. Clinical periodontology. 10th edition. St Louis (MO): Saunders Elsevier; 2006. p. 714–21.
3. Carranza FA, Carmago PM. The periodontal pocket. In: Newman MG, Takei HH, Klokkevold PR, et al, editors. Clinical periodontology. 10th edition. St Louis (MO): Saunders Elsevier; 2006. p. 434–51.
4. Niemiec BA. Fundamentals of endodontics. Vet Clin North Am Small Anim Pract 2005;35(4):837–68.
5. Fiani N, Arzi B. Diagnostic imaging in veterinary dental practice. J Am Vet Med Assoc 2009;235(3):271–3.
6. Hale FA. Localized intrinsic staining of teeth due to pulpitis and pulp necrosis in dogs. J Vet Dent 2001;18(1):14–20.
7. Duncan HL. Diagnostic imaging in veterinary dental practice. Dental caries. J Am Vet Med Assoc 2010;237(1):41–3.
8. DuPont GA, DeBowes LJ. Endodontic disease. In: DuPont GA, DeBowes LJ, editors. Atlas of dental radiography in dogs and cats. St Louis (MO): Saunders Elsevier; 2009. p. 5–133.
9. Hoover EA, Kahn DE. Experimentally induced feline calicivirus infection: clinical signs and lesions. J Am Vet Med Assoc 1975;166(5):463–8.
10. Johnson RP, Povey RC. Effect of diet on oral lesions of feline calicivirus infection. Vet Rec 1982;110(5):106–7.

11. Knowles JO, McArdle F, Dawson S, et al. Studies on the role of feline calicivirus in chronic stomatitis in cats. Vet Microbiol 1991;27(3–4):205–19.
12. Dawson S, Bennett D, Carter SD, et al. Acute arthritis of cats associated with feline calicivirus infection. Res Vet Sci 1994;56(2):133–43.
13. Pesavento PA, MacLachlan NJ, Dillard-Telm L, et al. Pathologic, immunohistochemical, and electron microscopic findings in naturally occurring virulent systemic feline calicivirus infection in cats. Vet Pathol 2004;41(3):257–63.
14. Suchy A, Bauder B, Gelbmann W, et al. Diagnosis of feline herpesvirus infection by immunohistochemistry, polymerase chain reaction, and in situ hybridization. J Vet Diagn Invest 2000;12(2):186–91.
15. Gaskell R, Dawson S, Radford A, et al. Feline herpesvirus. Vet Res 2007;38(2): 337–54.
16. Baker MK. Ulcerative glossitis. A facet of feline panleukopenia. J S Afr Vet Assoc 1975;46(3):295–7.
17. Tenorio AP, Franti CE, Madewell BR, et al. Chronic oral infections of cats and their relationship to persistent oral carriage of feline calici-, immunodeficiency, or leukemia viruses. Vet Immunol Immunopathol 1991;29(1–2):1–14.
18. Reubel GH, George JW, Higgins J, et al. Effect of chronic feline immunodeficiency virus infection on experimental feline calicivirus-induced disease. Vet Microbiol 1994;39(3–4):335–51.
19. Ishida T, Washizu T, Toriyabe K, et al. Feline immunodeficiency virus infection in cats of Japan. J Am Vet Med Assoc 1989;194(2):221–5.
20. Favrot C, Olivry T, Dunston SM, et al. Parvovirus infection of keratinocytes as a cause of canine erythema multiforme. Vet Pathol 2000;37(6):647–9.
21. Woldemeskel M, Liggett A, Ilha M, et al. Canine parvovirus-2b-associated erythema multiforme in a litter of English Setter dogs. J Vet Diagn Invest 2011;23(3): 576–80.
22. Jadhav VJ, Pal M. Canine mycotic stomatitis due to Candida albicans. Rev Iberoam Micol 2006;23(4):233–4.
23. Pal M. Role of Geotrichum candidum in canine oral ulcers. Rev Iberoam Micol 2005;22(3):183.
24. Maggs DJ, Nasisse MP, Kass PH. Efficacy of oral supplementation with L-lysine in cats latently infected with feline herpesvirus. Am J Vet Res 2003;64(1):37–42.
25. Stiles J, Townsend WM, Rogers QR, et al. Effect of oral administration of L-lysine on conjunctivitis caused by feline herpesvirus in cats. Am J Vet Res 2002;63(1): 99–103.
26. Hennet PR, Camy GA, McGahie DM, et al. Comparative efficacy of a recombinant feline interferon omega in refractory cases of calicivirus-positive cats with caudal stomatitis: a randomised, multi-centre, controlled, double-blind study in 39 cats. J Feline Med Surg 2011;13(8):577–87.
27. Domenech A, Miro G, Collado VM, et al. Use of recombinant interferon omega in feline retrovirosis: from theory to practice. Vet Immunol Immunopathol 2011; 143(3–4):301–6.
28. Bragg RF, Duffy AL, DeCecco FA, et al. Clinical evaluation of a single dose of immune plasma for treatment of canine parvovirus infection. J Am Vet Med Assoc 2012;240(6):700–4.
29. Malik R, Lessels NS, Webb S, et al. Treatment of feline herpesvirus-1 associated disease in cats with famciclovir and related drugs. J Feline Med Surg 2009;11(1):40–8.
30. Thomasy SM, Lim CC, Reilly CM, et al. Evaluation of orally administered famciclovir in cats experimentally infected with feline herpesvirus type-1. Am J Vet Res 2011;72(1):85–95.

31. Hartmann K, Stengel C, Klein D, et al. Efficacy and adverse effects of the antiviral compound plerixafor in feline immunodeficiency virus-infected cats. J Vet Intern Med 2012;26(3):483–90.
32. Taharaguchi S, Matsuhiro T, Harima H, et al. Suppression of feline calicivirus replication using small interfering RNA targeted to its polymerase gene. Biocontrol Sci 2012;17(2):87–91.
33. Knowles JO, Gaskell RM, Gaskell CJ, et al. Prevalence of feline calicivirus, feline leukaemia virus and antibodies to FIV in cats with chronic stomatitis. Vet Rec 1989;124(13):336–8.
34. Dawson S, McArdle F, Bennett M, et al. Typing of feline calicivirus isolates from different clinical groups by virus neutralisation tests. Vet Rec 1993;133(1): 13–7.
35. Quimby JM, Elston T, Hawley J, et al. Evaluation of the association of Bartonella species, feline herpesvirus 1, feline calicivirus, feline leukemia virus and feline immunodeficiency virus with chronic feline gingivostomatitis. J Feline Med Surg 2008;10(1):66–72.
36. Gaskell CJ, Gaskell RM, Dennis PE, et al. Efficacy of an inactivated feline calicivirus (FCV) vaccine against challenge with United Kingdom field strains and its interaction with the FCV carrier state. Res Vet Sci 1982;32(1):23–6.
37. Wardley RC, Povey RC. The clinical disease and patterns of excretion associated with three different strains of feline caliciviruses. Res Vet Sci 1977;23(1):7–14.
38. Love DN. Pathogenicity of a strain of feline calicivirus for domestic kittens. Aust Vet J 1975;51(12):541–6.
39. Belgard S, Truyen U, Thibault JC, et al. Relevance of feline calicivirus, feline immunodeficiency virus, feline leukemia virus, feline herpesvirus and Bartonella henselae in cats with chronic gingivostomatitis. Berl Munch Tierarztl Wochenschr 2010;123(9–10):369–76.
40. Lee M, Bosward KL, Norris JM. Immunohistological evaluation of feline herpesvirus-1 infection in feline eosinophilic dermatoses or stomatitis. J Feline Med Surg 2010;12(2):72–9.
41. Dowers KL, Hawley JR, Brewer MM, et al. Association of Bartonella species, feline calicivirus, and feline herpesvirus 1 infection with gingivostomatitis in cats. J Feline Med Surg 2010;12(4):314–21.
42. Sykes JE, Westropp JL, Kasten RW, et al. Association between Bartonella species infection and disease in pet cats as determined using serology and culture. J Feline Med Surg 2010;12(8):631–6.
43. Dolieslager SM, Riggio MP, Lennon A, et al. Identification of bacteria associated with feline chronic gingivostomatitis using culture-dependent and culture-independent methods. Vet Microbiol 2011;148(1):93–8.
44. Williams CA, Aller MS. Gingivitis/stomatitis in cats. Vet Clin North Am Small Anim Pract 1992;22(6):1361–83.
45. Johnessee JS, Hurvitz AI. Feline plasma cell gingivitis-pharyngitis. J Am Anim Hosp Assoc 1983;19(2):179–81.
46. White SD, Rosychuk RA, Janik TA, et al. Plasma cell stomatitis-pharyngitis in cats: 40 cases (1973-1991). J Am Vet Med Assoc 1992;200(9):1377–80.
47. Sato R, Inanami O, Tanaka Y, et al. Oral administration of bovine lactoferrin for treatment of intractable stomatitis in feline immunodeficiency virus (FIV)-positive and FIV-negative cats. Am J Vet Res 1996;57(10):1443–6.
48. Arzi B, Murphy B, Baumgarth N, et al. Analysis of immune cells within the healthy oral mucosa of specific pathogen-free cats. Anat Histol Embryol 2011;40(1): 1–10.

49. Harley R, Gruffydd-Jones TJ, Day MJ. Immunohistochemical characterization of oral mucosal lesions in cats with chronic gingivostomatitis. J Comp Pathol 2011;144(4):239–50.

50. Arzi B, Murphy B, Cox DP, et al. Presence and quantification of mast cells in the gingiva of cats with tooth resorption, periodontitis and chronic stomatitis. Arch Oral Biol 2010;55(2):148–54.

51. Harley R, Gruffydd-Jones TJ, Day MJ. Salivary and serum immunoglobulin levels in cats with chronic gingivostomatitis. Vet Rec 2003;152(5):125–9.

52. Harley R, Helps CR, Harbour DA, et al. Cytokine mRNA expression in lesions in cats with chronic gingivostomatitis. Clin Diagn Lab Immunol 1999;6(4):471–8.

53. Hennet P. Chronic gingivo-stomatitis in cats: long-term follow-up of 30 cases treated by dental extractions. J Vet Dent 1997;14:15–21.

54. Bellei E, Dalla F, Masetti L, et al. Surgical therapy in chronic feline gingivostomatitis (FCGS). Vet Res Commun 2008;32(Suppl 1):S231–4.

55. Lowe AD, Campbell KL, Graves T. Glucocorticoids in the cat. Vet Dermatol 2008; 19(6):340–7.

56. Lowe AD, Graves TK, Campbell KL, et al. A pilot study comparing the diabetogenic effects of dexamethasone and prednisolone in cats. J Am Anim Hosp Assoc 2009;45(5):215–24.

57. Lowe AD, Campbell KL, Barger A, et al. Clinical, clinicopathological and histological changes observed in 14 cats treated with glucocorticoids. Vet Rec 2008; 162(24):777–83.

58. Vercelli A, Raviri G, Cornegliani L. The use of oral cyclosporin to treat feline dermatoses: a retrospective analysis of 23 cases. Vet Dermatol 2006;17(3):201–6.

59. Lommer MJ. Efficacy of cyclosporine for the treatment of refractory gingivostomatitis in cats. J Vet Dent 2012.

60. Heinrich NA, McKeever PJ, Eisenschenk MC. Adverse events in 50 cats with allergic dermatitis receiving ciclosporin. Vet Dermatol 2011;22(6):511–20.

61. Barrs VR, Martin P, Beatty JA. Antemortem diagnosis and treatment of toxoplasmosis in two cats on cyclosporin therapy. Aust Vet J 2006;84(1–2):30–5.

62. Beatty J, Barrs V. Acute toxoplasmosis in two cats on cyclosporin therapy. Aust Vet J 2003;81(6):339.

63. Last RD, Suzuki Y, Manning T, et al. A case of fatal systemic toxoplasmosis in a cat being treated with cyclosporin A for feline atopy. Vet Dermatol 2004;15(3):194–8.

64. Boutoille F, Hennet P. Maxillary osteomyelitis in two Scottish terrier dogs with chronic ulcerative paradental stomatitis. J Vet Dent 2011;28(2):96–100.

65. Wiggs RB, Lobprise H. Clinical oral pathology. In: Wiggs RB, Lobprise H, editors. Veterinary dentistry: principles and practice. Philadelphia: Lippincott-Raven; 1997. p. 104–39.

66. Madewell BR, Stannard AA, Pulley LT, et al. Oral eosinophilic granuloma in Siberian husky dogs. J Am Vet Med Assoc 1980;177(8):701–3.

67. German AJ, Holden DJ, Hall EJ, et al. Eosinophilic diseases in two Cavalier King Charles spaniels. J Small Anim Pract 2002;43(12):533–8.

68. Bredal WP, Gunnes G, Vollset I, et al. Oral eosinophilic granuloma in three cavalier King Charles spaniels. J Small Anim Pract 1996;37(10):499–504.

69. Joffe DJ, Allen AL. Ulcerative eosinophilic stomatitis in three Cavalier King Charles spaniels. J Am Anim Hosp Assoc 1995;31(1):34–7.

70. Bloom PB. Canine and feline eosinophilic skin diseases. Vet Clin North Am Small Anim Pract 2006;36(1):141–60, vii.

71. Persico P, Roccabianca P, Corona A, et al. Detection of feline herpes virus 1 via polymerase chain reaction and immunohistochemistry in cats with ulcerative

facial dermatitis, eosinophilic granuloma complex reaction patterns and mosquito bite hypersensitivity. Vet Dermatol 2011;22(6):521–7.

72. Wildermuth BE, Griffin CE, Rosenkrantz WS. Response of feline eosinophilic plaques and lip ulcers to amoxicillin trihydrate-clavulanate potassium therapy: a randomized, double-blind placebo-controlled prospective study. Vet Dermatol 2012; 23(2):110–8, e24–5.

73. Voie KL, Campbell KL, Lavergne SN. Drug hypersensitivity reactions targeting the skin in dogs and cats. J Vet Intern Med 2012;26(4):863–74.

74. Byrne KP, Giger U. Use of human immunoglobulin for treatment of severe erythema multiforme in a cat. J Am Vet Med Assoc 2002;220(2):197–201, 183–94.

75. Scott DW, Miller WH. Erythema multiforme in dogs and cats: literature review and case material from the Cornell University College of Veterinary Medicine (1988-1996). Vet Dermatol 1999;10:297–309.

76. Nemec A, Zavodovskaya R, Affolter VK, et al. Erythema multiforme and epitheliotropic T-cell lymphoma in the oral cavity of dogs: 1989 to 2009. J Small Anim Pract 2012;53(8):445–52.

77. Olivry T. A review of autoimmune skin diseases in domestic animals: I—superficial pemphigus. Vet Dermatol 2006;17(5):291–305.

78. Mueller RS, Krebs I, Power HT, et al. Pemphigus foliaceus in 91 dogs. J Am Anim Hosp Assoc 2006;42(3):189–96.

79. Bizikova P, Dean GA, Hashimoto T, et al. Cloning and establishment of canine desmocollin-1 as a major autoantigen in canine pemphigus foliaceus. Vet Immunol Immunopathol 2012;149(3–4):197–207.

80. Olivry T, Linder KE. Dermatoses affecting desmosomes in animals: a mechanistic review of acantholytic blistering skin diseases. Vet Dermatol 2009;20(5–6): 313–26.

81. Pedersen NC. A review of immunologic diseases of the dog. Vet Immunol Immunopathol 1999;69(2–4):251–342.

82. Olivry T, Jackson HA. Diagnosing new autoimmune blistering skin diseases of dogs and cats. Clin Tech Small Anim Pract 2001;16(4):225–9.

83. Olivry T, Dunston SM, Schachter M, et al. A spontaneous canine model of mucous membrane (cicatricial) pemphigoid, an autoimmune blistering disease affecting mucosae and mucocutaneous junctions. J Autoimmun 2001;16(4):411–21.

84. Hofmeister AS, Heseltine JC, Sharp CR. Toxicosis associated with ingestion of quick-dissolve granulated chlorine in a dog. J Am Vet Med Assoc 2006;229(8): 1266–9.

85. Gieger TL, Correa SS, Taboada J, et al. Phenol poisoning in three dogs. J Am Anim Hosp Assoc 2000;36(4):317–21.

86. Snead E. Oral ulceration and bleeding associated with pancreatic enzyme supplementation in a German shepherd with pancreatic acinar atrophy. Can Vet J 2006;47(6):579–82.

87. Buelow ME, Marretta SM, Barger A, et al. Lingual lesions in the dog and cat: recognition, diagnosis, and treatment. J Vet Dent 2011;28(3):151–62.

88. El-Menoufy H, Aly LA, Aziz MT, et al. The role of bone marrow-derived mesenchymal stem cells in treating formocresol induced oral ulcers in dogs. J Oral Pathol Med 2010;39(4):281–9.

89. McManus LM, Pinckard RN. PAF: A putative mediator of oral inflammation. Crit Rev Oral Biol Med 2000;11(2):240–58.

Exodontics
Extraction of Teeth in the Dog and Cat

Bill Gengler, DVM*

KEYWORDS

- Exodontics • Tooth extraction • Dogs • Cats

KEY POINTS

- The identification and treatment or removal of diseased teeth are the responsibility of the veterinarian.
- When diseased teeth cannot be saved by specialized care, extraction of teeth is necessary.
- Proper extraction of teeth in dogs and cats can be challenging and frustrating, but with review of the oral anatomy, proper instrumentation, and gentle tissue-handling techniques, this can be a rewarding part of clinical practice.
- Making this investment has a positive impact on the patient's health, the respect of clients, and the success of a practice.

INTRODUCTION

Dental extractions in veterinary patients vary in difficulty across a wide range of conditions. In past years, dental education during the student years may have fallen short of producing graduates who were comfortable with and knowledgeable about treating oral disease, especially the extraction of a tooth solidly held in the alveolus. Despite the many anatomic and pathologic variations that are encountered, a consistent group of established principles is the basis of the skill set for performing these procedures effectively. A thorough understanding of the basic approach to surgical extractions is paramount for providing minimally invasive, efficient technique to minimize anesthetic time and maximize patient comfort and safety.[1–6] As the basic principles are mastered, it becomes obvious that these principles can be extended and applied in many ways to reduce pain and improve the oral health of our patients. As technique improves, confidence builds and joy is derived from tasks that were once a struggle. The intention of this article is to help surgeons to learn the basic principles and the instrumentation required to acquire the technique needed to perform tooth extraction in the dog and cat with skill.

University of Wisconsin, School of Veterinary Medicine, 4661 Signature Drive, Middleton, WI 53562, USA
* 10304 Countryside Drive, Denton, TX 76207.
E-mail address: wrgdvm@gmail.com

Vet Clin Small Anim 43 (2013) 573–585
http://dx.doi.org/10.1016/j.cvsm.2013.02.008
0195-5616/13/$ – see front matter © 2013 Elsevier Inc. All rights reserved.

GENERAL PRINCIPLES

Surgery in the oral cavity is a challenge. The surgical space is small, and other organs such as the tongue or equipment like endotracheal tubes, monitors, and so forth often get in the way. Bleeding is often significant and hemostasis can be difficult. Healing of oral surgery is similar to wound healing elsewhere in the body. However, there are modifying factors within the oral cavity that affect healing. The following factors all play a role in the healing process: the unique biochemical and anatomic function of the bones of the face and jaw; the protruding teeth; specialized tissue such as the gingiva; the constant exposure to contamination; and the specialized medium of saliva, food, and foreign material. Although these factors might retard healing in other areas of the body, healing in the oral cavity usually progresses rapidly, the major reason being the abundant vascular supply and antibody-rich saliva.

Extraction of teeth may be divided into 2 types: nonsurgical and surgical. The principles involved to break down the gingival attachment and separation of the periodontal ligament (PDL) fibers are the same for both types of extractions. The attached gingiva is nonelastic and firm in structure because of the heavy make-up of collagen. The attachment of the gingiva to the tooth creates significant holding power for the tooth and consequently should be the first tissue to be released from attachment to the tooth during extraction. This release may be accomplished with a number 15 scalpel blade or a sharp periosteal elevator. The PDL fibers crisscross the space between the bone and cementum and are attached firmly to these structures on each end of the ligament. The PDL holds or suspends the tooth within the alveolus. The PDL is a viable tissue receiving a blood supply from the surrounding bone and gingiva. Tension is applied to the PDL fibers by use of hand instruments such as a dental elevator, luxator, periotome, or other instrument using mechanical principles. Sustained tension on the tooth for 15 to 20 seconds in each direction in which the tooth can be moved causes the PDL to tear. Abrupt and jerking movements are not helpful when extracting teeth. Sustained tension causes the breakdown or shearing of the PDL fibers. The fibers withstand abrupt, sudden forces well but cannot tolerate sustained tension without shearing. Shearing forces or tearing of the PDL may be accomplished using a dental elevator (Cislak, Glenview, IL) (**Fig. 1**) in a fulcrum and lever arrangement (**Fig. 2**) and a wheel and lever position (**Fig. 3**). In addition, the attached gingiva may be severed and extraction forces applied to the PDL with the use of a luxator (**Figs. 4** and **5**). The most important principle is the lever principle. Hand instruments are excellent when using the lever principle. A lever gains its effect

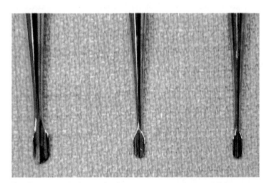

Fig. 1. Working end of winged dental elevators. Varying widths are used depending on special arrangement of teeth.

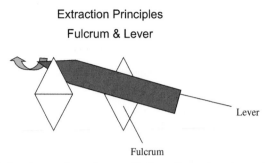

Extraction Principles
Fulcrum & Lever

Lever

Fulcrum

Fig. 2. The dental elevator used as a lever, with the adjacent tooth as a fulcrum. The tooth to be extracted may be moved laterally and displaced coronally by clockwise rotation of the elevator.

by using a fulcrum to maximize force. The fulcrum for tooth extraction can be an adjacent tooth, surrounding bone, and so forth. The lever may also maximize force when the elevator is rotated, as with the wheel and lever principle (see **Fig. 3**). Dental elevators are made in various widths to be inserted between the teeth and rotated. As the working edge of the elevator contacts the tooth, the instrument may be rotated to move the tooth in a lateral extruding direction. In addition, this movement may be coupled with the fulcrum principle. The luxator and periotome (Cislak) (**Fig. 6**) function when inserted along the long axis of the tooth between the tooth and bone severing

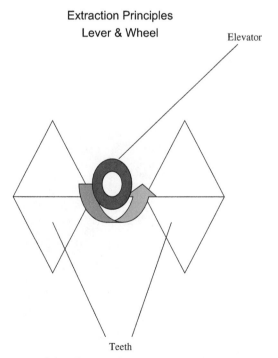

Extraction Principles
Lever & Wheel

Elevator

Teeth

Fig. 3. The cross section of the elevator shown rotating in a counterclockwise direction to displace the tooth laterally and coronally.

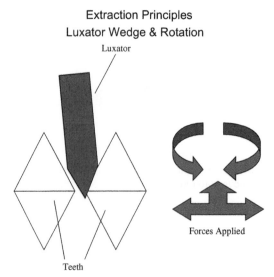

Fig. 4. The sharp end of the luxator is driven between the bone and the tooth to sever the PDL. Tooth displacement is achieved by multiple directional movement of the instrument.

the PDL. When the tooth is moved, the vascular supply to the PDL is torn along with the PDL fibers, creating hemorrhage. Dental forceps should be used once the tooth is sufficiently loose. Veterinary dentistry does not have the advantage of a wide array of extraction forceps so that an instrument can be selected that has jaws that perfectly fit

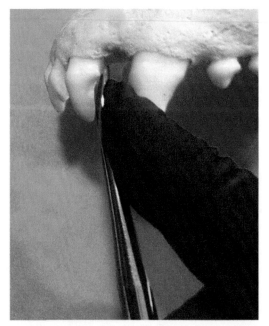

Fig. 5. The luxator is driven between bone and root to shear the PDL. Placing the index finger close to the working end of the instrument prevents patient trauma should the instrument slip.

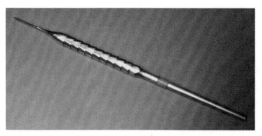

Fig. 6. The periotome provides a long slender sharp working end to shear the PDL when used as a luxator.

and engage all of the crown of the tooth. Animal dentistry encompasses a wide range of shapes and sizes of tooth crowns. Consequently, there is seldom an extraction forceps that fully engages all of the tooth crown. Often, only the tips of the forceps contact the crown of the tooth. When heavy force is placed on the forceps to grip the tooth, the pressure is concentrated in a small area, causing the crown to fracture. Therefore, it is recommended to use elevators and luxators to create substantial tooth mobility, whereby the tooth may simply be gently lifted from the alveolus using a small extraction forceps with short handles (Cislak) (**Fig. 7**), preventing crown fracture. Nonsurgical extraction involves severing only the gingival attachment in the sulcus and shearing of the PDL. When this procedure is performed without incising the gingiva and mucosa or exposing alveolar bone, it is termed a nonsurgical extraction. Surgical extractions involve creating exposure and potential removal of the alveolar bone to give greater access to the root portion of the tooth.[6]

Before attempting to perform oral surgery, it is important to have complete command of the oral anatomy. Some common principles that are critical in the success of oral surgery are:

1. Gingiva does not have elasticity but mucosa is elastic, therefore it is important in planning oral surgery to extend the incisions beyond the mucogingival line to take advantage of elasticity of the mucosa for tension-free wound closure.

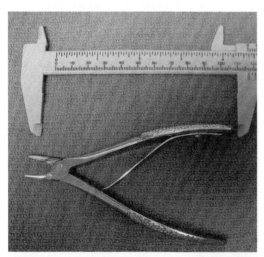

Fig. 7. Forceps measuring 10 to 12 cm (4–5 inches) are used to lift the loose tooth from the alveolus. Longer handles tend to exert excessive force and can crush the tooth.

2. Create incision lines with rounded corners, when possible, to avoid avascularity of the flap, gently elevating the flap from the periosteal attachment to the bone with a periosteal elevator (Cislak) **(Fig. 8)**.
3. Anticipate a healthy blood supply with the use of surgical suction. It helps ready identification of dental structures and saves surgery time.
4. Allow for deep tissue bites when suturing oral tissue.
5. Avoid tension on the suture line.
6. Plan the incision so closure of soft tissue is not over a bony void but is lying on supportive bone.
7. Use suture needles that do not cut or tear the soft tissue.
8. Use surgical technique to prevent cutting of soft tissue during closure by suture drag.
9. When suturing in the oral cavity, always try to begin with the unattached or flap portion of the tissue and advance toward the tissue that is attached to the bone by the periosteum.

Wound healing for most healthy oral soft tissue occurs within 5 to 7 days. The suture of choice for healthy oral soft tissue is one that is nonreactive, monofilament, absorbable in 10 to 14 days in a 5/0 to 3/0 size when suture removal is to be avoided. Poliglecaprone 25 (Monosyn, B. Braun Melsungen, Melsungen, Germany), a synthetic polyester composed of glycolide dioxanone and trimethylene carbonate (Biosyn, Covidien, Mansfield, MA), polyglyconate (Maxon, Covidien), Polyglacton 910 (Vicryl Rapide, Ethicon, New Brunswick, NJ), or other similar synthetic absorbable monofilament sutures. Most of these sutures require 2 to 3 weeks or more to absorb in the mouth and are the suture of choice when delayed healing is anticipated. Polyglacton 910 (Vicryl Rapide) is a coated braided suture, which, according to the manufacturer, behaves like a monofilament and is the quickest of the synthetic sutures to absorb (7–10 days). Chromic gut may be used in a noninfected/noninflamed site, in which normal healing is anticipated. Chromic gut is an absorbable, sterile surgical suture composed of purified connective tissue (mostly collagen) derived from either the serosal layer of beef (bovine) or the submucosal fibrous layer of sheep (ovine) intestines. Nonabsorbable sutures may be used intraorally but often require patient sedation or anesthesia for removal or slough with tissue turnover.

The most common suture pattern used is a simple interrupted pattern, but a vertical mattress is beneficial when extra tissue-holding strength is anticipated. When the vertical mattress is used, it should be combined with a simple interrupted pattern to produce precise tissue alignment to the incision. A simple or interlocking continuous

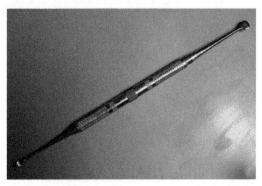

Fig. 8. Cislak EX9 periosteal elevator used to create mucogingival flaps.

pattern may be used when closing large incisions, such as full mouth extractions, in which time under general anesthesia is critical but the risk of wound dehiscence may be greater.

SIMPLE FLAP DESIGN

Surgical flaps are usually used for single tooth surgical extractions, gingival repositioning, surgical endodontics or small mass excisions.[7] The flap configuration includes a horizontal incision with a single or double vertical releasing incision (**Figs. 9** and **10**). For tooth extraction purposes, the horizontal incision is usually made within the sulcus and continuing in the interdental spaces at the crest of the gingiva. The vertical releasing incision, when extended beyond the mucogingival line, gives the flap elasticity from the mucosa, therefore any flap that requires transposition or added stretch or coverage must have a vertical release into the mucosa. If bony voids are created with extraction or en bloc removal of a mass, the flap should be planned so the closure of the soft tissue is not suspended over the bony void, but instead, underlying bone supports the incision. The vertical releasing incision should be made boldly, attempting to make 1 clean incision from the surface epithelium completely through the soft tissue to the bone. A clean single incision allows the surgeon to more easily identify the proper tissue plane when elevating the periosteum and accompanying gingiva or mucosa. If the flap is created to cover a void, it should be made approximately 1.5 times larger than the anticipated void when possible. If double vertical releasing incisions are made and the expectation is that the flap is transposed some distance from the origin, the 2 vertical releasing incisions should be made in a divergent coronal to apical pattern to allow for narrowing of the flap as it is elongated or stretched to extend over the void. In cases in which the marginal gingival has a poor integrity, it may be easier to begin elevating the soft tissue at the apical end of the incision rather than the gingival margin. The periosteum resists separation from bone when forces are more in a coronal to apical direction than the reverse (eg, chewing). Using this technique often prevents tearing or shredding of the marginal gingiva.

SURGICAL EXTRACTIONS

Maxillary third incisor and canine teeth should always be extracted surgically, not simply because of the degree of difficulty of extraction, but primarily because of the close proximity to the nasal cavity (**Fig. 11**A, B). The alveoli should always be sutured, entrapping a healthy blood clot when possible to prevent alveolitis. In addition, the extraction site heals quickly by first intention, preventing an oronasal fistula should

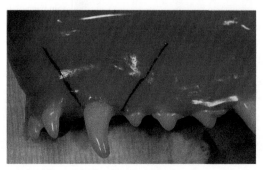

Fig. 9. The divergent double vertical releasing incision for surgical extraction of a left maxillary canine tooth.

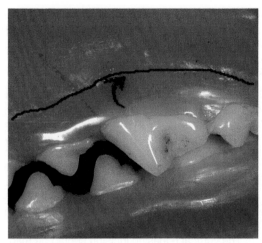

Fig. 10. The single vertical releasing incision (*red*) for extraction of the left fourth maxillary premolar tooth. The blue line indicates the mucogingival line and the black arrow shows the direction of flap elevation.

the thin layer of bone separating the alveolus from the nasal cavity be perforated. Other multirooted teeth usually require surgical extraction to perform a buccocortical osteotomy and sectioning of the crown (**Fig. 12**) into individual root components. A dental radiograph should always be taken before extraction to determine the morphology and integrity of the root and to determine the degree, if any, of ankylosis. These factors help you prepare a more accurate treatment plan and estimate of cost.

Once the flap design has been completed, a releasing incision(s) is/are made, the flap may be elevated with a periosteal elevator (Cislak) (see **Fig. 8**), and the bone over the buccal (or vestibular) 180° of the circumference of the root is removed using a round or pear-shaped carbide bur in a water-cooled high-speed handpiece.[8,9] Often, the coronal one-third of buccal bone is removed, but more may be removed depending on the morphology and integrity of the root(s). A common mistake in performing the buccocortical osteotomy for tooth extraction is to remove less than a full 180° of buccal bone. A shelf of bone at the edge of the tooth root can have excellent

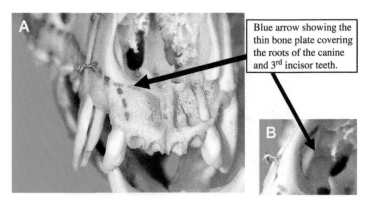

Blue arrow showing the thin bone plate covering the roots of the canine and 3rd incisor teeth.

Fig. 11. (*A, B*) Photograph and insert showing the proximity of the root of the third incisor and the canine tooth to the nasal cavity.

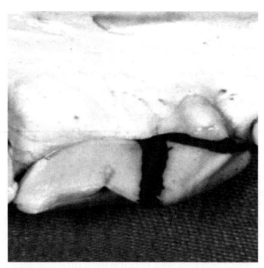

Fig. 12. Incisal view. Dark lines indicate sectioning of a maxillary fourth premolar tooth at the rostral and vestibular furcations, dividing it into 3 crown/root segments to eliminate the divergent root retention capabilities and allow each segment to be extracted like a single rooted tooth.

holding strength and prevents gaining the mobility needed to shear the PDL fibers. The removal of buccal bone assists in moving the tooth to shear the PDL. The direction of force for the hand instrument (lever) should always be toward the area of bone removal. The removal of buccal bone from multirooted teeth also exposes the furcation(s). The furcation is the starting point for crown sectioning. A cross-cut carbide bur, such as a 701, on a high-speed handpiece is used to produce 2 or 3 single root-crown components, depending if the tooth is 2 or 3 rooted. Roots of teeth are usually divergent. This root configuration helps maintain the stability of the teeth in the jaw. Sectioning eliminates the divergent root retention capabilities and allows the segment to be extracted like a single rooted tooth with the use of elevators and luxators (see **Fig. 1**). As stated earlier, the most important consideration in using elevators, luxators, periotomes, and so forth is to provide tension on the tooth for 15 to 20 seconds to allow the PDL to tear and hemorrhage. Abrupt and jerking movements are not helpful when extracting teeth. Sustained tension causes the breakdown or shearing of the PDL fibers.

Most veterinarians find the extraction of a maxillary fourth premolar tooth to be the most challenging. Follow these steps to make extraction of this tooth a more predictable procedure:

1. Create a vertical releasing incision beginning at the rostral sulcus of the mesiobuccal root, extending the incision in a rostrodorsal direction to avoid the juga of the underlying root (see **Fig. 10**). The incision should not lie over the void you later create by removing buccal bone but rostral to it.
2. Once the buccal bone is removed over the mesiobuccal (also named mesiovestibular) and distal root, the furcation of the roots become visible.
3. Section the crown into thirds with a cross-cut bur in a water-cooled high-speed handpiece, beginning at the furcation and extending the vertical cut to the cusp of the tooth (see **Fig. 12**). A 701 carbide cross-cut or similar bur is most suitable for this task.

4. Dental elevators may be used as a lever, with the third premolar or first molar as a fulcrum. Elevators may also be placed between the teeth and rotated in a wheel and lever principle to displace the tooth segment and produce shearing of the PDL fibers. As the space widens, wider elevators are used to displace the tooth. Luxators may be used to wedge between the root and alveolar bone to move the tooth (see **Fig. 4**). It is important to hold the luxator with the index finger a few millimeters from the tip of the luxator to prevent inadvertent trauma to the tissues, should the luxator slip from position (see **Fig. 5**). Always attempt to move the tooth/root toward the area of bone removal to maximize surgical extraction technique.

5. If the distal crown is contacting the first molar, making it difficult to elevate the distal portion, cut a small notch with the bur in the distal crown of PM4 to allow for an elevator purchase point.

6. Once both the mesiobuccal and distal segments are loosened, use extraction forceps to lift the mesiobuccal segment from the alveolus, but leave the distal segment to use as a fulcrum for elevating the mesiopalatal root-crown segment.

7. Remove interradicular bone from the buccal side of the mesiopalatal root with a round or pear-shaped bur.

8. Use the distal root-crown segment and the third premolar as a fulcrum to elevate the mesiopalatal root buccally. Once this tooth segment is loosened, use a small extraction forceps (Cislak) (see **Fig. 7**) to lift the 2 remaining segments from their alveoli.

9. Curette the alveoli and surgical site to remove any diseased bone.

10. Remove any sharp bony points (alveoloplasty) with a carbide bur.

11. Irrigate liberally with saline or a dilute chlorhexidine solution.

12. Make horizontal releasing incisions in the mucoperiosteum (or a buccinator muscle release) to allow the mucosa to stretch, releasing tension on your subsequent closure with absorbable suture.

13. Close the alveolar gingival, making certain that there is good adaptation with the gingiva of the adjacent teeth.

14. Close the remaining gingiva followed by the more elastic mucosa.

By following this sequence, fracture of the smallest (mesiopalatal) root is avoided, because it is never used as a fulcrum to attempt to displace a larger root.

Release for the Maxillary Canine and Maxillary Fourth Premolar Extraction

Eliminating tension on mucoperiosteal flap closure is the key to successful healing of surgical extraction sites. Defects left from extracted teeth require increased tissue volume to close adequately. An effective and efficient method of providing considerable flap mobility is the use of the mucoperiosteal release. This release may be performed routinely in surgical extractions of any teeth when an increased area of tissue is needed to cover a defect. After the proper mesial vertical releasing incision, the mucoperiosteum is identified lying superficial to the bone. A scalpel or Metzenbaum scissors can be used to begin dissection between the bone and mucosa. With the flap held with forceps, horizontal incisions are made next to the bone to release the attachment of the mucosa to the bone. This effort produces 2 to 7 mm of additional mucosal length, which may be used to complete the tension-free closure. Alternatively, the buccinator muscle release provides a similar benefit.[7] This release may be performed routinely in surgical maxillary canine and maxillary fourth premolar extractions. After the proper mesial vertical releasing incision, the buccinator muscle is identified just palatal to the palatal aspect of the alveolar mucosa. Metzenbaum scissors are used to begin dissection parallel and between the 2 tissue planes. Once

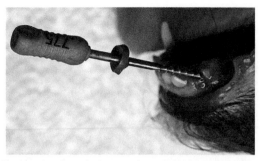

Fig. 13. Hedstrom files can be threaded into a fractured root and used to displace the root, shearing the PDL for extraction. (*Courtesy of* Dr Brett Beckman.)

adequate separation has occurred, scissors are used to excise the buccinator muscle, separating it from the rostral portion of the palatal aspect of the gingival mucosa adjacent to the tooth.

Additional Techniques

Use of a periotome for extraction of deciduous canines
A periotome (Cislak) (see **Fig. 6**) is an instrument designed to sever the PDL to aid in tooth extraction. It is not as sharp as a scalpel but is thinner than a luxator. The flat shape makes it particularly adapted to placement in alveoli adjacent to anatomically flat roots like the vestibular, lingual, and palatal root surfaces of the deciduous canines. Careful placement and manipulation of a periotome on these surfaces can decrease extraction time and decrease the chance of root fractures.[7]

Endodontic files to dislodge partially mobile root tips
Root tip fractures occur occasionally and require complete removal. If fractures occur when little mobility is present at the root tip, additional exposure is generally recommended. However, if extraction was almost complete when the fracture occurred, a Hedstrom root canal file can aid in retrieval without additional tissue removal or trauma (**Figs. 13–15**). ISO size is selected based on radiographic evaluation of the canal. The root canal file is advanced to the root tip to enter and engage the coronal canal. Gentle pressure and a clockwise motion allow the flutes of the canal to grasp the wall of the canal, and the root tip may be pulled from the alveolus.[10]

Feline full mouth extractions
This procedure is often required for the treatment of chronic mucositis (formerly called lymphocytic-plasmacytic gingivostomatitis) and may be simplified by making 3 large

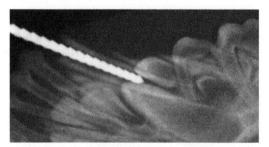

Fig. 14. Radiograph showing the Hedstrom file threaded into the pulp canal of a fracture root of a deciduous canine tooth. (*Courtesy of* Dr Brett Beckman.)

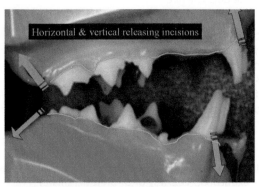

Fig. 15. A model shows the position of the vertical releasing incisions (*orange*), and the blue line shows the horizontal interdental releasing incisions.

flaps with the use of 2 vertical releasing incisions on each jaw between the third incisor and canine tooth. Horizontal incisions are made at the alveolar crest interdentally from canine to molar tooth and across the incisor teeth. Three large flaps are created (see **Fig. 12**) by making vertical releasing incisions between the canine and third incisor teeth with horizontal interdental incisions at the gingival crest, then elevating the gingiva and mucosa from the buccal bone over the cheek and incisor teeth. It may be necessary to extend the horizontal incision slightly distal to the molar tooth to increase exposure and access. Buccal bone is removed using a round or pear-shaped carbide bur on a high-speed handpiece, as previously described for sectioning multirooted teeth into single root components then elevating for complete removal. When chronic mucositus is the reason for full mouth extractions, some surgeons are more aggressive in bone removal and tend to remove any bone that seems to be less than normal. Once the bone has been removed, a diamond bur is used to perform an alveoloplasty to smooth sharp edges of bone. The site is irrigated with sterile saline, and suction may be used. Closure of the surgical flaps is made with 5/0 monofilament absorbable suture in a simple interrupted, simple continuous pattern or a combination of the 2 patterns.

SUMMARY

Dental disease can have a profound affect on the comfort and well-being of pets. Oral disease can be difficult to detect. Patients often hide their discomfort. The identification and treatment or removal of diseased teeth are the responsibility of the veterinarian. When diseased teeth cannot be saved by specialized care, extraction of teeth is necessary. Proper extraction of teeth in dogs and cats can be challenging and frustrating, but with review of the oral anatomy, proper instrumentation, and gentle tissue-handling techniques, this can be a rewarding part of clinical practice. Making this investment has a positive impact on the patient's health, the respect of clients, and the success of a practice.

REFERENCES

1. Wiggs RB, Lobprise HB. Veterinary dentistry principles and practice. Philadelphia: Lippincott; 1997.
2. Holmstrom SE, Eisner ER, Frost-Fitch P. Veterinary dental techniques for the small animal practitioner. 3rd edition. Philadelphia: Elsevier Health Sciences; 2004.

3. Harvey CE, Emily PP. Small animal dentistry. New York: Elsevier; 1993.
4. Bellows J. Small animal dental equipment, materials and techniques: a primer. Hoboken (NJ): Wiley-Blackwell; 2004.
5. Carmichael DT. Surgical extraction of the maxillary fourth premolar tooth in the dog. J Vet Dent 2002;19(4):231–3.
6. Scheels JL, Howard PE. Principles of dental extraction. Semin Vet Med Surg (Small Anim) 1993;8(3):146–54.
7. Beckman B. How to extract a maxillary canine in dogs. Vet Med 2012;107(2).
8. Knaake F, van Foreest A. Surgical extraction techniques for companion animals. Tijdschr Diergeneeskd 2005;130(20):618–23 [in Dutch].
9. Niemiec BA. Extraction techniques. Top Companion Anim Med 2008;23(2): 97–105.
10. Beckman B, Smith MM. Alternative extraction techniques in the dog and cat. J Vet Dent 2011;28(2):134–8.

Equipment for Oral Surgery in Small Animals

Alexander M. Reiter, Dipl Tzt, Dr med vet, DAVDC, DEVDC

KEYWORDS

- Oral surgery • Equipment • Instruments • Materials

KEY POINTS

- Three basic requirements will help to achieve success in oral surgery: (1) presence of a skilled oral surgeon, (2) provision of treatment that has been thoroughly planned and is carefully executed, and (3) availability of good instruments and materials.
- To avoid damage and wear, instruments must be cared for to prevent corrosion, pitting, and discoloration, and must only be used for the purposes for which they were designed.
- Oral surgery is performed in patients that are intubated with a cuffed and wire-reinforced tube to prevent collapse of the tube when bent.

INTRODUCTION

There is a wide variety of instruments and materials available in oral surgery, the use of which greatly depends on the oral disease present and the type of procedure performed. Operators likely have developed or will develop a personal preference for a particular instrument or material during their careers.

Three basic requirements will help to achieve success in oral surgery: (1) presence of a skilled oral surgeon, (2) provision of treatment that has been thoroughly planned and is carefully executed, and (3) availability of good instruments and materials. To avoid damage and wear, instruments must be cared for to prevent corrosion, pitting, and discoloration, and must only be used for the purposes for which they were designed.[1] Oral surgery is performed in patients that are intubated with a cuffed and wire-reinforced tube to prevent collapse of the tube when bent.

SURGICAL LOUPE AND HEADLAMP

A surgical loupe (3-powered magnification with 15–18 in [38–46 cm] of focal distance) is recommended for delicate surgery.[2] A headlamp is especially useful for procedures in the caudal aspect of the oral cavity, where it may be difficult to obtain good illumination with standard dental and surgical lighting.[3]

Department of Clinical Studies, School of Veterinary Medicine, University of Pennsylvania, 3900 Delancey Street, Philadelphia, PA 19104, USA
E-mail address: reiter@vet.upenn.edu

Vet Clin Small Anim 43 (2013) 587–608
http://dx.doi.org/10.1016/j.cvsm.2013.02.005
0195-5616/13/$ – see front matter © 2013 Elsevier Inc. All rights reserved.

vetsmall.theclinics.com

ORAL EXAMINATION

Wedge props and mouth gags keep the mouth open to allow access to the oral cavity and oropharynx. Props are designed to be wedged between the maxillary and mandibular premolars and molars. Gags are made of metal and are spring-loaded, and often placed between maxillary and mandibular canine teeth. Various sizes and shapes are available.[1] Custom-made devices (such as needle caps and syringe cases) are also helpful. Keeping the mouth stretched open wide for prolonged periods of times may cause strain to masticatory muscles and injury to temporomandibular joints, and could affect maxillary arterial blood flow (particularly in cats). Therefore, it is recommended to exercise caution during procedures whereby wide mouth opening is necessary, and to do so only for the shortest periods of time possible.[4,5]

A dental mirror is useful in visualizing lesions that are not approachable for inspection from the front or side of the mouth; it also can be used as a retraction tool to hold the cheeks to the side, push the tongue medially or ventrally, and lift the soft palate dorsally or gently pull it rostrally. Tissue retraction can also be accomplished with a moistened wooden tongue depressor.

The structural integrity of teeth is assessed with a dental explorer (**Fig. 1**) whose pointed tip can detect fine irregularities of the crown and exposed root surface. It is also used to determine the presence of pulp exposure in a fractured tooth.[6] The periodontal probe (**Fig. 2**) is invaluable for an accurate periodontal examination. It is gently inserted into the gingival sulcus, and measurements are obtained at several locations around the entire circumference of each tooth. The gingival sulcus should not be deeper than 0.5 mm in cats and 3 mm in dogs. Greater measurements indicate

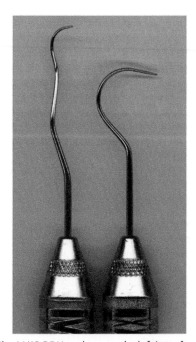

Fig. 1. Dental explorers. The 11/12 ODU explorer on the left is preferred for use in cat teeth, and the shepherd's hook on the right is for exploration of dog teeth. (*Courtesy of* Alexander M. Reiter, Dipl Tzt, Dr med vet, Dipl AVDC, Dipl EVDC, Philadelphia, PA. Copyright ©2012; with permission.)

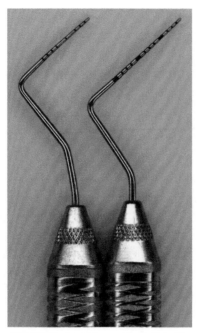

Fig. 2. Periodontal probes. The Williams probe on the left (with markings at 1, 2, 3, then 5, then 7, 8, 9, and 10 mm) is used for cat teeth, and the CP-15 UNC on the right (with millimeter markings and a wide, black marking at 5, 10, and 15 mm) is used to probe dog teeth. (*Courtesy of* Alexander M. Reiter, Dipl Tzt, Dr med vet, Dipl AVDC, Dipl EVDC, Philadelphia, PA. Copyright ©2012; with permission.)

the presence of a periodontal pocket or, in the case of gingival enlargement, a pseudopocket.[6] The probe is also used to assess furcation exposure of multirooted teeth and explore sinus tracts (often located near the mucogingival junction), which may indicate endodontic disease.

DIAGNOSTIC IMAGING

Radiographic equipment includes a portable or wall-mounted dental radiography machine and dental films or digital systems. For the processing of dental films, a chairside darkroom, developer and fixer solutions, and a view box are required. Indirect (phosphor plates) and direct (sensor pads) digital systems require less radiation to produce an image, which is transferred to a computer and can be modified with software programs. Most commonly used dental film and phosphor plate sizes are 0, 2, and 4 (**Fig. 3**). A size 4 is very useful for evaluating diseases present and monitoring procedures performed in the nasal cavity, orbit, zygomatic arch, upper jaw, lower jaw, temporomandibular joint, and tympanic bulla.[6] Sensor pads do not come in size 4. Gauze or paper may be used to hold films, plates and pads in the proper position within the mouth of a patient. Exposure time often is the only adjustment to be made and depends on the size of the patient and tissue thickness to be imaged. Processing of dental films takes place within the chairside darkroom. Films dried overnight are stored in a labeled envelope and kept as part of the patient's medical record. In the case of indirect imaging, phosphor plates are inserted into an appropriate reading machine that transfers the image to a computer. In the case of direct imaging, the image will automatically be transferred to a computer.[6]

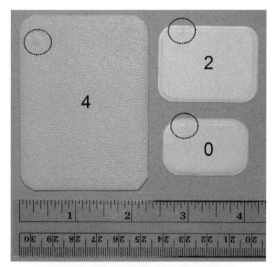

Fig. 3. Sizes 0, 2, and 4 dental film. The convex surface of the dimple (*circled*) must face the radiographic beam during exposure. (*Courtesy of* Alexander M. Reiter, Dipl Tzt, Dr med vet, Dipl AVDC, Dipl EVDC, Philadelphia, PA. Copyright ©2012; with permission.)

Computed tomography is the principal imaging tool for the diagnosis and treatment planning of oral trauma, neoplasia, and uncertain head abnormality (**Fig. 4**). It allows exploration of a large volume of soft and hard tissue in a significantly shorter examination time than with magnetic resonance imaging. Three-dimensional reconstruction images facilitate understanding of the overall picture. Computed tomography also helps guidance of a needle to obtain a cytologic diagnosis.[7]

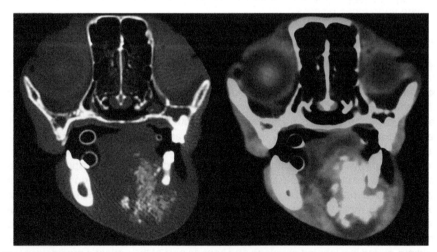

Fig. 4. Transverse sections of a computed tomography scan in a cat with left mandibular squamous cell carcinoma, showing a bone algorithm image on the left and a post-contrast soft-tissue algorithm image on the right. (*Courtesy of* Alexander M. Reiter, Dipl Tzt, Dr med vet, Dipl AVDC, Dipl EVDC, Philadelphia, PA. Copyright ©2012; with permission.)

LOCAL AND REGIONAL ANESTHESIA

Local anesthesia (such as infiltration anesthesia, use of topical anesthetic gels, and splash block) is less commonly performed in oral surgery. Topical anesthetic gels may provide temporary relief from superficial pain, but their effects are short lived. Splash block (wound irrigation) refers to dropping a local anesthetic solution directly onto an incision or wound, for example into the nasal cavity after a maxillectomy before closure of the surgical site. Regional anesthesia (nerve blocks) refers to injection of a local anesthetic solution around a major nerve, using 27-gauge, 1½-inch (4 cm) needles on 1-mL syringes (22-gauge needles when going through skin).[6]

Commonly used local anesthetics in dentistry and oral surgery include bupivacaine 0.5% (effective for 6–10 hours) and lidocaine 2% (effective for less than 2 hours). The onset time for analgesia is longer with longer-acting local anesthetics (a few minutes for lidocaine, up to 30 minutes for bupivacaine). The total maximum dose of bupivacaine in cats and dogs is 2 mg/kg, and that of lidocaine 5 mg/kg in the dog and 1 mg/kg in the cat. There is 5 mg of active agent in 1 mL of a 0.5% solution. Regional anesthesia is most commonly performed for the maxillary nerve, infraorbital nerve, major palatine nerve, inferior alveolar nerve, and middle mental nerve.[6]

ORAL BIOPSY

Fine-needle cytologic techniques are often performed with a 22-gauge needle by means of a needle biopsy ("woodpecker method") or needle aspiration. Impression smears and scrapings may only be of value if obtained from the cut surface of a tumor.[8]

Instruments for histologic sampling include tissue grasping forceps (used for less accessible pharyngeal and nasal lesions), rongeurs (very useful for obtaining samples from firm or bony tissue), disposable open-ended biopsy punches (for obtaining deeper tissue samples), and cold scalpel blades for incisional (to obtain a wedge of tissue) or excisional biopsy (for smaller masses and lymph nodes). Hemostasis is achieved by digital pressure, and biopsy sites of more deeply invading tumors are sutured. For adequate fixation, the specimen is placed in 10% buffered formalin at 1 part tissue to 10 parts fixative.[8]

DENTAL LUXATORS, ELEVATORS, AND EXTRACTION FORCEPS

Dental luxators have sharp, flat-tipped blades that can penetrate into and cut the periodontal ligament between the tooth and alveolar bone. Dental elevators have less sharp, more curved blades that should fit the circumference of the tooth and are designed to exert a rotational force, thus fatiguing the periodontal ligament.[6] Many oral surgeons prefer winged elevators that combine the benefits of conventional dental luxators and elevators, having short shafts and large-diameter handles for improved control and comfort for operators with smaller hands and thin, sharp, and winged blades that conform to the roots of various circumferences.[3] Dental luxators and elevators are grasped with the butt of the handle seated in the palm, and the index finger is extended along the blade to act as a stop in case the instrument slips. Extraction forceps should only be used when the tooth is already mobile and is applied as far apically as possible to reduce the chances of tooth fracture. Smaller-sized luxating elevators, root-tip-teasers, root-tip forceps, and extraction forceps are available for use in cats and small dogs, and for the removal of root remnants.[7]

POWERED SYSTEMS

Electrical-powered and air-powered systems are available for polishing teeth and cutting teeth and bone. Electrical-powered systems operate at lower speeds and have higher torque, and some of them are equipped with irrigating mechanisms.[2] Air-powered systems, using compressed gas from a cylinder or air produced in a compressor, are preferred, as they run at higher speeds and are supplied with various irrigating mechanisms. A battery-powered unit may also be useful.[3]

HANDPIECES, ATTACHMENTS, AND BURS

Low-speed handpieces are used for polishing teeth, cutting bone, and performing various other procedures. Contra-angle and prophy-angle attachments can be secured to low-speed handpieces. A prophy cup is attached to a prophy angle to polish teeth or resin splints that have been applied to teeth.[2]

High-speed handpieces are equipped with water-cooling systems and are primarily used for cutting holes into teeth for endodontic access, preparing dental defects for restoration, sectioning multirooted teeth into single-rooted crown-root segments in preparation for extraction, removing and shaping alveolar bone, and making precise cuts into bony structures during mandibulectomy and maxillectomy procedures.[2]

Various shapes, sizes, and lengths of burs are available for low- and/or high-speed handpieces, including round carbide, round diamond, fissure and cross-cut fissure, tapered diamond, 12-fluted, and acrylic burs. An osteotomy bur attached to an autoclavable straight or contra-angle handpiece, with built-in lactated Ringer's irrigation, is useful for bone cutting in oral surgery.[3]

EQUIPMENT FOR PROFESSIONAL DENTAL CLEANING

Professional dental cleaning is performed with power sonic or ultrasonic scalers, followed by the use of hand scalers to remove residual calculus in pits, fissures, and developmental grooves of the crowns supragingivally, and hand curettes to clean and plane exposed root surfaces subgingivally (**Fig. 5**). Hand curettes can also be used for gingival curettage that removes the inflamed and infected soft-tissue lining of the periodontal pocket.[6] Once scaling is completed, the tooth surfaces are polished with fine polishing paste and a rubber cup on a prophy angle that is attached to a low-speed handpiece. Debris and polishing paste are rinsed from the tooth surface with water from a 3-way syringe that has two buttons, one for air and one for water; a mist is created if both buttons are pushed at the same time.[2]

DRAPES

Before surgery, clipping the hair from the skin, cleansing and aseptically preparing the skin, followed by irrigating the oral and oropharyngeal mucosa with 0.12% chlorhexidine gluconate or 10% povidone-iodine and draping the surrounding areas (4-drape system), are useful in preventing contamination of cut surfaces.[1,3] Disposable synthetic or reusable cloth drapes may be used, secured in position with Backhaus towel clamps (**Fig. 6**). A single large drape with a central fenestration may also be placed over the entire surgical field. Once in place, a drape must not be repositioned.[1]

SURGICAL PACK

Instruments are cleaned, autoclaved, and stored in closed cassettes, which are then placed on a sterile field and opened ready for use.[3] The basic contents of a surgical

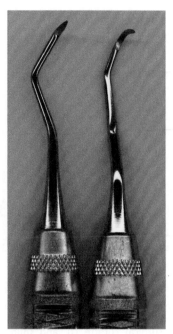

Fig. 5. Scaler with pointed tip on the left and curette with rounded toe on the right. (*Courtesy of* Alexander M. Reiter, Dipl Tzt, Dr med vet, Dipl AVDC, Dipl EVDC, Philadelphia, PA. Copyright ©2012; with permission.)

pack include towel clamps, scalpel handles, retractors, thumb forceps, tissue forceps, hemostatic forceps, periosteal elevators, surgical curettes, tissue scissors, needle holders, and suture scissors (**Fig. 7**). In addition, there may be cassettes for specific procedures, such as tooth extraction and periodontal surgery (**Fig. 8**). Infrequently used instruments are individually packed, stored, and opened as needed.[3] Many of the basic surgical instruments come in long-handled versions (17–23 cm) and are

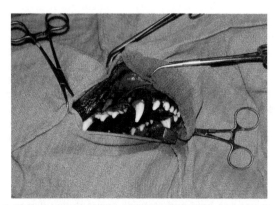

Fig. 6. Reusable cloth drapes secured in position with Backhaus towel clamps in a dog with previously debulked malignant melanoma in the area of a supernumerary right maxillary first premolar tooth. (*Courtesy of* Alexander M. Reiter, Dipl Tzt, Dr med vet, Dipl AVDC, Dipl EVDC, Philadelphia, PA. Copyright ©2012; with permission.)

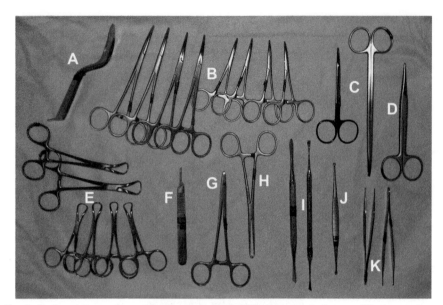

Fig. 7. Basic contents of a surgical pack. Retractor (*A*), hemostatic forceps (*B*), tissue scissors (*C*), suture scissors (*D*), towel clamps (*E*), scalpel handle (*F*), needle holder (*G*), tissue forceps (*H*), periosteal elevators (*I*), surgical curette (*J*), and thumb forceps (*K*). (*Courtesy of* Alexander M. Reiter, Dipl Tzt, Dr med vet, Dipl AVDC, Dipl EVDC, Philadelphia, PA. Copyright ©2012; with permission.)

used when working deep inside the mouth and oropharynx (soft palate, palatine tonsils, pharyngeal walls, and so forth) (**Fig. 9**).

SCALPEL HANDLE AND BLADES

Numbers 3 (with metric ruler markings) and 5 scalpel handles are typically used in oral surgery and accept blade sizes #10, #11, #15, and #15C.[1]

SCISSORS

Oral surgeons prefer Metzenbaum scissors for fine cutting and blunt dissection of soft tissues. These scissors come in several types, shapes, and lengths.[9] Smaller-sized, curved, blunt-ended versions with serrated blades are most useful in oral surgery but should never be used to cut suture material, as the blades become blunt and will loosen.[1] Iris scissors are small, sharp-pointed, straight, or curved scissors, allowing very precise small cuts to be made.[3] Mayo scissors are either curved or straight and come in a variety of sizes. These robust instruments are used for cutting firm soft tissue and cartilage. In the absence of specific suture scissors, a designated pair of Mayo scissors should be reserved for cutting sutures.[1]

THUMB FORCEPS

Thumb forceps are used to hold and stabilize tissue during dissection and suturing, and should be able to grasp tissue securely without traumatizing delicate tissue. Thumb forceps should not be used to grasp needles, as this may damage their fine tips. The tips should meet, and any intermeshing striations or teeth should align

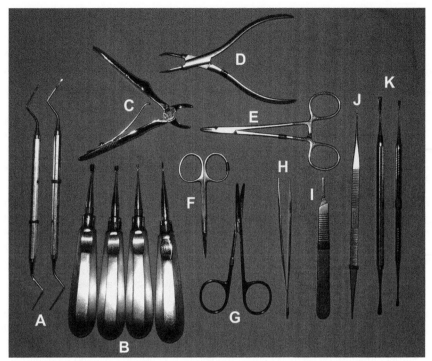

Fig. 8. Set of smaller-sized instruments for tooth extraction and periodontal surgery in cats and small dogs. Root-tip "teasers" (*A*), smaller-sized winged elevators (*B*), extraction forceps (*C*), root-tip forceps (*D*), needle holder (*E*), suture scissors (*F*), small curved Metzenbaum scissors (*G*), Adson thumb forceps (*H*), scalpel handle (*I*), spoon curette (*J*), and periosteal elevators (*K*). (*Courtesy of* Alexander M. Reiter, Dipl Tzt, Dr med vet, Dipl AVDC, Dipl EVDC, Philadelphia, PA. Copyright ©2012; with permission.)

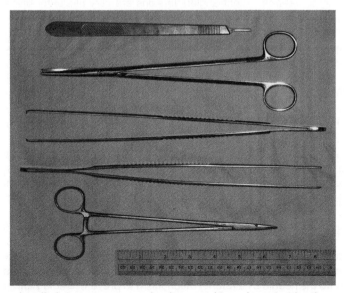

Fig. 9. Long-handled instruments used when working deep inside the mouth and oropharynx. (*Courtesy of* Alexander M. Reiter, Dipl Tzt, Dr med vet, Dipl AVDC, Dipl EVDC, Philadelphia, PA. Copyright ©2012; with permission.)

perfectly. Delicate Adson 1 × 2 forceps have a fine rat-tooth grip, which causes minimal trauma to mucosal and submucosal tissue.[9] Adson forceps are preferred over DeBakey and other thumb forceps in oral surgery.[1]

TISSUE FORCEPS

Tissue forceps are used to hold larger volumes of tissue. Allis forceps have traumatic gripping teeth, and may be used on tissue that is definitely going to be excised, or to secure suction, diathermy, and power lines to drapes.[1]

TOWEL CLAMPS

Penetrating Backhaus towel clamps end in a fine point, and are usually used to secure drapes and towels to the skin.[9] Once they have been placed they are nonsterile. In the absence of specific bone-holding or tissue forceps, they may also be used to hold on to smaller-sized bones or grasp skin flaps for manipulation during elevation and apposition before suturing.[1]

HEMOSTATIC FORCEPS

Hemostatic forceps are used to hold delicate tissue, gently separate tissue, or compress a bleeding vessel; they must not be used as needle holders.[1] Several types are available in varying sizes, shapes, and extent of serration of their jaws. Commonly used versions in oral surgery include the relatively small, regular, or fine-tipped Halstead mosquito and the larger Kelly hemostatic forceps.[9] Both have ratchets and transverse serrations, but Kelly hemostatic forceps have serrations only over the distal half of the jaw.

ANGLED FORCEPS

Mixter forceps are dissecting tools with transversely serrated, standard, or delicate tips of varying curvatures.[1] Right-angled versions are very useful for dissecting free and encompassing the inferior alveolar neurovascular bundle as it enters the mandibular canal through the mandibular foramen at the caudomedial aspect of the mandible, in preparation for ligation (**Fig. 10**). A Mixter, Rochester-Carmalt, or Schnidt forceps can also be used for placement of an esophagostomy tube by advancing the instrument from the oral cavity into the midcervical esophagus and pushing its curved tips laterally, which can be seen and felt on the skin to be incised.[3]

NONCRUSHING TISSUE FORCEPS

DeBakey tangential vascular clamps can be placed on the elongated soft palate for resection of excess tissue, or along the attachments of the palatine tonsil for tonsillectomy. Doyen intestinal forceps and other noncrushing tissue forceps are useful for clamping the body of the tongue to provide temporary hemostasis while the distal tissue portion is resected and the cutting edge repaired (**Fig. 11**).

NEEDLE HOLDERS

Needle holders are used to grasp and manipulate curved needles, choosing the correct size for the needle being used.[9] The author prefers needle holders that can be locked onto the needle by a ratchet mechanism to prevent needle slippage. Halsey (sturdier) and DeBakey (more delicate) needle holders with serrated jaws are often used in oral surgery.[1]

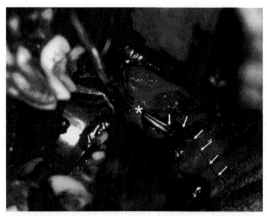

Fig. 10. Right-angled forceps encompassing the dissected free inferior alveolar neurovascular bundle (*asterisk*) on the medial aspect of the right mandible in a dog in preparation for vessel ligation with a synthetic absorbable monofilament suture material (*arrows*). (*Courtesy of* Alexander M. Reiter, Dipl Tzt, Dr med vet, Dipl AVDC, Dipl EVDC, Philadelphia, PA. Copyright ©2012; with permission.)

RETRACTORS

Appropriate tissue retraction will improve visualization of the surgical site,[9] thus decreasing surgical time and reducing the risk of complications. Hand-held versions

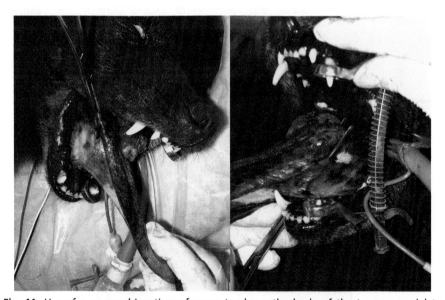

Fig. 11. Use of a noncrushing tissue forceps to clamp the body of the tongue caudal to a malignant melanoma on the dorsal aspect of the tongue in a dog. Note the insertion of one blade of the forceps through a stab incision in the sublingual mucosa (*left*) and emergence of that blade through another stab incision on the other side (*right*). (*Courtesy of* Alexander M. Reiter, Dipl Tzt, Dr med vet, Dipl AVDC, Dipl EVDC, Philadelphia, PA. Copyright ©2012; with permission.)

used in oral surgery include the Seldin (also useful for breaking remaining bony attachments after osteotomy during mandibulectomy and maxillectomy procedures), Senn (with 3 sharp prongs at one end and a right-angled fingerplate at the other), and Cawood-Minnesota (useful for retraction of the tongue, lip, and cheek) retractors.[3] Skin hooks may also be used, and stay sutures attached to a hemostatic forceps are highly effective in tissue retraction. Self-retaining versions are able to maintain themselves in a spread position. Gelpi retractors come in small and large sizes and have single-pronged, outwardly turning pointed or blunt tips, maintaining tension by using a grip-lock mechanism.[1] Other self-retaining systems come as rings with elastic stay hooks, available in different sizes, shapes, and materials (**Fig. 12**).

PERIOSTEAL ELEVATORS

Periosteal elevators come in various sizes and blade shapes. Sharp and narrow-tipped (2–6 mm) periosteal elevators (such as Mead #3 or Periosteal #EX-9 for midsized and larger dogs, Glickman #24G or Periosteal #EX-9 for small dogs and cats) are very useful in reflecting the mucoperiosteum during periodontal flap procedures, mandibulectomies, maxillectomies, and hard-palate surgery. The blade portion is used with the flat side against the bone and the convex side against the soft tissue, reducing the chance of tearing or puncturing the elevated soft tissue.[1]

RONGEURS

Rongeurs (straight or curved) are not only useful for biopsy of firm soft tissue and bone, but can also be used for condylectomy, partial zygomectomy, partial coronoidectomy, smoothing of sharp alveolar bone margins after tooth extraction or mandibulectomy and maxillectomy procedures, and resection of excess bone in the case of

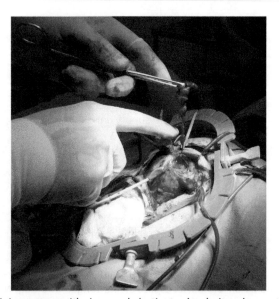

Fig. 12. Self-retaining system with rings and elastic stay hooks in a dog; note also the use of an Allis forceps during resection of the mandibular and sublingual salivary glands. (*Courtesy of* Alexander M. Reiter, Dipl Tzt, Dr med vet, Dipl AVDC, Dipl EVDC, Philadelphia, PA. Copyright ©2012; with permission.)

temporomandibular joint ankylosis. Double-action rongeurs (such as Ruskin with 3-, 5-, or 7-mm wide jaws) are more powerful and have a smoother action than single-action rongeurs (such as Lempert with 2–3-mm wide jaws).[1,9]

SURGICAL CURETTES

Surgical curettes are used for removal of debris and granulation tissue from a soft-tissue wound, a bone surface or defect, or an alveolar socket after tooth extraction. Various shapes and sizes are available, including Spratt (single-ended with round cups), Volkmann (double-ended with round or oval cups), and Miller (with spoon-shaped working tips) curettes.[1]

POCKET-MARKING FORCEPS

The blunt tip of the pocket-marking forceps is inserted into the pocket. The forceps is closed, causing the right-angled, pointed tip to create a bleeding point on the labial or buccal side of the attached gingiva at the level of the base of the pocket, thus indicating the proposed line of incision for gingivectomy.

GINGIVECTOMY KNIVES

Gingivectomy knives have mostly been replaced by other means of gingivectomy and gingivoplasty such as cold scalpel blade, electrosurgery and radiosurgery, laser, and 12-fluted burs.[10] The Orban knife is spear shaped, with cutting edges on both sides of the blade. Its double-ended or single-ended blades are used for fine delicate procedures, such as the removal of tissue in interdental areas. The Kirkland knife is kidney shaped. Its double-ended or single-ended blades are used for removal of large amounts of firm tissue, as the entire periphery is the cutting edge.[1] The blades of both of these knives must be kept sharp to be effective.

COTTON-TIPPED APPLICATORS

These applicators, which have long wooden handles with a cotton-bud tip on one end, are useful for absorbing blood from delicate tissue or for applying a topical astringent (such as aluminum chloride) or tissue protectant (such as tincture of myrrh and benzoin) to cut gingival surfaces.[10] When moistened, they can be used as a gentle dissecting tool, such as when freeing the medial retropharyngeal lymph node or the ducts of salivary glands.[1]

SWABS

Laparotomy swabs can be useful for temporary packing of the pharynx of large dogs during surgical procedures of the oral cavity and surrounding structures, as they provide additional protection against aspiration of foreign material. Gauze swabs and small sponges can be used for the same purpose in smaller dogs and cats. A cord attaches the swab(s) or sponge(s) to the endotracheal tube, ensuring that none is left in the throat once the procedure is completed and before the patient has recovered from anesthesia. Alternatively, it is wise to count the number of swabs or sponges placed, and visually inspect the throat before extubation to ensure none is remaining. Gauze swabs 3 by 3 inches (7.6 × 7.6 cm) in size are commonly used for absorption of blood and tissue fluid during oral surgical procedures.[1]

MAYO BOWL AND BULB SYRINGE

Wound-rinsing solutions in a stainless-steel Mayo bowl can be applied to exposed tissues by means of a bulb syringe. Smaller-sized bulb syringes or larger catheters attached to a disposable syringe with plunger can also be used to flush nasal passages. Keeping tissues moist is particularly important when large flaps are raised for the repair of defects in or surrounding the mouth. Wound rinsing often improves visibility during dissection, and cold lavage can occasionally provide excellent hemostasis.[1]

SUTURE MATERIAL

Even though there are many synthetic absorbable suture materials available, including polyglycolic acid and polyglactin 910, a monofilament suture material (3-0, 4-0, and 5-0, depending on the size of the animal and type of procedure performed) with a swaged-on, noncutting, taper-point round needle is preferred for wound closure in the oral cavity and oropharynx, thus avoiding chemical restraint for potential suture removal in the future, minimizing an inflammatory oral tissue reaction around sutures, and reducing trauma to already inflamed or friable tissues.[1] Many oral surgeons prefer Polyglecaprone 25 for suturing connective tissue and oral and oropharyngeal mucosa, persisting in the oral cavity for about 3 to 5 weeks.[11,12] Polydioxanone is used if prolonged suture strength is required, such as for palate surgery and ligation of larger vessels, persisting in the oral cavity for about 6 to 8 weeks. Nylon with a swaged-on, reverse cutting needle is preferred for skin sutures. Alternatives for skin closure include polybutester and polypropylene. Square or surgeon's knots should be followed by at least 3 more throws to ensure knot security.[1]

POWER SAWS

Power saws whose variably sized blades move in an arc of 5° or 6° parallel (sagittal) or at a right angle (oscillating) to the drive shaft are most commonly used in oral surgery. The cutting teeth only move a small distance on the bone, and adjacent soft tissues are usually unaffected.[1] Piezoelectric surgery (also called piezosurgery) uses microvibrations when cutting hard tissue while leaving soft tissue untouched by the process. The cutting tip vibrates within a range of 60 to 200 μm, allowing clean cutting with precise incisions. The heat produced by friction may cause bone necrosis, which is minimized by cooling the cutting tool with a sterile rinsing solution.[1]

MALLET, CHISEL, AND OSTEOTOME

A mallet, chisel (beveled on one side), or osteotome (double beveled) may be needed to separate the two mandibles in the mandibular symphysis when performing mandibulectomies.[1] In the absence of available power equipment, these instruments may also be useful during maxillectomy procedures.

ORTHOPEDIC WIRE

Excessive manipulation and kinking of orthopedic wire should be avoided, as it can lead to wire fatigue and breakage. Thus the author prefers precut surgical steel wire sutures (**Fig. 13**) over spool wire. Orthopedic wire is used for circumferential, interdental, and intraosseous wiring. A 22-gauge wire is appropriate for circumferential wiring to treat mandibular symphyseal separation or parasymphyseal fracture in dogs and cats. Depending on the size of the animal, a 22- to 26-gauge wire can be

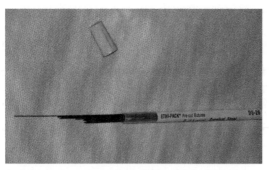

Fig. 13. Precut surgical steel wire sutures (18 in [46 cm] long) that have never been kinked, supplied in straight plastic tubes. (*Courtesy of* Alexander M. Reiter, Dipl Tzt, Dr med vet, Dipl AVDC, Dipl EVDC, Philadelphia, PA. Copyright ©2012; with permission.)

used for interdental and intraosseous wiring in dogs, whereas a 24- to 28-gauge wire may be more suitable for cats. Stout multiple loop is the most commonly used interdental wiring technique, followed by a modified Risdon. Hypodermic needles (18, 20, and 22 gauge) are used to place wire as close to the bone as possible during circumferential wiring and intragingivally in between teeth during interdental wiring.

ORTHOPEDIC PINS

A trocar-tipped Kirschner (K)-wire can be used for drilling intraosseous wire holes by hand. Holes through bone away from the mandibular canal may be drilled with a smooth-tipped K-wire, which less likely damages the neurovascular bundle that runs within this tubular structure.[3] K-wires or small Steinmann pins can also be used in external skeletal fixation for jaw-fracture repair. At least 2 of the wires/pins are percutaneously placed into each bone-fracture segment, carefully avoiding tooth roots and neurovascular bundles in the infraorbital or mandibular canal. A plastic tube is placed over the exposed cut ends of the wires/pins, and while normal occlusion is maintained with the jaws closed the tube is filled with self-curing acrylic or custom tray material.[13] To remove the device, the wires/pins are cut close to the acrylic bar and then pulled from the bone. External skeletal fixation systems that include fixation pins, clamps, and connecting bars are available.[3]

WIRE TWISTER AND CUTTER

Many oral surgeons tighten wire by means of a twist knot. The first 2 or 3 twists are formed by hand. Then the loose twist is grasped with a wire twister (or old large needle holder), and further twists are formed.[13] It is essential that the wire be applied tightly to ensure a stable fixation. As the twist knot is tightened, tension must be applied by pulling up on the wire and away from bone ("pull and twist"). The wire is cut with a wire cutter (maintaining at least 3 twists), and bent over against the bone and away from the gingival margin.

BONE PLATES AND SCREWS

Bone plating provides rigid fracture stabilization and rapid return to normal function. Healing occurs with little or no callus formation.[14] However, specialized and expensive equipment is required, and significant soft-tissue elevation is necessary for the placement of bone plates and screws. Trauma to tooth roots and neurovascular structures and mucosal erosion with plate and screw exposure could complicate bone healing and adds to postoperative morbidity. The development of monocortical screws and low-profile miniplates made of titanium greatly reduces the occurrence of complications.

A craniomaxillofacial instrument set may include locking reconstruction plates, locking and nonlocking miniplates (straight, curved, L-, T-, H-, Y-, and X-shaped), meshes, locking-head screws, self-tapping and nonself-tapping screws, bending screws for locking plates, drill bits and battery-operated unit, drill guides, countersink with handle, depth gauge, bending template, bending pliers, bending press, bending irons, plate cutter, bone tap, and screwdrivers with handles.[15]

RESIN MATERIALS

Wire slippage from teeth (in particular the teeth of cats) can be prevented by placing drops of light-activated flowable composite at the gingival third of the mesial and distal crown surfaces of the cheek teeth and labial and palatal/lingual surfaces of the canine teeth, to create overhangs that allow the wire to remain in position during wire placement and tightening.[7]

Plaque and calculus should first be removed, and the enamel surface roughened with coarse pumice and etched with 40% phosphoric acid.[6] Placing a layer of light-activated unfilled resin onto the cleaned, etched, rinsed, and dried tooth surface before composite application likely will improve the composite's bonding qualities, but may complicate its removal on completion of treatment (potential iatrogenic tooth fracture). The self-hardening powder-liquid form of polymethylmethacrylate is inexpensive but exothermic (possible thermal injury to the pulp of teeth) and produces a noxious odor during setting. Light-activated resin sheets, ropes, or gel that can be molded to the teeth are also available. Self-hardening bis-acrylate composites are most commonly used in oral surgery and come in double-barreled, automix delivery systems, allowing for easy splint fabrication without noxious odors that are harmful to the operator or exothermic reaction that is irritating to the oral tissues.[3,6]

SURGICAL MARKER PEN AND PLASTIC RULER

A sterile surgical marker pen is used for outlining skin or oral mucosa incisions in preparation for creating flaps, repairing defects, and excising suspicious lesions.[3] The plastic ruler accompanying the marker pen allows measurement of the required length of flaps and careful planning of incisions sufficiently away from the gross tumor margins.

WOODEN DOWEL

Reduction of rostrodorsal temporomandibular joint luxation in the cat is obtained by placing a wooden dowel (such as a hexagonal pencil) between the maxillary fourth premolar and mandibular first molar teeth on the affected side only (the dowel acts as a fulcrum), and closing the lower jaw against the pencil while simultaneously easing the jaw caudally.[7]

TAPE

Bandage tape can be used to fabricate a custom-made muzzle that is placed in cats and dogs for management of mandibular body fractures occurring in young animals, manually reduced temporomandibular joint luxation and open-mouth jaw locking, minimally displaced mandibular ramus fractures, pathologic mandibular fractures while awaiting definitive treatment, and provision of additional support in active patients where the healing mandible may be subjected to excessive forces.[6] A double-layered adhesive tape muzzle is applied snugly enough to maintain a dental interlock, but loosely enough (leaving a gap of about 5–8 mm in cats and 10–15 mm in dogs between the incisal edges of the maxillary and mandibular incisors) to permit the tongue to protrude and lap water and semiliquid food. Bandage tape may also be used for securing the upper and lower jaws to fluid poles, the operating table, or a metal frame spanning over the head of the patient, and for keeping fluid lines and anesthesia tubes away from the surgical field (**Fig. 14**).

Moistened 6-mm umbilical tape can be used for isolation and temporary occlusion of the carotid artery preemptively in patients undergoing major oral, maxillofacial, palatal, and nasal surgery, or when severe bleeding cannot be controlled by conventional means. A Rumel tourniquet for such a purpose has been described.[3]

DIATHERMY

Surgical diathermy is the application of a high-frequency electric current through tissue, which generates heat that coagulates and seals a bleeding vessel (arteries up to 1 mm in diameter and veins up to 2 mm in diameter). Its application in oral surgery should be limited as much as possible, as indiscriminate use of diathermy could prolong wound healing. Monopolar (handpiece is brought in contact with a forceps that has been applied to a bleeding vessel) or bipolar (tips of the handpiece are held about 1 mm apart so the current can flow from one side through the tissue to the opposite side) diathermy is available, and can be activated by hand or foot switch.[1]

ELECTROSURGERY AND RADIOSURGERY

The greatest advantage of electrosurgery and radiosurgery is good hemostasis when cutting through soft tissues. Their use is limited to treatment of gingival enlargement (and perhaps removal of small masses such as papillomas). Using a loop, needle-shaped, or diamond-shaped electrode in a fully rectified mode (cutting and coagulating), the excess free gingiva is shaved off while contouring the remaining attached

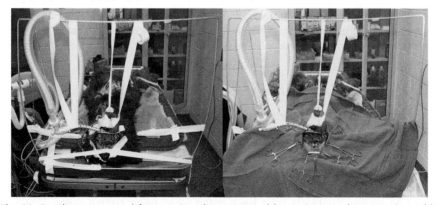

Fig. 14. Bandage tape used for securing the upper and lower jaws to the operating table and a metal frame spanning over the head of a patient prepared for palatal surgery, also keeping the lips, tongue, fluid lines, and anesthesia tubes away from the surgical field, before draping (*left*) and after draping (*right*). (*Courtesy of* Alexander M. Reiter, Dipl Tzt, Dr med vet, Dipl AVDC, Dipl EVDC, Philadelphia, PA. Copyright ©2012; with permission.)

gingiva. It is important to avoid contact of the electrode with the crown, root, or alveolar bone, as irreparable thermal tissue damage and delayed wound healing can occur.[10]

LASER

Carbon dioxide (CO_2) lasers are most commonly used for incision, excision, and ablation of oral and oropharyngeal soft tissues. Water, hemoglobin, melanin, and some proteins absorb varying wavelengths of laser light, resulting in tissue heating, necrosis, and vaporization. Smoke evacuators are therefore essential in preventing inhalation of the laser plume.[1] The CO_2 wavelength is absorbed by the water content of oral tissues. Thermal necrosis zones of 100 to 300 µm at cut tissue edges are less deep than those of diode and other lasers.[1]

The CO_2 laser may be used for gingivectomy and gingivoplasty, frenoplasty, ablation of stomatitis ulcers, marsupialization of sublingual sialoceles, tonsillectomy, reduction of elongated soft palates, and various surgeries of the nose, lips, cheeks, tongue, and pharynx.[16–18] Fibrosis formation after laser treatment of patients with feline stomatitis is enhanced when treated areas are left to heal by second intention. Follow-up oral examination typically shows granulation tissue and striations of fibrous tissue spanning the previously treated areas. Laser treatments are repeated at intervals of several weeks to months, increasing the amount of fibrous tissue and decreasing interspersed areas of continued inflammation.[7]

SUCTION

Suctioning allows removal of fluid and blood from the wound during a surgical procedure or the throat before extubation. Smaller Frasier or disposable plastic suction tips with a single end hole are most suitable in oral surgery. These tips come in varying sizes, with a wire stylet that is used for unblocking a clogged tip and a decompression opening that can be covered or uncovered to regulate suction pressure at the tip.[1,3]

DRAINS

Sublingual foreign-body penetration, severe lower lip avulsion, and excessive dissection of tissue planes during mandibulectomy procedures and resection of mandibular and medial retropharyngeal lymph nodes or mandibular and sublingual salivary glands may sometimes warrant the use of Penrose drains to allow the withdrawal of fluids and discharges from the wound.[1]

RINSING SOLUTIONS AND CULTURE MEDIUM

A concentration of 0.12% chlorhexidine gluconate is recommended for irrigating the mucosal surfaces of the oral cavity and oropharynx before surgery. Higher concentrations of this antimicrobial agent are to be avoided, as they may elicit epithelial desquamation and wound-healing complications.[1] An alternative is 10% povidone-iodine applied with a swab to intact oral mucosa surfaces (diluted by 10-fold if mucosa is not intact).[3] The use of normal saline for wound lavage is discouraged. Cytotoxic effects on canine fibroblasts have been noted when using normal saline, whereas phosphate-buffered saline and lactated Ringer solution were found to induce no significant fibroblast injury in an in vitro model.[19] Hank's balanced salt solution is a commercial tissue culture medium for temporary storage of avulsed teeth until they are replanted.

BONE REPLACEMENT MATERIALS

Bone grafting is a surgical procedure whereby bone or a bone substitute is used to take the place of a removed piece of bone or bony defect. Bone-graft substitutes include allograft-based (demineralized allograft bone; used alone or in combination with other materials), factor-based (natural and recombinant growth factors; used alone or in combination with other materials), cell-based (mesenchymal stem cells; used to generate new tissue alone or seeded onto a support matrix), ceramic-based (calcium phosphate, calcium sulfate, and bioglass; used alone or in combination with other materials) and polymer-based (degradable and nondegradable polymers; used alone or in combination with other materials) materials.

Autogenous bone can be harvested in many ways from areas local or distant to the oral surgical site, using rongeurs with narrow jaws to collect marginal and septal alveolar bone, manual trephines or trephine burs to retrieve larger blocks of cortical and cancellous bone, and sharp periodontal or surgical curettes, back-action chisels, or cortical bone collectors whose blades are scraped along an exposed bone surface (**Fig. 15**). The harvested autogenous bone is collected in a sterile dappen dish and reduced to chips as needed. Commonly used bone-graft substitutes in oral surgery include natural, real bone allografts, consisting of osteoinductive demineralized bone matrix (DBM) and osteoconductive cancellous bone chips, and synthetic, bioactive, osteoconductive ceramics, containing salts of calcium, sodium, silica, and phosphorus ceramics.

BARRIER MEMBRANES

Guided tissue regeneration is a procedure using an absorbable or nonabsorbable barrier membrane to direct the growth of periodontal ligament, alveolar bone, and gingival tissue at sites having insufficient volumes or dimensions of these tissues.

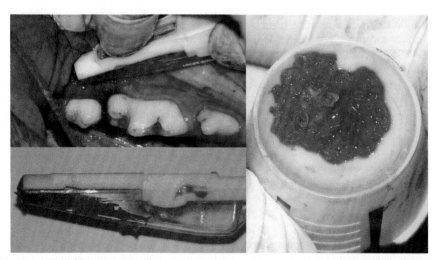

Fig. 15. (*Top left*) Harvesting of autogenous bone with a cortical bone collector at the caudobuccal aspect of the left mandible in a dog. (*Bottom left*) Side view of frontal aspect of the cortical bone collector, showing transparent chamber filled with cortical bone chips. (*Right*) Dappen dish filled with cortical bone chips. (*Courtesy of* Alexander M. Reiter, Dipl Tzt, Dr med vet, Dipl AVDC, Dipl EVDC, Philadelphia, PA. Copyright ©2012; with permission.)

The custom-fitted barrier membrane is placed between the prepared and treated bone defect and the covering mucoperiosteal flap, thus inhibiting the growth of gingival epithelium and gingival connective tissue into the defect and allowing time for the more slowly growing tissues (periodontal ligament, cementum, and alveolar bone) to occupy the defect and reestablish normal periodontal architecture.[3] A nonabsorbable expanded polytetrafluoroethylene membrane may be impractical in veterinary patients because a second procedure is required for removal of the membrane. Absorbable membranes are not approved for use in veterinary patients, thus requiring client-informed consent before their use; they can be synthetic or natural.[3] An alternative may be a flexible bone membrane that is made of a thin sheet of natural, demineralized cortical bone.

TOPICAL HEMOSTATIC AGENTS

Lavage with refrigerated lactated Ringer, normal saline, or 0.12% chlorhexidine gluconate may provide good hemostasis during maxillectomies and other surgical procedures that expose bleeding nasal mucosa.[1] Aluminum chloride is an astringent which, when applied to cut gingival surfaces after gingivectomy and gingivoplasty, produces tissue shrinkage and reduces minor hemorrhage. Bone wax is a sterile beeswax-based compound that is very useful for control of bleeding from alveolar sockets after tooth extraction, cut bony surfaces after maxillectomies and mandibulectomies, and exposed tubular structures such as the mandibular and infraorbital canals.[1]

Oxidized regenerated cellulose is a dry, absorbable sterile mesh that can be applied directly to an area of bleeding. Gelatin matrix comes in sponge (sheets that may be cut into appropriately sized pieces) or powder form, and is effective for placement in excessively bleeding alveolar sockets. Microporous polysaccharide spheres (powder is liberally applied onto a bleeding site) are derived from potato starch, which accelerates clot formation by acting as a molecular sieve to absorb water and concentrate platelets and blood proteins.[3] Microfibrillar collagen (available as powder or sheets) is an absorbable acid salt obtained from bovine collagen, acting as a scaffold for clot formation and activating platelets.

Topical thrombin in a gelatin matrix can be applied with a needle and syringe to a specific area of bleeding and may be indicated when hemostasis by any other means is ineffective or impractical. Fibrin sealants are a 2-component system that includes (a) a solution of concentrated fibrinogen and factor XII and (b) a solution of thrombin and calcium. When mixed together just before use, a fibrin clot forms; in some preparations, an antifibrinolytic agent is included to prevent lysis of the clot. Cyanoacrylate tissue adhesives are liquid monomers that change to strong polymers with exposure to moisture and may be used for closure of minor wounds and to seal small bleeding sites. Diffuse bleeding from nasal mucosa may respond to wound irrigation with a mixture (0.05–0.1 mL/kg in cats; 0.1–0.2 mL/kg in dogs) of 0.25 mL phenylephrine 1% and 50 mL lidocaine 2%.[7]

MICROSURGERY

Microvascular free tissue transfer from distant sites of the body to oral sites requires delicate tissue handling and vessel anastomosis, with or without nerve repair. Equipment needed includes a dual-headed surgical microscope, jeweler's forceps, fine-needle holders, vessel dilators, straight dissecting scissors, curved adventitial scissors, vessel approximation clamps (with or without frame), bipolar diathermy, hemoclips, and 10-0 monofilament suture material.[3,9]

FEEDING TUBES

Feeding tubes are preferably made of polyurethane or silicone.[3] Polyurethane is stronger than silicone (which is softer and more flexible), allowing for a tube of this material to have thinner walls and thus a larger internal diameter, despite the same French size. Less optimal material choices for feeding tubes include polyvinylchloride or red rubber.

The French (F) unit measures the outer lumen diameter of a tube (1 F unit is equal to 0.33 mm).[3] For nasoesophageal tubes, a size 5F to 7F is recommended for cats and dogs weighing less than 15 kg, and size 8F to 10F is suitable for dogs weighing 15 kg and more. For esophagostomy tubes, size 10F to 14F is recommended for use in cats and small dogs less than 10 kg, 15F to 17F for dogs between 10 and 15 kg, and 18F to 20F for larger dogs. The length of tube to be inserted into the distal esophagus is determined by measuring the distance from the tip of the nose (for nasoesophageal tubes) or midcervical esophagus (for esophagostomy tubes) to the eighth intercostal space, avoiding reflux esophagitis from incorrect placement of the tube in the stomach.

HOME ORAL CARE

An Elizabethan collar may be placed to prevent the patient from self-mutilating the surgical site. Plaque control is a critical component in the prevention of oral disease and the maintenance of treatment success. The owner is given instructions on the postoperative use of oral rinses and gels containing 0.12% chlorhexidine gluconate and, once healing has occurred, daily tooth brushing with a soft-bristled toothbrush and pet dentifrice.[6] Cats seem to tolerate the taste of zinc ascorbate gel better than that of chlorhexidine products.[3] In addition, oral hygiene is enhanced by the use of treats, diets, and products that meet preset criteria for effectiveness in mechanically and/or chemically controlling plaque or calculus deposition. A list of approved products is available at the web site of the Veterinary Oral Health Council (http://vohc.org).[6]

SANITATION, DISINFECTION, AND STERILIZATION

Sanitization refers to cleansing an object or area free from any dirt or dust. Disinfection is accomplished by application of a disinfectant to an inanimate object or an antiseptic to a living tissue. Sterilization refers to the removal of all living microorganisms and bacterial endospores from an object or instrument and is achieved by steam or chemical vapor under pressure, dry heat, and low-temperature sterilization processes (ethylene oxide gas, plasma sterilization).[3]

Before sterilizing, instruments are soaked in hot water then scrubbed with detergent and rinsed, or they are laid in an ultrasonic cleaning bath containing special solutions to enhance its cleaning activity. Selected instruments may be arranged into cassettes, which are then covered with steam-permeable wrappers and sealed with tape.[3] Packs should be evenly distributed within the sterilization chamber to allow circulation of heat and moisture. The use of steam in gravity displacement type sterilizers (15–30 minutes at 121.5°C) and high-speed prevacuum sterilizers (4–5 minutes at 132°C) tends to dull and rust carbon steel instrument cutting edges; thus, the use of a rust inhibitor is advised to prevent corrosion. Dry-heat sterilizers (60 minutes at 160°C) can be used for delicate instruments that might be damaged or corroded by moist heat. Heat-sensitive objects such as powders, plastics, rubber, and acrylic resin materials with low melting points may be treated with ethylene oxide gas or other low-temperature sterilization processes.[3]

REFERENCES

1. Lipscomb V, Reiter AM. Surgical materials and instrumentation. In: Brockman DJ, Holt DE, editors. BSAVA manual of canine and feline head, neck and thoracic surgery. Gloucester (United Kingdom): BSAVA; 2005. p. 16–24.
2. Holmstrom SE. Dental instruments and equipment. In: Holmstrom SE, editor. Veterinary dentistry for the technician & office staff. Philadelphia: Saunders; 2000. p. 65–95.
3. Terpak CH, Verstraete FJ. Instrumentation, patient positioning and aseptic technique. In: Verstraete FJ, Lommer MJ, editors. Oral and maxillofacial surgery in dogs and cats. Philadelphia: Saunders; 2012. p. 55–68.
4. Stevens-Sparks CK, Strain GM. Post-anesthesia deafness in dogs and cats following dental and ear cleaning procedures. Vet Anaesth Analg 2010;37: 347–51.
5. Stiles J, Weil AB, Packer RA, et al. Post-anesthetic cortical blindness in cats: twenty cases. Vet J 2012;193:367–73.
6. Reiter AM, Lewis JR, Harvey CE. Dentistry for the surgeon. In: Tobias KM, Johnston SA, editors. Veterinary surgery: small animal. St Louis (MO): Saunders Elsevier; 2012. p. 1037–53.
7. Reiter AM. Dental and oral diseases. In: Little SE, editor. The cat: clinical medicine and management. St Louis (MO): Saunders Elsevier; 2012. p. 329–70.
8. Reiter AM, Smith MM. The oral cavity and oropharynx. In: Brockman DJ, Holt DE, editors. BSAVA manual of canine and feline head, neck and thoracic surgery. Gloucester (United Kingdom): BSAVA; 2005. p. 25–43.
9. Boothe HW. Instrumentation. In: Tobias KM, Johnston SA, editors. Veterinary surgery: small animal. St Louis (MO): Saunders Elsevier; 2012. p. 152–63.
10. Lewis JR, Reiter AM. Management of generalized gingival enlargement in a dog—case report and review of the literature. J Vet Dent 2005;22:160–9.
11. LaBagnara J. A review of absorbable suture materials in head and neck surgery and introduction of monocryl: a new absorbable suture. Ear Nose Throat J 1995; 74:409–15.
12. Trimbos JB, Niggebrugge A, Trimbos R, et al. Knotting abilities of a new absorbable monofilament suture: poligecaprone 25 (Monocryl). Eur J Surg 1995;161: 319–22.
13. Roe SC. External fixators, pins, nails, and wires. In: Johnson AL, Houlton JE, Vannini R, editors. AO principles of fracture management in the dog and cat. Stuttgart (Germany): Thieme; 2005. p. 53–70.
14. Griffon DJ. Fracture healing. In: Johnson AL, Houlton JE, Vannini R, editors. AO principles of fracture management in the dog and cat. Stuttgart (Germany): Thieme; 2005. p. 73–98.
15. Koch D. Screws and plates. In: Johnson AL, Houlton JE, Vannini R, editors. AO principles of fracture management in the dog and cat. Stuttgart (Germany): Thieme; 2005. p. 27–50.
16. Bellows J. Laser use in veterinary dentistry. Vet Clin North Am Small Anim Pract 2002;32:673–92.
17. Holt TL, Mann FA. Soft tissue application of lasers. Vet Clin North Am Small Anim Pract 2002;32:569–99.
18. Lewis JR, Tsugawa AJ, Reiter AM. Use of CO_2 laser as an adjunctive treatment for caudal stomatitis in a cat. J Vet Dent 2007;24:240–9.
19. Buffa EA, Lubbe AM, Verstraete FJ, et al. The effects of wound lavage solutions on canine fibroblasts: an in vitro study. Vet Surg 1997;26:460–6.

Oral and Maxillofacial Surgery in Dogs and Cats

Amalia M. Zacher, DVM[a,b],*,
Sandra Manfra Marretta, DVM, DACVS, DAVDC[c]

KEYWORDS

- Oral and maxillofacial surgery • Dogs • Cats

KEY POINTS

- Establish a definitive diagnosis before treatment planning.
- Assess the patient for multiple and concurrent problems.
- Apply fundamental surgical principles.
- Provide appropriate follow-up to detect complications early.

The field of oral and maxillofacial surgery in dogs and cats has expanded significantly in the past 10 to 20 years,[1,2] prompting the publication of a textbook[3] devoted solely to the topic. Advancements in diagnostic and treatment modalities have allowed veterinarians to offer clients a range of alternatives for their pets. Categories of oral and maxillofacial surgery reviewed in this article include jaw fracture management, management of palatal/oronasal defects, recognition and treatment of oral masses, and management of several miscellaneous pathologic conditions. Miscellaneous oral lesions discussed in this article include odontogenic cysts, osteonecrosis and osteomyelitis, and lesions of the tongue and lips.

JAW FRACTURE MANAGEMENT

Head trauma is a common cause of jaw fractures in small animal patients. Car accidents are the most common cause of traumatic jaw fractures, but other causes include fighting with other animals, falls, blunt force trauma, and gunshot wounds.[4,5] Predisposing conditions that may lead to atraumatic/pathologic jaw fractures include

Disclosures: None.
Conflicts of Interest: None.
[a] Dentistry and Oral Surgery, Department of Veterinary Clinical Medicine, University of Illinois, Urbana, IL, USA; [b] VCA San Francisco Veterinary Specialists, 600 Alabama Street, San Francisco, CA 94110, USA; [c] Department of Veterinary Clinical Medicine, University of Illinois Veterinary Teaching Hospital, University of Illinois, 1008 West Hazelwood Drive, Urbana, IL 61801, USA
* Corresponding author. VCA San Francisco Veterinary Specialists, 600 Alabama Street, San Francisco, CA 94110.
E-mail addresses: amalia.zacher@gmail.com; amalia.zacher@vcahospitals.com

Vet Clin Small Anim 43 (2013) 609–649
http://dx.doi.org/10.1016/j.cvsm.2013.02.010
0195-5616/13/$ – see front matter © 2013 Elsevier Inc. All rights reserved.

severe periodontal disease, neoplasia, and metabolic abnormalities.[4,6] Before performing advanced diagnostics and definitive treatment of jaw fractures, the clinician must assess and stabilize the patient.[4,6]

After stabilizing the patient, an extraoral examination should be performed to assess facial symmetry, occlusion, ability to open and close the mouth, hemorrhagic oral/nasal discharge, and signs of instability or discomfort.[7] After the extraoral examination, the patient may be sedated or anesthetized for a thorough intraoral examination including assessment of instability of the maxillae and mandibles, fractured teeth, open wounds, and other injuries involving the palate, zygomatic arch, and frontal sinus.[4,8] Patients who have experienced head trauma may have multiple maxillofacial injuries (**Fig. 1**).[5] Dental radiographs are useful for identifying dentoalveolar injuries and disease in patients with maxillofacial fractures.[7] Computed tomography is particularly useful for assessing maxillary fractures and caudal mandibular fractures (**Fig. 2**).[7] Feeding tube placement may be indicated to maintain body condition in patients with severe maxillofacial injuries or repairs that restrict function during healing.[4,7]

The main goals of maxillofacial fracture repair, regardless of technique used, are as follows:

- Provide appropriate pain management
- Restore normal/preoperative occlusion[4,6,9]
- Restore normal function as soon as possible[6–8]
- Avoid/minimize vascular and nerve impairment during fracture repair[4,6,9–11]
- Avoid/minimize dental trauma during fracture repair[4,6,9–11]
- Extract diseased teeth in fracture sites[6,7,9,10,12]
- Provide appropriate antibiotic therapy[4,11]
- Maintain adequate nutrition during healing[4,7,13]

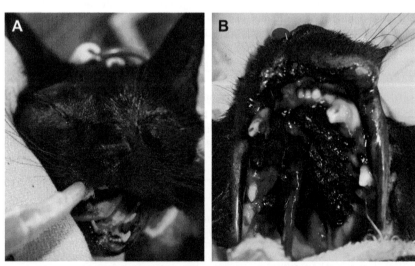

Fig. 1. A 4-year-old cat was presented with multiple maxillofacial fractures after vehicular trauma. (*A*) The right eye had been partially proptosed and was treated with a temporary tarsorrhaphy. Note the nasal hemorrhage, the severe right periorbital swelling, and the incongruity of the rostral mandibles. An esophagostomy feeding tube can be seen in the background. (*B*) A large palatal defect was present beneath a dried layer of mucus and blood. (*Courtesy of* University of Illinois Dentistry Service, Urbana, IL.)

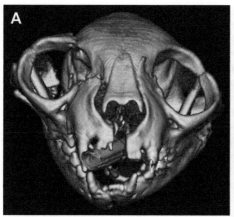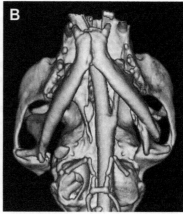

Fig. 2. Three-dimensional reconstructions of the computed tomography scan of the cat from **Fig. 1** show multiple maxillofacial fractures. In (*A*) and (*B*), note the separation of the right zygoma and temporomandibular joint from the skull, the midline palatal fracture, and the mandibular symphyseal separation/fracture. (*A*) Note also the dorsal right maxillary fracture. (*B*) On this view, note the caudal left mandibular fracture and the collapsed right bulla. (*Courtesy of* University of Illinois Dentistry Service, Urbana, IL.)

- Maintain adequate respiration/thermoregulation during healing[6,10]
- Provide long-term follow-up to monitor the success of therapy and treat dental complications[4,11]

Three broad categories of jaw fracture management include noninvasive to minimally invasive management, open/surgical fracture management, and salvage procedures. Developing an appropriate treatment plan involves selecting the least invasive technique that will achieve a successful outcome.[9] No matter which treatment modality is selected, it is imperative to provide appropriate perioperative and postoperative care for patients with maxillofacial trauma. Regular oral and radiographic evaluations are indicated in the months after jaw fracture repair to ensure early detection and management of complications.[4,6,14,15]

Various complications associated with jaw fractures include:

- Dental trauma
- Malocclusion
- Oronasal fistulas/palatal defects
- Osteomyelitis and bone sequestration
- Delayed union
- Nonunion
- Facial deformities
- Abormalities in dental eruption and development

Noninvasive to Minimally Invasive Management of Jaw Fractures

Noninvasive to minimally invasive techniques for management of jaw fractures include muzzles,[4,9,10,16] symphyseal wires,[4,5,9,17] interdental/intraoral wires and splints,[4,9,10,18] intercanine bonding,[4,9,10] labial reverse suture through buttons,[17] and bignathic encircling and retaining device (BEARD)/cerclage suture.[19] Muzzles, intercanine bonding, labial reverse suture through buttons, and BEARD/cerclage suture are 4 types of maxillomandibular fixation (MMF); muzzles are the most easily applied and removed. Several factors, including history, signalment, and fracture type/location, help to determine the appropriate technique for each case. The various indications, contraindications, and potential complications of noninvasive and minimally invasive fracture stabilization techniques are described in **Table 1**. Intraoral or facial soft tissue injuries should be addressed during the initial procedure.[20]

Tape or cloth muzzles are often the only means of fracture repair required in young patients[9,10,16] due to their potential for rapid healing. Using muzzles to achieve stabilization in young patients avoids further disruption of tooth and skeletal development (**Fig. 3**).[4]

Acute mandibular symphyseal separations are common in dogs and cats.[4,5] Open symphyseal separations require debridement, flushing, and soft tissue closure before reduction and stabilization with a circumferential wire of appropriate size (**Fig. 4**).[5,9,17]

Interdental wires and splints are most suitable in animals with healthy teeth and fractures rostral to the first molar teeth without large fracture gaps (**Fig. 5**).[4,9,10,16,18] Hemisection[21] or root resection with appropriate endodontic therapy can be used for multirooted teeth when a diseased tooth root is located in the fracture site. Circumferential intraoral wires around the body of the mandible can be incorporated into composite or acrylic in edentulous regions for splint application.

MMF[9,10,16] stabilizes fractures by temporarily connecting the maxillae and mandibles and maintaining occlusion. Less restrictive techniques are preferable because they allow earlier return to function; however, MMF techniques are indicated when alternative techniques do not achieve adequate stabilization and occlusion. Tape muzzles, intercanine bonding, labial reverse suture through buttons, and BEARDs/cerclage sutures are 4 types of MMF that have been used in cats and dogs (**Fig. 6**).[9,10,17,19] Arch-bar wiring has also been used for this purpose, but is more difficult to apply and to remove. MMF can limit a patient's ability to eat and respire or pant. Maintaining adequate nutrition may be difficult in patients treated with MMF. This complication may be circumvented by a preplaced feeding tube. Vomiting or regurgitation during MMF increases the risk of aspiration pneumonia.[9,10] Although intercanine bonding can hamper the natural swallowing reflex, it maintains a slightly open but rigid MMF position and may present a lower risk of aspiration pneumonia by allowing expulsion of vomitus. An Elizabethan collar may need to be applied concurrently with MMF until the animal becomes accustomed to the restrictive nature of the device.

Open/Surgical Management of Jaw Fractures

Open or surgical techniques for management of jaw fractures include intraosseous wires,[4,8,16,22] external fixators,[8,16,23] and mini-plates (**Table 2**).[8,11] Open/surgical management of jaw fractures can be technically challenging and require thorough understanding of anatomy,[7,24] biomechanics,[8,22] and repair techniques. Various surgical approaches may be indicated when other techniques have not been successful, or in patients with edentulous regions, comminuted fractures, or fracture gaps.

Intraosseous wires are indicated for simple, relatively stable fractures.[4,8,16,22] The bone fragments must reduce perfectly to allow the wires to share stresses with the bone rather than bear them. Careful planning of wire placement is important. The initial wire should lie perpendicular to the fracture line, near the alveolar margin, along the lines of tension to neutralize bending forces. A second wire may be placed several millimeters apically, usually parallel to the bone cortex, to reduce shear and rotational forces. Additional wires may be needed based on the fracture type and location. Before wire placement, holes should be made at least 5 to 10 mm from the fracture

Table 1
Noninvasive to minimally invasive jaw fracture stabilization techniques

Stabilization Technique	Indications	Contraindications	Potential Complications	Follow-up
Muzzle (cloth or tape)	Temporary stabilization until definitive repair Patients <6 mo of age Minimally displaced fractures Adjunct stabilization for other techniques TMJ luxation	Brachycephalic breeds ↓ air flow Emesis/regurgitation	Dermatitis beneath the muzzle Difficulty breathing ↓ ability to pant (hyperthermia) ↓ range of motion Risk of aspiration	Reevaluate every 1–2 wk Radiograph at 4–6 wk If not healed, radiograph at 8–12 wk Remove muzzle when stable
Symphyseal wire	Acute symphyseal separation	None	Dermatitis at wire exit site Minimal bone resorption under the wire Mucosal erosion over the wire	Reevaluate at 4 wk Radiograph at 6–8 wk Remove wire when stable
Interdental/intraoral wires and splints	Fractures rostral to first molars	Fractures caudal to first molars Comminuted fractures and fractures with gaps	Inflammation adjacent to splint Premature loosening or fracture of splint Risk of tooth fracture during removal	Reevaluate at 3 wk and 6 wk Radiograph at 6 wk and 12 wk Remove splint when healed
Intercanine bonding	Unstable TMJ luxation Caudal mandibular fractures	Brachycephalic breeds Canine teeth absent	Risk of canine tooth fracture during removal Difficulty eating	TMJ luxation stabilization: radiograph after 4 wk Caudal mandibular fracture repair: radiograph after 6–8 wk Remove acrylic when stable
Labial reverse suture through buttons	Caudoversion of canine teeth Unstable TMJ luxation Caudal mandibular fractures	Brachycephalic breeds ↓ air flow Emesis/regurgitation	Swelling or discharge from needle holes in skin Difficulty eating Difficulty breathing ↓ ability to pant (hyperthermia) Risk of aspiration	Monitor for 24–48 h after placement Radiograph at 1–3 wk postoperatively Remove suture when stable
Bignathic encircling and retaining device (BEARD)/cerclage suture	Unstable TMJ luxation Caudal mandibular fractures	Brachycephalic breeds ↓ air flow Emesis/regurgitation Concurrent nasal bone fractures	Swelling or discharge from needle holes in skin BEARD loosening Difficulty eating Difficulty breathing ↓ ability to pant (hyperthermia) ↓ range of motion Risk of aspiration	Monitor for 24–48 h after placement Radiograph at 2–4 wk postoperatively Remove suture when stable

Abbreviation: TMJ, temporomandibular joint.

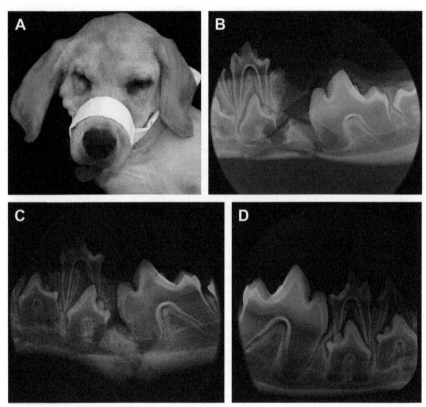

Fig. 3. (*A*) A 4-month-old Labrador retriever puppy was presented for blood-tinged saliva and oral pain after playing with a larger dog. (*B*) On the preoperative radiograph, an irregular butterfly fracture is evident between the permanent tooth buds of the left mandibular fourth premolar and the first molar. There was limited bone available for internal fixation because of the developing permanent teeth. (*C*) This radiograph of the left mandibular fracture was acquired after 3.5 weeks of continuous use of a tape muzzle. A bony callus is present on the ventral aspect of the fracture site and the fracture was stable on palpation. The development and eruption of the left mandibular fourth premolar and first molar teeth seem delayed in comparison with the unaffected right side (*D*). Continued monitoring and the potential need for tooth extraction were discussed with the client. (*Courtesy of* University of Illinois Dentistry Service, Urbana, IL.)

site. Hand drilling increases tactile perception, which can help prevent trauma to tooth roots. Wire ends are placed through the predrilled holes and gently pulled taut. The ends are twisted together under tension to achieve even tightening and stable fracture fixation.

External fixators are indicated for comminuted fractures and fractures with gaps, or in patients with severe soft tissue injuries, to avoid further compromise of neurovascular supply.[8,16,23] Positive-profile, end-threaded pins are recommended to improve pin retention and fracture stability. The pins are placed percutaneously through stab incisions in the skin. Predrilling of pilot holes may be required if self-threading pins are not used. A minimum of 2 pins should be placed on each side of the fracture line. While the fracture is held in reduction, a bar is placed over the pins to achieve stabilization (**Fig. 7**).

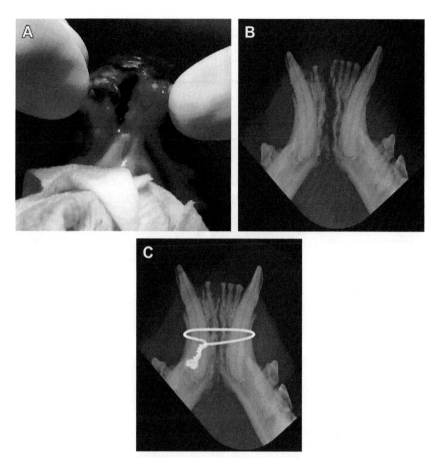

Fig. 4. Mandibular symphyseal separation in a cat after vehicular trauma. (*A*) The wound after debridement, before closure. (*B*) The preoperative radiograph demonstrates the symphyseal separation. (*C*) The postoperative radiograph demonstrates reduction of the separation and stabilization using a symphyseal cerclage wire. (*Courtesy of* University of Illinois Dentistry Service, Urbana, IL.)

Mini-plates have been shown to be efficacious in the repair of maxillofacial fractures in dogs and cats, and are especially useful for repairing caudal mandibular fractures.[8,11,25] There are various types of nonlocking and locking mini-plates. Nonlocking mini-plates are load sharing and, like intraosseous wires, are applied using tension-band principles. Locking mini-plates are load bearing and can be applied in severely comminuted fractures or fractures with gaps, but may be too large for use in very small patients. Mini-plates can be contoured to the morphology of the bone using specialized tools. The small screw size and fine thread pitch enable secure placement of mini-plates, even in areas of thin bone. The screws used with nonlocking mini-plates can be angled to avoid tooth roots. Locking plates do not allow the screws to be angled to avoid tooth roots, thus limiting their use in tooth-bearing regions of bone. Hands-on laboratory courses are available and are highly recommended before application of mini-plates.[26–28]

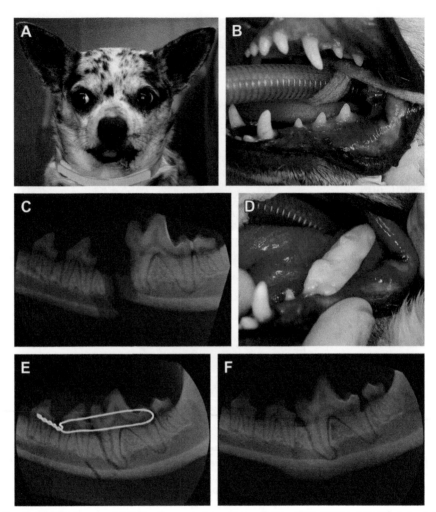

Fig. 5. (*A*) This 2-year-old Chihuahua was injured in a fight with another dog. (*B*) A caudal left mandibular fracture is evident on oral examination. (*C*) The preoperative radiograph shows an irregular fracture at the mesial aspect of the left mandibular first molar tooth. (*D*) The postoperative photograph shows the interdental acrylic splint in place from the third premolar to the second molar. (*E*) The immediate postoperative radiograph shows good fracture reduction and stabilization using an interdental wire and splint. (*F*) The 3-month postoperative radiograph shows a healed fracture with a ventral bony callus. (*Courtesy of* University of Illinois Dentistry Service, Urbana, IL.)

Salvage Procedures in the Management of Jaw Fractures

Salvage procedures can be used in the management of mandibular fractures when extensive trauma or infection/necrosis precludes reduction or adequate fixation. These techniques should be limited to cases in which primary fracture repair is likely to fail or cases in which unsuccessful primary fracture repair has resulted in the inability to eat and drink.[14,15] Salvage procedures include various partial maxillectomy or mandibulectomy techniques. In addition, a unique salvage procedure has been

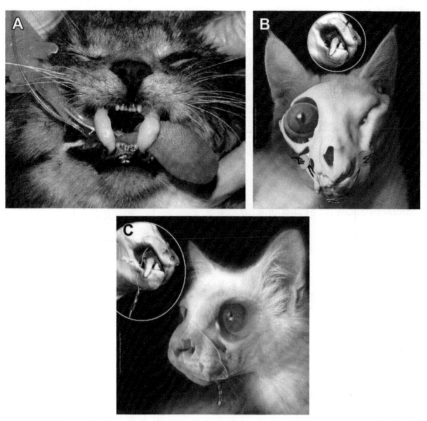

Fig. 6. (*A*) Intercanine bonding was used to treat an unstable temporomandibular joint luxation in a cat. (*B*) Labial reverse suture through buttons technique and (*C*) bignathic encircling and retaining devices (BEARDs)/cerclage sutures. (*Courtesy of* University of Illinois Dentistry Service, Urbana, IL.)

described for dogs with bilateral pathologic mandibular fractures secondary to end-stage periodontal disease in the region of the first molar teeth.[15] This technique involves opening the fracture site, removing all periodontally diseased teeth, debridement and osteoplasty of the fracture ends, and bilateral cheiloplasties to advance the commissures of the lips to the level of the canine teeth (**Fig. 8**). Additional tension-relieving sutures, incorporating buttons or rubber stents, may be used at the rostral aspect of the cheiloplasty to prevent dehiscence.

MANAGEMENT OF PALATAL/ORONASAL DEFECTS

Palatal/oronasal defects can be congenital or acquired. Clinical signs of congenital or acquired palatal defects include nasal (± ocular) discharge, coughing/gagging/sneezing while eating, and occasionally aspiration pneumonia.[29–31] Selection of the most appropriate repair technique is based on the cause of the lesion, size, location, and previous repair attempts (**Tables 3** and **4**). Developing an appropriate treatment plan involves selecting the least invasive technique that will achieve a successful outcome. Properly planned and executed surgical repairs of palatal/oronasal defects in veterinary patients generally have a good to excellent prognosis.

Table 2
Open/surgical jaw fracture stabilization techniques

Stabilization Technique	Indications	Contraindications	Potential Complications	Follow-up
Intraosseous wires	Edentulous regions Simple, relatively stable fractures Well-interdigitating fracture fragments	Comminuted fractures and fractures with gaps Severe periodontal disease, very small breeds	Implant/reduction failure Mucosal erosion over the wires Damage to tooth roots and neurovascular structures	Reevaluate at 3 wk and 6 wk Radiograph at 6 wk and 12 wk Remove wires when healed (may leave wires in place if no complications arise)
External fixators	Comminuted fractures and fractures with gaps Edentulous regions Stabilization of nonunions with concurrent bone graft	Mandibular fractures caudal to first molars Patients <6 mo of age Insufficient bone to hold fixation pins Severe periodontal disease, very small breeds	Implant failure Mucosal erosion over the pins Damage to tooth roots and neurovascular structures	Reevaluate twice weekly for first 2 wk, then weekly until fixator removal Radiograph at 6 wk and 12 wk Remove pins when healed
Mini-plates	Comminuted fractures and fractures with gaps Rigid support for maxillofacial structures Edentulous region Bone thickness ≥1–2 mm	Rostral mandibular fractures Locking plates along the alveolar margin (unless edentulous) Inadequate soft tissue coverage	Implant failure Soft tissue erosion over the plates Damage to tooth roots and neurovascular structures	Reevaluate soft tissue healing at 2 wk and 4 wk Radiograph at 6 wk and 12 wk (may leave mini-plates in place if no complications arise)

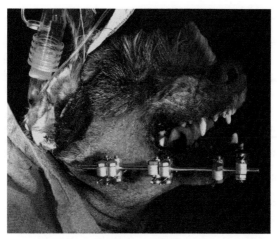

Fig. 7. An external fixator was used for repair of comminuted mandibular fractures in this patient. Note the pharyngostomy intubation caudally. (*Courtesy of* University of Illinois Dentistry Service, Urbana, IL.)

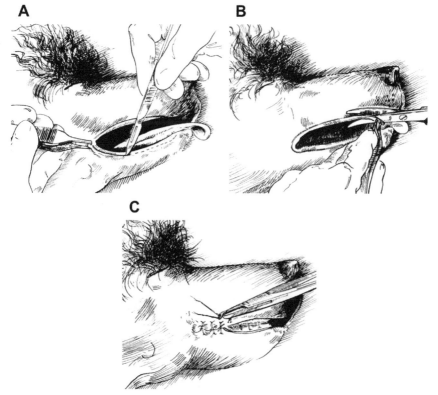

Fig. 8. Cheiloplasty for advancing the commissure of the lip. (*A*) An incision is made along the entire lip margin, from the commissure of the lip to the level of the extracted canine teeth. (*B*) The lip margin is excised. (*C*) The commissure is advanced rostrally and sutured in 2 layers. The oral mucosa is sutured in a simple interrupted pattern with the knots in the oral cavity using an absorbable suture material, and the skin is closed routinely. (*Courtesy of* University of Illinois Dentistry Service, Urbana, IL.)

Table 3
Treatment of congenital defects of the palate

Palatal Defect	Repair Technique	Contraindications	Potential Complications
Wide hard palate defects	Overlapping flap (± full-thickness release incision)	Extremely wide defects	Dehiscence Chronic rhinitis Persistent clinical signs
Narrow hard palate defects	Medially repositioned double flap	Wide defects	Damage to local neurovascular structures
Midline soft palate defects	Double-layer appositional flap (± partial thickness relief incisions)	Bilateral soft palate hypoplasia	
Unilateral soft palate defects			
Midline soft palate defects	Bilateral overlapping single-pedicle flaps	Bilateral soft palate hypoplasia When appositional technique adequate	
Bilateral soft palate hypoplasia	Bilateral tonsillectomy and pharyngeal flaps Bilateral buccal mucosal flaps	Clinical signs alleviated with dietary management and intermittent medical therapy	

Recommendations for postoperative care after surgical repair of palatal/oronasal defects are as follows:[29,32]

- Appropriate pain management
- Broad-spectrum antibiotic therapy for 10 to 14 days
- Intravenous fluid therapy for 24 hours or until the patient resumes eating/drinking
- Blenderized diet for 2 weeks; soft-food diet for 4 additional weeks
- Consider placing esophagostomy or gastrostomy feeding tubes in selected cases
- No chew toys, restrict activities (such as grooming and rough play) until healed; consider basket muzzle or Elizabethan collar for noncompliant patients
- Reevaluation of surgical sites 2 and 6 weeks postoperatively; sedation or anesthesia may be required

Management of Congenital Defects of the Palate

Congenital defects of the palate range from complete defects through the hard and soft palates to defects involving only the soft palate.[29,31] If a congenital hard palate defect is present, then the defect extends from the incisive papilla to the caudal edge of the hard palate, and along the entire length of the soft palate. Even if areas of the hard palate appear intact, a defect will be detectable on probing. Soft palate defects often appear V-shaped as a result of muscle traction from both sides. Congenital defects of the soft palate can occur independently from defects of the hard palate and can be difficult to diagnose without sedation. They may appear as midline or unilateral clefts, or as bilateral/hypoplastic defects.

When managing congenital palatal defects, ideally the initial repair should be performed when the animal is 3 to 4 months of age.[29,31] Until the repair procedure can be performed, adequate nutrition may be provided by intermittent bottle or orogastric tube feeding, or in rare cases esophagostomy/gastrostomy tube feeding. Animals with

Table 4
Treatment of acquired palatal/oronasal defects

Palatal/Oronasal Defect	Repair Technique	Contraindications	Potential Complications
Acute midline palate defects	Primary appositional closure with or without releasing incisions	Wide chronic defects	Dehiscence Chronic rhinitis Persistent clinical signs Damage to local neurovascular tissues
Marginal defects in edentulous regions	Single-layer vestibular mucosal flap	Recurrent defects	
	Double-layer vestibular mucosal/ hard palatal flap	Previously untreated defects that may respond to single-layer closure	
	Double-layer vestibular mucosal/ perifistular flap		
Small hard palate defects lateral to midline	Transposition flap	Large caudal defects	
Wide midline caudal palate defects	Advancement flap	Large rostral defects	
Midline defects at the junction of the hard and soft palates			
Central palate defects at the level of the fourth premolar teeth	Split palatal U-flap	Lateral and caudal defects	
Caudal palate defects with deficient local tissues	Island axial pattern flap	Marginal defects Local tissues available for repair	
Large midline palate defects	Bilateral vestibular mucosal overlapping flaps (staged procedure if teeth present)	Previously untreated defects that may respond to simpler techniques	
Large rostral palate defects	Tongue flap	When alternatives available	
Large palate defects when multiple procedures with local tissues unsuccessful	Myoperitoneal microvascular free flaps	When alternatives available	
	Obturators	When alternatives available	

congenital palatal defects should be evaluated for other congenital anomalies to plan appropriate treatment of the whole patient, and to discuss prognosis and treatment options with clients. Animals with large palate defects may require multiple corrective surgeries.

The overlapping flap technique may be used in patients presenting with relatively wide, congenital, hard palatal defects.[29,31] This technique involves making an initial incision 2 to 3 mm palatal to the maxillary teeth on 1 side. Perpendicular releasing incisions are made at the rostral and caudal ends of the incision, extending to the cleft. A separate incision is made in the mucoperiosteum along the edge of the cleft on the opposite side. The first mucoperiosteal flap is elevated carefully to avoid damaging the major palatine artery. The flap is then folded with the attached artery over the defect and inserted beneath the mucoperiosteum on the opposite side. The flap is sutured in place using preplaced, simple interrupted, vest-over-pants sutures. If tension is encountered, a full-thickness releasing incision can be made as needed through the palatal mucoperiosteum on the intact side, 2 to 3 mm palatal to the teeth (**Fig. 9**). The overlapping flap technique is generally preferred for treatment of wide hard palatal defects over the medially repositioned double flap. It is associated with less tension on the suture line and increased strength due to the overlapping construct and support of the underlying bone.

Narrower congenital hard palatal defects may be repaired using the medially repositioned double flap (von Langenbeck technique).[29,31,33] For this technique, the epithelial margins of the cleft are removed using a scalpel blade or diamond bur. Bilateral full-thickness releasing incisions are made along the maxillary arch, 2 mm palatal to the teeth. The mucoperiosteum is undermined bilaterally on each side of the defect, carefully avoiding the major palatine arteries as they exit the hard palate through the major palatine foramina, located halfway between the midline and the maxillary fourth

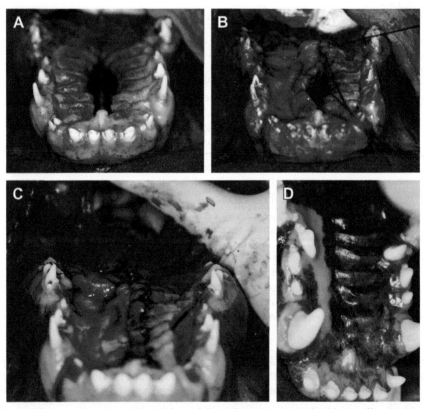

Fig. 9. A large congenital midline defect of the palate in a 4-month-old Mastiff was treated using the overlapping flap technique. (*A*) Note the initial incision in the palatal mucoperiosteum along the dental arch. (*B*) The flap is raised with the major palatine artery, folded, and inserted beneath the mucoperiosteum on the opposite side. In this case, a full-thickness releasing incision was made along the dental arch on the opposite side. (*C*) The immediate postoperative image shows the completed repair of the hard and soft palate. (*D*) The intact repair 3 years postoperatively. (*Courtesy of* University of Illinois Dentistry Service, Urbana, IL.)

premolar teeth. The undermined flaps can then be repositioned medially and sutured over the defect using a simple interrupted pattern.

Congenital defects of the soft palate can occur as unilateral clefts (**Fig. 10**), midline clefts (**Fig. 11A**), or as bilateral/hypoplastic defects.[29,31] When assessing midline or unilateral cleft soft palates preoperatively, the tissues at the edges of the defect are manually apposed to evaluate the amount of tension along the proposed repair.[34] If no tension is present, then partial thickness relief incisions may not be required, and the defect may be repaired solely with a double-layer appositional flap. This procedure involves incising along the entire length of the cleft, including the rostral aspect. A small pair of blunt-ended scissors is used to separate the soft palate into 2 layers: the nasopharyngeal mucosa and the oral mucosa. The nasopharyngeal mucosa of the soft palate is then apposed and closed using a simple interrupted suture pattern, with the knots lying in the nasopharynx. A second layer of simple interrupted sutures is placed in the oral mucosa, with the knots lying in the oral cavity. During the procedure, it is important to plan the final length of the soft palate so that it extends caudally to the tip of the epiglottis (see **Fig. 11**). An alternate technique has been described to repair midline soft palate defects using bilateral overlapping single-pedicle flaps. This technically challenging procedure is usually unnecessary for repair of most midline soft palate defects (see **Table 3**).[29,35]

Bilateral hypoplasia of the soft palate is an uncommon congenital defect that presents as a significantly shortened soft palate with a small uvula-like structure. The epiglottis and nasopharynx are clearly visible during sedated oral examination, confirming the presence of a hypoplastic soft palate. Treatment of this condition is controversial. Options for treatment include medical management ± surgical correction, or possibly euthanasia.[29,36] If medical management is successful, surgical correction is not warranted. Medical management involves reliance on normal compensatory mechanisms, providing an elevated mounted water bottle for drinking, feeding the patient from an elevated bowl, and selecting a diet that can be easily directed to the esophagus, such as small meatballs or hard kibble. Intermittent antibiotic therapy may be indicated for episodes of rhinitis.[36] Surgical correction can be technically challenging and may not restore normal function[31] of the soft palate. Previously described surgical techniques for treatment of bilateral hypoplasia of the soft palate include bilateral tonsillectomy and pharyngeal flaps and bilateral buccal mucosal flaps (see **Table 3**).[29]

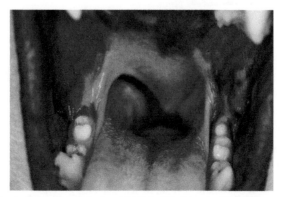

Fig. 10. A unilateral cleft soft palate is evident in this 5-year-old dog presented for chronic, intermittent nasal discharge. (*Courtesy of* University of Illinois Dentistry Service, Urbana, IL.)

Management of Acquired Palatal/Oronasal Defects

Acquired palatal/oronasal defects may occur at any age secondary to severe chronic periodontal disease, tooth extraction, trauma, electric cord injury, foreign body penetration, pressure necrosis, neoplasia, radiation necrosis, or dehiscence of a surgical wound.[31,32] Selection of an appropriate repair technique is based on the cause of the lesion, size, location, and previous repair attempts (see **Table 4**). Care should be taken to create flaps that are larger than the defects to be covered to ensure adequate closure without tension,[31] and to position the suture line over bone whenever possible.

Acute midline palatal defects, commonly associated with high-rise syndrome in cats, may be successfully repaired using primary appositional closure after debridement, with or without releasing incisions.[5] A transpalatal figure-of-eight wire between the maxillary canine teeth may be indicated to reduce and stabilize rostral palatal defects (**Fig. 12**).

Single-layer vestibular mucosal flaps, also referred to as labial-based mucoperiosteal flaps, are most frequently performed for repair of marginal defects in edentulous regions and are similar to flaps designed for surgical extractions. This technique is used to repair oronasal fistulas associated with chronic periodontal disease and defects occurring after maxillectomy procedures.[30–32] Before using this technique to repair oronasal fistulas, the perifistular epithelium needs to be removed. Incising tissues at the rostral and caudal aspects of the defect and creating 2 full-thickness divergent incisions buccally creates a trapezoid-shaped mucoperiosteal flap. The flap is elevated from the bone and advanced to cover the defect. Closure of the mucosa is performed using a simple interrupted suture pattern in a single layer, or, when possible, a double layer. Before closure, the flap should be assessed for tension.[34]

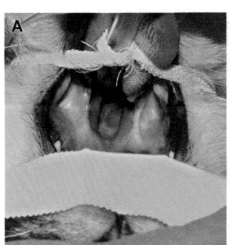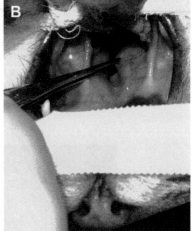

Fig. 11. A 3-year-old cat was presented for chronic nasal discharge since birth. (*A*) Note the large cleft of the soft palate, diagnosed as a congenital midline palatal defect. (*B*) Gentle traction was used to evaluate the amount of tissue available for closure without tension. Adequate tissue was found to be present for appositional closure. (*C*) An incision has been made along the edge of the cleft to remove epithelium; 2 stay sutures on either side of the defect facilitate placement of sutures for closure. (*D*) Three intranasal sutures have been preplaced to close the first layer. (*E*) The surgical repair is completed with a second layer of simple interrupted sutures. (*Courtesy of* University of Illinois Dentistry Service, Urbana, IL.)

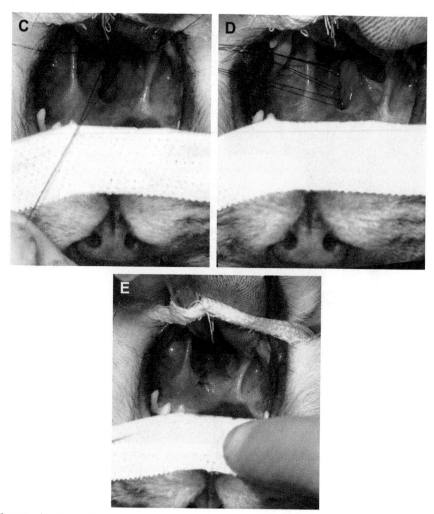

Fig. 11. (*continued*)

Options for relieving vestibular mucosal flap tension are to:

- Extend releasing incisions apically
- Perform periosteal fenestration/release[37,38]
- Reduce alveolar bone height
- Bluntly separate mucosa/submucosa from the skin to the mucocutaneous junction, if necessary (may be indicated for large maxillectomy procedures or large defects)

Double-layer vestibular mucosal/hard palatal and double-layer vestibular mucosal/perifistular flaps have been previously described[14,30–32] and are used to repair palatal/oronasal defects that have recurred despite properly performed single-layer vestibular mucosal flap repairs. These techniques involve creating a hinged flap from the palatal or perifistular mucosa that is folded over the defect so that the oral epithelial surface faces the nasal cavity. The flap is sutured in place using simple interrupted sutures of

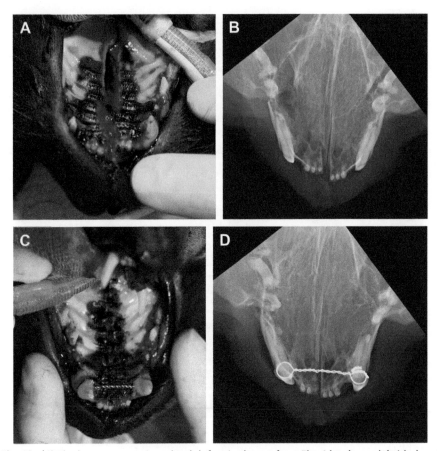

Fig. 12. (*A*) The large, traumatic, palatal defect in the cat from **Fig. 1** has been debrided and prepared for closure. (*B*) The preoperative radiograph shows the midline palatal fracture. (*C*) Appositional/primary closure has been used to close the defect. A figure-of-eight wire was positioned between the maxillary canine teeth to aid in reduction and stabilization. Composite material was used to attach the wire to the canine teeth. (*D*) The postoperative radiograph shows reduction of the midline defect. (*Courtesy of* University of Illinois Dentistry Service, Urbana, IL.)

absorbable material. The second layer is derived from a pedicle flap from the vestibular mucosa, which is rotated or advanced to cover both the defect and the harvest site of the first flap, and sutured in place.

Transposition flaps (or rotational flaps) can be used to repair small hard palate defects located lateral to the midline.[30,32] The transposition flap must be designed to be significantly larger than the defect. To prepare the receiving site for the transposition flap, the epithelium must be removed from the defect and from the surrounding area to be covered by the flap. The flap is created by a full-thickness, U-shaped incision in the palatal mucosa adjacent to the defect. The U-shape is oriented so that the caudal aspect remains attached. If possible, the major palatine artery should be elevated and moved with the flap to provide good vascular supply. The major palatine artery must be ligated at the rostral border of the flap. The transposition flap is shifted laterally (transposed) to cover the defect, with the flap margins overlying bone for support.

The flap is then sutured in place using a simple interrupted suture pattern. The exposed palatal bone at the donor site of the flap heals by second intention.

The major indications for palatal advancement flaps in dogs and cats are wide caudal midline defects of the palate.[30,32,39] The perifistular epithelium is debrided, and a large pedicle flap is created caudal to the defect. The flap is then advanced rostrally to cover the defect, with the margins of the flap situated over bone for support. The flap is sutured in place without tension using 1 or 2 layers of simple interrupted sutures, depending on the size of the patient.

The split palatal U-flap is a relatively specialized flap technique for repair of central hard palate defects in the region of the fourth premolar teeth.[31,32,40,41] Mucosa around the rim of the fistula is excised in preparation for the flaps. A large, full-thickness, U-shaped flap is created rostral to the defect and divided along the midline. The flaps may be made as far laterally as a few millimeters from the dental arch, as dictated by the size of the defect. The major palatine arteries require ligation at the rostral margins of the flaps. When elevating the flaps, care should be taken to avoid traumatizing the major palatine arteries, which should remain with the flap. One flap is rotated approximately 90° toward the midline to cover the defect and sutured in place caudally using a simple interrupted pattern. The other flap is also rotated 90° toward the midline and sutured in place just rostral to the initial flap. The exposed bone of the hard palate at the flap harvest site is allowed to heal by second intention.

The island axial pattern flap, a variation of the split palatal U-flap, is useful for repair of caudal palate defects with deficient local tissues.[31,32,42,43] The edges of the defect are excised in preparation for flap placement. A large, full-thickness, oblong flap is created in healthy palatal mucosa. The length of the flap should be centered over 1 of the major palatine arteries and should extend caudally to include tissues around the major palatine foramen. The major palatine artery requires ligation at the rostral margin of the flap. Most of the artery is elevated and harvested as the sole pedicle with the flap. Extra care must be taken when elevating the flap caudally to avoid transecting the artery as it exits the major palatine foramen.

A new technique specially designed for repair of very large midline palate defects has been successfully used at the authors' institution. This technique, named bilateral vestibular mucosal overlapping flaps, has not been previously described. A staged procedure is required in patients with teeth in the region from which the vestibular mucosal flaps are to be harvested. The maxillary and mandibular teeth in the region of the proposed vestibular flaps are surgically extracted, and alveoloplasties are performed to reduce alveolar bone height. Approximately 8 weeks later, the definitive surgical repair of the large palatal defect is performed. Large, bilateral vestibular flaps are created by making 2 divergent releasing mucosal incisions from the alveolar margin to the mucocutaneous junction. Blunt dissection is used to separate the vestibular mucosa from the skin to the level of the mucocutaneous junction. The palatal mucosa is not elevated, thereby leaving the major palatine arteries intact. Any palatal mucosa that will be located beneath the flaps must be debrided of all epithelium using a diamond bur to permit proper healing. The diamond bur can also be used to reduce and smooth the palatine rugae[44] for better flap apposition. In addition, it is important to remove the epithelium from the region of the first vestibular flap that will be covered by the second vestibular flap. After preparing and pretesting the flaps for apposition without tension, the flaps are sutured in place to the debrided palatal tissue. The overlapping construct of these vestibular flaps increases the strength of the repair by providing double-layer closure over the defect (**Fig. 13**).

A tongue flap has been described in the repair of large rostral defects of the palate.[45] This technique has a high incidence of dehiscence, restricts function, and may not be

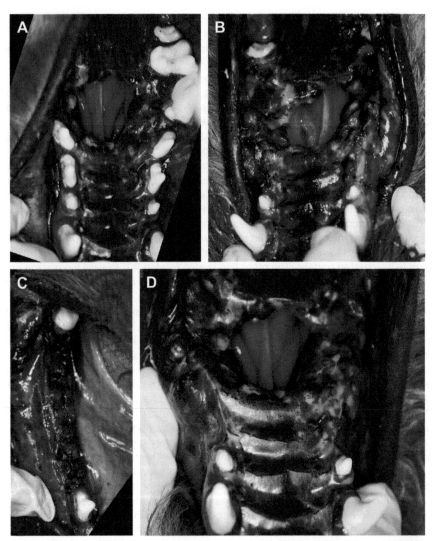

Fig. 13. A 4-year-old dog was referred for treatment of a large acquired defect of the caudal hard palate. A previous attempt to repair the defect with a single-layer vestibular flap was unsuccessful. Bilateral vestibular mucosal overlapping flaps were used to repair the defect. (*A*) The preoperative view shows the extent of the defect. (*B, C*) The maxillary second premolars to the first molars and mandibular third premolars to the first molars were extracted bilaterally in preparation for the definitive repair. (*D*) The healed extraction sites 8 weeks later. (*E–G*) Large, divergent, vestibular mucosal flaps were created bilaterally. (*H, I*) The flaps were temporarily positioned over the defect to assess appropriate coverage without tension. (*J, K*) A diamond bur was used to remove the epithelium from the edges of the palatal defect and the area of the palatal mucosa to be covered by the flaps. (*L, M*) A diamond bur has been used to remove the epithelium from the surface of the first flap, which will be covered by the second flap. The first vestibular flap was positioned over the defect and sutured in place. (*N*) The second vestibular flap was positioned over the defect and a portion of the first flap, and sutured in place. (*O*) Appropriate healing was evident at the 4-week follow-up, and the surgical repair remained intact at the 4-month follow-up, with resolution of clinical signs. (*Courtesy of* University of Illinois Dentistry Service, Urbana, IL.)

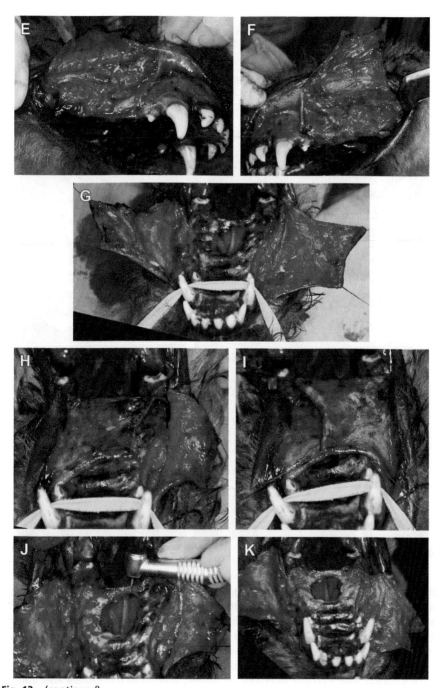

Fig. 13. (*continued*)

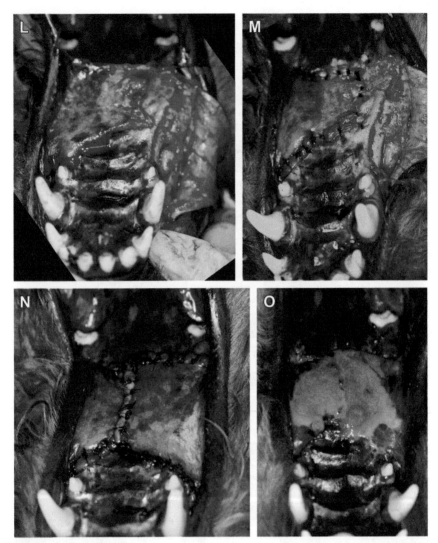

Fig. 13. (*continued*)

tolerated well by patients.[32] The procedure involves removing epithelium around the palatal defect and the rostral edges of the tongue, and elevating the perifistular soft tissues from the bone. The tongue is rotated 180° on its axis (so that the papillae of the tongue face ventrally) and positioned between the elevated perifistular soft tissues and the palatal bone. The rostral portion of the tongue is sutured in place using a simple interrupted pattern. Concurrent use of MMF and an esophagostomy feeding tube may improve results with this technique. However, alternative techniques are strongly recommended before resorting to this procedure.

Myoperitoneal microvascular free flaps have been described for repair of large palatal defects in which local tissue flaps have been unsuccessful.[32,46,47] For this procedure, a myoperitoneal flap is harvested from the body wall along with associated vessels. Microvascular surgical techniques are used to anastomose flap vessels to local arteries and veins. The free flap is positioned under the elevated edges of the palatal mucosa and sutured in place.

Obturators can help control clinical signs in patients with palatal defects that cannot be repaired. Reports have described direct, chair-side construction of obturators, as well as fabrication by external laboratories.[32,48–52] Another alternative for reducing the clinical signs associated with unresolved palatal defects is the placement of long-term feeding tubes, such as low-profile gastrostomy tubes (**Fig. 14**).[13]

MANAGEMENT OF ORAL MASSES

Oral masses in dogs and cats may be benign or malignant. Benign oral masses are common in dogs.[53,54] In dogs, malignant oral neoplasia accounts for 6% of cancer cases; in cats, malignant oral neoplasia accounts for 3% of cancer cases.[54] The most common malignant oral masses in dogs are malignant melanoma, squamous cell carcinoma (SCC), and fibrosarcoma.[54] Male dogs have 2.4 times greater risk of developing oral cancer than female dogs. The most common malignant oral neoplasia in cats is SCC, followed by fibrosarcoma.[54] Infectious and inflammatory oral lesions and nonneoplastic growths such as gingival hyperplasia may be mistaken for neoplastic lesions (**Figs. 15** and **16**).[55–57]

Some common causes of oral swellings/masses include:[58]

- Sequelae secondary to periodontal disease
- Sequelae secondary to endodontic disease
- Developmental abnormalities
- Trauma

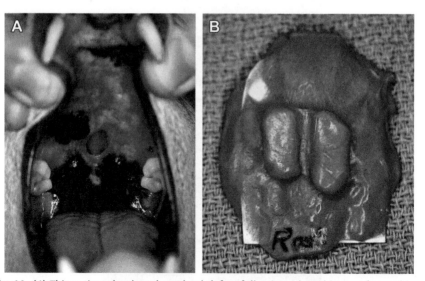

Fig. 14. (*A*) This patient developed a palatal defect following a long history of pemphigus vulgaris. An attempt to repair the defect was unsuccessful due to thin, friable local tissues. (*B*) An obturator was fabricated from this impression of the defect. With the obturator in place, the patient was able to eat normally. However, due to the lack of normal palatal structures, the obturator seal did not prevent water passage into the nasal cavity so it was removed. The patient was managed successfully for many years with a low-profile gastrostomy tube. (*Courtesy of* University of Illinois Dentistry Service, Urbana, IL.)

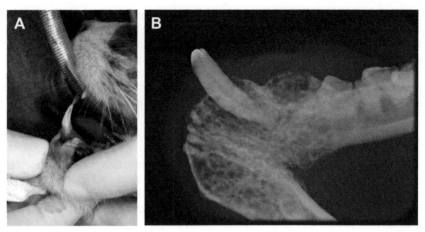

Fig. 15. A 10-year-old cat was presented for decreased appetite and rostral mandibular swelling. (*A*) The left mandibular canine tooth shows marked gingival recession. The periodontal probing depth adjacent to this tooth was 10 mm. (*B*) The preoperative radiograph shows perialveolar osteitis surrounding the periodontally diseased left mandibular canine tooth. Root resorption is also evident. (*Courtesy of* University of Illinois Dentistry Service, Urbana, IL.)

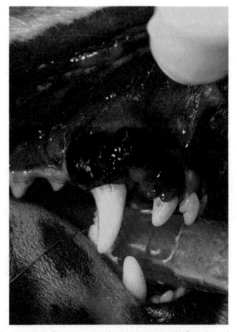

Fig. 16. This dark red, raised, inflammatory lesion was multifocal and was diagnosed as Wegener syndrome, an autoimmune vasculitis, in a 4-year-old dog. (*From* Krug W, Marretta SM, de Lorimier LP, et al. Diagnosis and management of Wegener's granulomatosis in a dog. J Vet Dent 2006;23:231–6; with permission.)

- Primary infection of bone or soft tissues caused by fungal or bacterial organisms
- Cysts
- Benign masses
- Malignant masses

The gross appearance of oral masses and swellings should be assessed for benign or malignant characteristics, bearing in mind that the diagnosis must be confirmed with histopathology. The initial gross assessment facilitates diagnostic and treatment planning.

General gross characteristics of oral masses and swellings	
Benign Characteristics	Malignant Characteristics
• Pedunculation	• Broad-based attachment
• Slow growth	• Rapid growth (± necrosis)
• Bilateral symmetry of lesions	• No association with diseased teeth
• Association with a diseased tooth	• Focal mobility of tooth or teeth in an otherwise healthy mouth[58]

The use of dental radiography is invaluable in the initial assessment of oral masses.[59] Radiographs of focal benign oral masses/swellings may reveal primary dental disease at the affected site. Radiographs of malignant oral masses may reveal irregular bone destructive and productive patterns inconsistent with underlying dental disease.[60] Destructive boney lesions may appear to be motheaten. Productive periosteal reactions to malignant lesions may appear as spiculated new bone formed at right angles to the outer cortex, or as radiating sunburst patterns (**Fig. 17**).[58,61]

A simple preliminary evaluation of exfoliating masses may be obtained using fine-needle aspirates and cytologic examination.[62] However, the definitive diagnosis of oral masses is based on a biopsy of the tissue followed by histopathologic examination. Small tumors or pedunculated lesions may be marginally resected. Attempts to

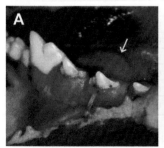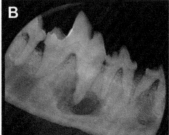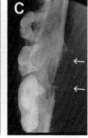

Fig. 17. An older canine patient was presented with a painful right mandibular swelling. Oral examination revealed no evidence of fractured teeth or significant periodontal pockets. (A) Note the submucosal hemorrhage buccally and the firm swelling lingually (*yellow arrow*). (B) On this intraoral parallel view of the caudal right mandible, a large lytic lesion is centered around the apex of the mesial root of the first molar tooth. Fine spicules of bone project from the ventral cortex. (C) This intraoral ventrodorsal/occlusal view of the caudal right mandible shows irregular bone lysis of the lingual cortex, with fine linear bone spicules at right angles to the cortex. Fibrosarcoma was diagnosed with histopathology. (*Courtesy of* University of Illinois Dentistry Service, Urbana, IL.)

remove large oral masses with excisional biopsies are not recommended until a histopathologic diagnosis is available for surgical treatment planning.[54,59] Superficial biopsies may reveal only inflammation or gingival hyperplasia,[54] and obtaining multiple biopsies from different parts of the lesion is recommended.[62] Tissue sampling methods include punch biopsy, deep Tru-cut biopsy, Jamshidi core biopsy, and deep wedge incisional biopsy. The use of electrosurgery to obtain oral tumor biopsies is not recommended because of the risk of specimen distortion.[14,54]

After the histologic diagnosis of oral malignancy, clinical staging should include a complete blood count, serum biochemistry profile, urinalysis, fine-needle aspirates of regional lymph nodes, and thoracic radiographs.[14] Abdominal ultrasonography should be considered to rule out concurrent or metastatic disease.[62,63] Advanced imaging techniques provide a more precise evaluation of the primary tumor site and facilitate surgical and radiation treatment planning. Computed tomography is often required to evaluate the full extent of invasion of maxillary masses and caudal mandibular masses.[62] Magnetic resonance imaging can reveal the extent of deep soft tissue infiltration and lymph node involvement.[62] These diagnostic results are used for therapeutic decision making.

Factors to consider before recommending surgery are:

- Oral examination findings
- Diagnostic imaging results
- Histopathologic diagnosis
- Recommended surgical margins based on tumor type and size[54,64,65]
- Intent of surgery (curative or palliative debulking)
- Availability of local tissues for surgical closure

Malignant or benign but invasive oral masses require a proactive surgical approach to achieve complete excision and prevent local recurrence. Procedure selection depends on the location and extent of the tumor. A wide variety of mandibulectomy[54,55,66] and maxillectomy techniques[54,55,67] have been described for the surgical management of malignant oral tumors (**Fig. 18**).

Mandibulectomy Techniques	Maxillectomy Techniques
• Unilateral rostral mandibulectomy	• Unilateral incisivectomy
• Bilateral rostral mandibulectomy	• Bilateral incisivectomy
• Rim excision/mandibulectomy	• Unilateral rostral maxillectomy
• Segmental mandibulectomy	• Bilateral rostral maxillectomy
• Caudal mandibulectomy	• Central/segmental maxillectomy
• Total mandibulectomy	• Caudal maxillectomy
• One-and-a-half mandibulectomy	• Unilateral (complete) maxillectomy

Regardless of the procedure to be performed, adherence to fundamental surgical principles can improve surgical outcome and reduce postoperative complications.

Important surgical principles for planning mandibulectomies and maxillectomies include:[66,67]

- Planning for adequate surgical margins
- Planning for complete mucosal closure
- Preserving local blood supply and minimizing trauma
- Using sharp dissection rather than electrosurgery to minimize postoperative dehiscence[30]

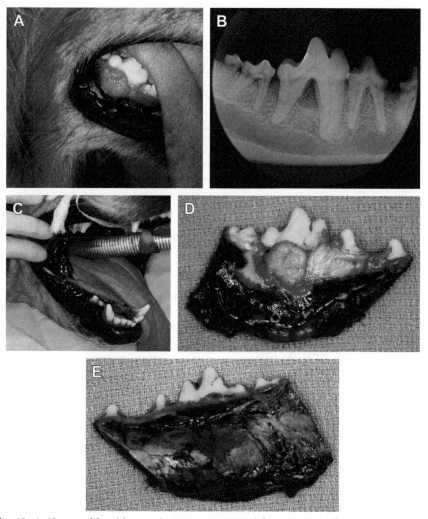

Fig. 18. A 10-year-old golden retriever was presented for resection of an acanthomatous ameloblastoma which had recurred 3 times following marginal resection. (*A*) The preoperative photograph shows a large irregular soft tissue mass on the gingiva and alveolar mucosa in the region of the right mandibular first molar tooth. (*B*) The preoperative radiograph shows a decrease in bone density in the region of the mass. (*C*) A definitive cure was achieved using a segmental mandibulectomy with 1-cm margins, which included en bloc resection of the right mandibular third and fourth premolars and the first and second molars. (*D, E*) These buccal and lingual views show the inked resected specimen. (*Courtesy of* University of Illinois Dentistry Service, Urbana, IL.)

- Harvesting/undermining large mucosal flaps to avoid tension on the suture line
- Positioning the suture line over bone when possible
- Using 2-layer closure when possible

Marking or inking the margins of the resected surgical specimen facilitate margin evaluation by the pathologist (see **Fig. 18**D, E). Immediate postoperative radiographs of the surgical site provide a baseline for future monitoring.

Recommendations for postoperative care after maxillectomy and mandibulectomy procedures include:[66,67]

- Provide appropriate pain management
- Provide intravenous fluid therapy for 24 hours or until the patient resumes eating/drinking
- Administer a soft-food diet for 2 to 4 weeks
- Consider placing esophagostomy or gastrostomy feeding tubes in selected cases
- Remove chew toys and restrict activities (such as grooming and rough play) until healed; consider basket muzzle or Elizabethan collar for noncompliant patients
- Reevaluate surgical sites 2 weeks postoperatively for skin suture removal
- Initiate adjunct oncologic therapy (if indicated) after surgical sites have healed
- Reevaluate 6 weeks postoperatively, remove any residual oral sutures, and treat traumatic dental occlusion as needed
- Reexamine surgical site every 3 months for 1 year with thoracic radiographs for patients diagnosed with malignant oral neoplasia

MANAGEMENT OF MISCELLANEOUS ORAL LESIONS

Dogs and cats can develop a range of miscellaneous oral lesions, including odontogenic cysts, osteonecrosis and osteomyelitis, and lesions of the tongue and lips. The surgical approaches to treating these lesions are discussed in this section.

Management of Odontogenic Cysts

Cysts are defined as pathologic cavities lined with epithelium that contain fluid or semisolid material. Odontogenic cysts form within tooth-bearing regions of the jaws after hyperplasia of odontogenic epithelial rests or remnants.[68–70] These epithelial rests are normal tissues that begin proliferating abnormally after an inflammatory or developmental stimulus (**Table 5**). Odontogenic cysts are uncommon in dogs and cats and are generally considered benign but can cause local destruction of bone and teeth. Regardless of cyst type, treatment typically involves extraction of affected teeth, complete enucleation of the cyst wall, curettage, and osteoplasty (**Fig. 19**).[69,70] Endodontic therapy for teeth associated with periapical cysts is an option, but apicoectomy, surgical curettage, and osteoplasty must also be performed to remove the inciting irritants.[69] Incomplete removal of the cyst lining results in recurrence and requires retreatment. Bone grafts may be placed if cyst defects are large. Surgical sites should be monitored radiographically until the cystic void has ossified.[69]

Table 5			
Origins of odontogenic cysts			
Odontogenic Cyst Type	**Inciting Stimulus**	**Origin of Epithelial Rests**	**Name of Rests**
Dentigerous cyst	Unerupted or malformed tooth	Enamel organ	Reduced enamel epithelium
Periapical cyst (radicular cyst)	Nonvital tooth	Epithelial root sheath	Rests of Malassez
Odontogenic parakeratinized cyst–like lesion in dogs	Unknown	Epithelial connection between the mucosa and enamel organ	Rests of Serres (rests of dental lamina)

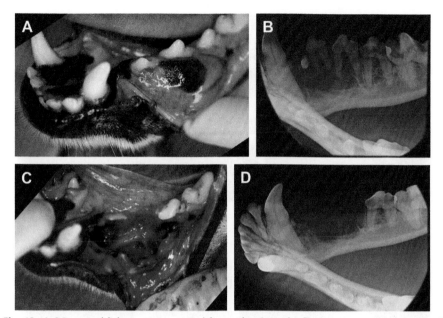

Fig. 19. A 6.5-year-old dog was presented for evaluation of a fluctuant, nonpainful, rostral left mandibular swelling. (*A*) The swelling is evident in the region of the absent left mandibular first premolar tooth. The overlying mucosa appears blue, a feature often seen in association with dentigerous cysts. (*B*) The preoperative radiograph of this region shows a large radiolucency with smooth borders affecting the alveolar bone of the canine tooth and the first, second, and third premolars. Note the unerupted and rotated left mandibular first premolar tooth contained within the radiolucency. (*C*) Surgical treatment of the cyst involved extraction of the first to third premolar teeth, enucleation of the cyst wall, curettage, and osteoplasty. (*D*) A demineralized, freeze-dried, bone allograft was placed at the distal aspect of the canine tooth root. (*Courtesy of* University of Illinois Dentistry Service, Urbana, IL.)

Management of Osteonecrosis

Osteonecrosis of the maxillae or mandibles is defined as exposed necrotic bone that fails to heal after 6 to 8 weeks in patients with no history of radiation therapy.[71] Osteoradionecrosis is defined as devitalized bone after radiation therapy for neoplasia.[71] Causes of osteonecrosis not induced by radiation include maxillofacial injuries, traumatic tooth extraction, and chronic infection. Chronic steroid administration and inflammatory processes have been associated with maxillary osteonecrosis in dogs.[72] In some cases, the cause of the osteonecrosis may remain unidentified.[71] Recently, high-dose bisphosphonate therapy in humans with cancer has increased the incidence of maxillofacial osteonecrosis in people. Use of bisphosphonates in companion animals may increase the incidence of osteonecrosis in veterinary patients.[71,73]

Patients with osteonecrosis may present with fetid breath, severe oral pain, facial swelling, reluctance or inability to eat, purulent discharge, regional lymphadenopathy, pyrexia, malaise, and exophthalmos.[14,72] Oral examination of these patients may reveal missing teeth, severe oral soft tissue inflammation, mucosal defects/deep ulcerations, and exposed, necrotic bone. Intraoral dental radiographs or other imaging modalities may reveal bone sequestra or sclerotic bone with a fine granular appearance (**Fig. 20**).[71]

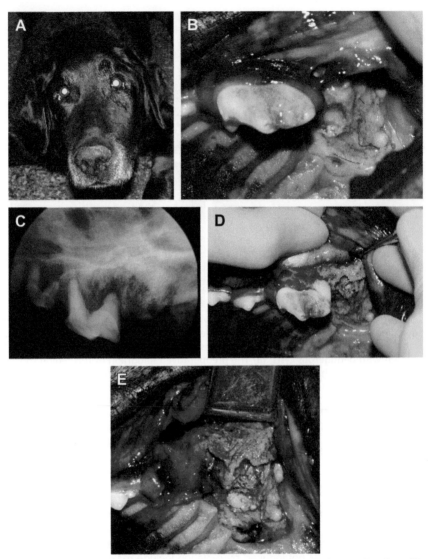

Fig. 20. A 10-year-old dog was referred for purulent left nasal discharge, facial swelling, weight loss, and difficulty chewing for 3 months after extraction of the left maxillary first and second molar teeth. Prednisone and cephalexin administered during this period did not resolve the clinical signs. (A) On presentation, a firm painful swelling was visible and palpable ventral to the left eye. (B) Intraoral examination revealed a large area of necrotic bone in the region of the previous extractions. (C) The dental radiograph of the caudal left maxilla showed an area of motheaten bone around the distal root of the fourth premolar and the previous extraction sites. (D–G) Surgical treatment involved a large vestibular flap, extraction of the fourth premolar, and removal of the necrotic bone with rongeurs and curettes until healthy bleeding bone was encountered. The surgical site was flushed and closed using a simple interrupted suture pattern. (H, I) At the 4-month postoperative follow-up, the facial swelling and clinical signs had resolved and the surgical site had healed. (*Courtesy of* University of Illinois Dentistry Service, Urbana, IL.)

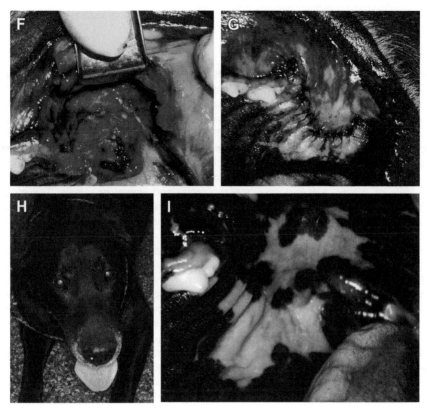

Fig. 20. (*continued*)

General principles for surgical management of osteonecrosis include the following:[14,71]

- Use a large mucoperiosteal flap around the site
- Excise the draining tract if present
- Extract any teeth remaining in necrotic bone
- Remove necrotic bone en bloc or with rongeurs (if attached) until healthy bleeding bone remains
- Perform partial maxillectomy or mandibulectomy as an alternative
- Flush the surgical area liberally with sterile saline
- Collect samples for cytology, culture and sensitivity, and histopathology
- Close the mucoperiosteal flap using a simple interrupted suture pattern
- Provide appropriate perioperative pain management
- Provide long-term broad-spectrum antibiotic therapy for 6 to 8 weeks postoperatively

The prognosis after surgical and medical management of maxillofacial osteonecrosis depends on the underlying cause. For patients with osteoradionecrosis, the prognosis is fair to guarded, with a high potential for local recurrence. For patients with osteonecrosis secondary to trauma or infection, the prognosis is generally excellent after appropriate surgical and medical management. For animals with idiopathic osteonecrosis, the prognosis is fair to good, although additional lesions may occur in other areas of the mouth.

Management of Tongue Lesions

Dogs and cats may be affected by a variety of lingual lesions due to traumatic, metabolic, idiopathic, infectious, immune-mediated, hereditary, and neoplastic causes.[74] Many lingual lesions require medical management, and some require surgical management. A lingual biopsy may be necessary to determine the definitive diagnosis and appropriate therapy. Biopsy techniques are similar to those discussed previously regarding oral masses.[74] Lingual lesions that may require surgical management include electrical cord injury, acute mechanical trauma, sublingual linear foreign body entrapment, severe sublingual hyperplasia secondary to self-trauma, sublingual sialocele or ranula, ankyloglossia, macroglossia, and lingual neoplasia. The most common indication for glossectomy is lingual neoplasia. Malignant melanoma and SCC are reported to be the 2 most common malignant lingual masses in dogs and cats.[54,74–77]

Electrical cord injury and other types of acute trauma may cause necrosis of lingual tissues. However, oral tissues have a large capacity for healing and may recover without surgical intervention, despite significant injury. Emergency management of severe injuries requires supportive medical therapy to address pain, anorexia, and risk of infection. The tissues should be monitored, allowing the full extent of necrosis or healing to occur before performing definitive surgical debridement.[74]

Acute mechanical trauma to the tongue may be caused by licking or chewing sharp objects, or by encounters with devices such as paper shredders.[74] Severe lingual hemorrhage caused by mechanical trauma may require surgical intervention for hemostasis. The degree of tissue trauma dictates the extent of surgical repair. Surgical approaches may range from traditional debridement, disinfection, and laceration repair, to tongue amputation.[74]

Sublingual linear foreign body entrapment may occur after ingestion of linear materials. Patients may present with systemic signs including vomiting, anorexia, and depression.[78] Diagnosis is based on visualization of the sublingual linear foreign body during oral examination. This is facilitated by elevating the patient's head, applying digital pressure to the ventral aspect of the intermandibular space, opening the mouth, and gently elevating and displacing the tongue to expose the sublingual area.[74] Treatment for a linear foreign body is surgical removal. In most cases, the linear material has descended from the base of the tongue to the gastrointestinal tract, necessitating abdominal surgery.[74]

Severe sublingual hyperplasia may develop after repeated trauma to sublingual tissues by the patient's own teeth. Differential diagnoses include neoplasia, so a biopsy is recommended for a definitive diagnosis. Large lesions are more easily traumatized, causing discomfort. These cases often respond well to surgical resection of the hyperplastic tissue. Care should be taken to avoid major vessels, nerves, and salivary ducts during resection.[74] Chronic recurrent lesions may require selective tooth extraction in rare cases.

Sialoceles or ranulas are caused by extravasation of saliva within surrounding tissues secondary to a rupture in the salivary glands or ducts. Definitive treatment of sublingual sialoceles or ranulas typically involves removal of the mandibular and sublingual salivary glands. Some success has been reported after marsupialization of ranulas, but recurrence rates are higher with this treatment.[74,79]

Ankyloglossia is a rare hereditary lingual condition that requires surgical intervention. Also known as tongue-tie, ankyloglossia has been reported in young dogs presented for ptyalism and poor weight gain. Patients with ankyloglossia have reduced lingual range of motion caused by increased rostroventral attachment, and may have a W-shaped tongue tip.[80] Surgical frenuloplasty relieves the tongue of its abnormal attachment and permits a more normal range of motion.

Macroglossia is another rare hereditary lingual abnormality that may require surgical intervention. Dogs with true macroglossia have increased susceptibility to lingual dessication and trauma secondary to exposure, as well as decreased lingual function.[74] Surgical resection of the excessive rostral lingual tissue provides good clinical results.[81] Care should be taken not to overdiagnose this condition in brachycephalic dogs whose tongues appear large but have normal function.

Surgical resection is recommended for lingual neoplasia.[54] Determination of the appropriate surgical technique is based on the location and size of the lesion, and histopathology and staging results.[82] Benign tumors can be removed conservatively using marginal excision. Malignant tumors require full-thickness glossectomy. The goal of glossectomy procedures in patients with malignant lingual masses is to achieve surgical cure while preserving as much tongue function as possible. For malignant masses such as SCC and melanoma, margins of at least 2 cm are recommended.[54] Various glossectomy techniques can be used in the removal of tongue masses, including marginal excision, wedge glossectomy, longitudinal glossectomy,[82] and transverse glossectomy.[75,83] Transverse glossectomies may be categorized as partial (removal of the free portion of tongue), subtotal (removal of the entire free tongue and portion of the genioglossus and geniohyoid muscles), near total (removal of >75% of tongue), and total (removal of 100% of tongue) (**Fig. 21**).[30,75,83] In general, dogs tolerate and adapt to major glossectomy,[83] whereas cats do not adapt as well to major changes in oral structure.[74,82,84] Placement of feeding tubes is recommended when major glossectomy is perfumed. Tubes should be maintained until patients can take in adequate nutrition and hydration orally (**Table 6**).

Management of Lip Avulsions, Lip Fold Pyoderma, and Neoplasia of the Lip

Lip avulsions may be caused by vehicular accidents, fights with other animals, or other trauma, and may involve the lower or upper lip. Lip avulsions usually occur at the mucogingival line,[20] and extend apically and caudally. These injuries are typically treated by wound cleansing and debridement (including removal of exuberant granulation tissue), followed by primary closure (**Fig. 22**).[20] When incisor teeth are present, interrupted horizontal mattress sutures may be passed interdentally, looped around each tooth, and tied rostrally.[20] In edentulous regions, small holes may be created in alveolar bone to facilitate suture passage/placement. Alternatively, deep tissue bites into the periosteum may provide adequate holding strength along the suture line. If extensive dead space or contamination is present, drain placement may be indicated. Animals recovering from lip avulsions should be prevented from grooming to avoid stress on the suture line during repetitive licking or chewing. Elizabethan collars are recommended postoperatively[20] for 4 to 6 weeks to prevent recurrence. Broad-spectrum systemic antibiotic therapy is often indicated because of the contaminated/infected nature of these wounds.[20]

In some dog breeds, the natural folds of the lower lips may create moisture or friction dermatitis that is exacerbated by trapped secretions and surface bacteria (**Fig. 23**). Severe lip fold pyoderma may require cheiloplasty to eliminate the underlying anatomic cause.[85] Medical management is recommended before cheiloplasty to reduce local tissue infection and inflammation. The surgical approach for cheiloplasty involves an elliptical incision to remove the affected and redundant tissue, including a rim of normal skin. The surgical site is closed in 2 layers.[85]

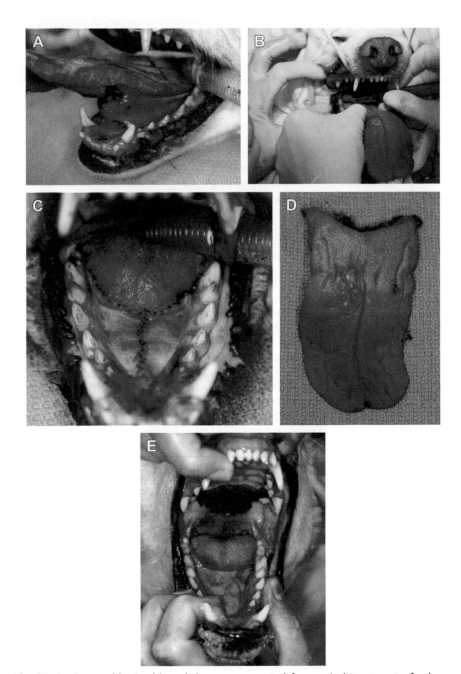

Fig. 21. An 8-year-old mixed breed dog was presented for surgical treatment of a large lingual SCC. (*A, B*) Note the large, ulcerated mass involving the ventral surface of the tongue and frenulum, and extending to the dorsal surface. In (*A*), the blue line on the dorsal surface of the tongue indicates the proposed glossectomy site to achieve 2-cm margins. (*B*) A U-shaped incision is made on the dorsal surface of the tongue while palpating the caudal extent of the mass to ensure adequate margins. (*C*) The immediate postoperative image shows simple interrupted suture closure along the glossectomy site. (*D*) The excised specimen was submitted for histopathology; the margins were free of neoplastic cells. (*E*) The 6-week postoperative follow-up showed a well-healed surgical site. The patient was being hand-fed canned food formed into meatballs and was able to drink without assistance. (*Courtesy of* University of Illinois Dentistry Service, Urbana, IL.)

Table 6
Glossectomy techniques

Glossectomy Type	Indications	Procedure	Potential Sequelae	Follow-up
Marginal excision	Benign masses	Partial thickness elliptical incision around the mass Simple interrupted or simple continuous closure	Rare	Reevaluate at 2 wk and 6 wk, all patients
Wedge glossectomy	Benign masses Small malignant masses at the lateral tongue edge	Full-thickness wedge-shaped incision around the mass Transverse or longitudinal closure[a,b] Preserves both lingual arteries	Transverse closure → deviation of tongue Longitudinal closure → narrowing of tongue	For malignant masses: Adjunct oncologic therapy as needed Reexamine every 3 mo for 1 y with thoracic radiographs
Longitudinal glossectomy	Rostral unilateral masses Surgical margin indicates ligation of 1 lingual artery	Full-thickness incision along the midline from the tongue tip to the caudal aspect of the mass Longitudinal closure[b] Preserves 1 lingual artery	Narrowing of rostral aspect of tongue	
Transverse glossectomy	Malignant masses on the midline or approaching midline	Full-thickness incision transversely across the tongue to the caudal aspect of the mass Incision may be straight, U-shaped, or V-shaped Straight or U-shaped incision → dorsal-to-ventral closure V-shaped incision → transverse closure[a] Both lingual arteries ligated	Shortening of tongue Ptyalism Difficulty eating and drinking orally Difficulty maintaining nutrition without feeding tube	Feeding tube maintenance/removal

[a] Transverse closure, dorsal-to-dorsal and ventral-to-ventral mucosal apposition.
[b] Longitudinal closure, dorsal-to-ventral mucosal apposition.

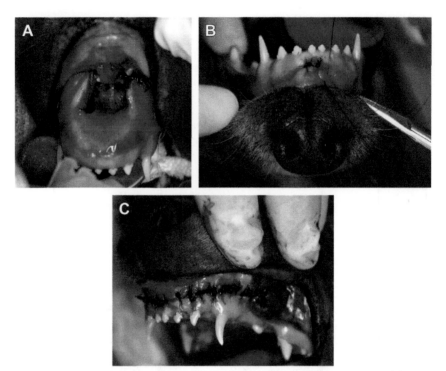

Fig. 22. A 3-month-old puppy was presented for repair of a traumatic avulsion of the upper lip. (*A*) The lip avulsion had exposed the nasal cavity and collected debris. (*B*) The area was debrided, flushed, and closed with simple interrupted sutures, taking care to incorporate the periosteum. (*C*) The immediate postoperative image showed the extent of the repair. (*Courtesy of* University of Illinois Dentistry Service, Urbana, IL.)

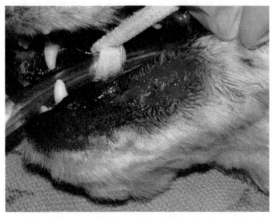

Fig. 23. A cocker spaniel was presented for severe halitosis. The animal was aggressive and in pain. Oral examination under anesthesia revealed severe, bilateral, lip fold pyoderma. Preoperative medical management was not possible in this case because of the patient's temperament. The redundant lip folds were clipped, surgically prepared, and resected. The subcutaneous tissues and skin were closed routinely in 2 layers. The resected tissue was submitted for histopathology and was found to be consistent with chronic pyoderma. (*Courtesy of* University of Illinois Dentistry Service, Urbana, IL.)

As in other regions of the mouth, surgical resection is recommended for neoplasms of the lip. In dogs and cats, the lips are not used in prehension of food, so resection or innervation defects postoperatively do not significantly affect quality of life.[82] However, ptyalism or decreased cosmesis can be complications of lip resection.[82] The surgical approach depends on the location and size of the lesion, and histopathology and staging results. Malignant lip masses require full-thickness excision for complete resection. Small malignant masses may be removed using a wedge resection at the border of the lip. Larger masses may be removed using a rectangular excision. Depending on the size and location, the rectangular defect resulting from the excision may be closed using one of several reconstructive techniques described previously.[82,86]

REFERENCES

1. Hoffman SL, Kressin DL, Verstraete FJ. Myths and misconceptions in veterinary dentistry. J Am Vet Med Assoc 2007;231:1818–24.
2. Pogrel MA. Foreword. In: Verstraete FJ, Lommer MJ, editors. Oral and maxillofacial surgery in dogs and cats. Philadelphia: Saunders Elsevier; 2012. p. ix.
3. Verstraete FJ, Lommer MJ. Oral and maxillofacial surgery in dogs and cats. 1st edition. Philadelphia: Saunders Elsevier; 2012. p. 1–567.
4. Legendre L. Maxillofacial fracture repairs. Vet Clin North Am Small Anim Pract 2005;35:985–1008.
5. Bonner SE, Reiter AM, Lewis JR. Orofacial manifestations of high-rise syndrome in cats: a retrospective study of 84 cases. J Vet Dent 2012;29:10–8.
6. Manfra Marretta S, Schrader SC, Matthiesen DT. Problems associated with the management and treatment of jaw fractures. In: Manfra Marretta S, editor. Problems in veterinary medicine. Philadelphia: JB Lippincott; 1990.
7. Boudrieau RJ, Verstraete FJ. Principles of maxillofacial trauma repair. In: Verstraete FJ, Lommer MJ, editors. Oral and maxillofacial surgery in dogs and cats. Philadelphia: Saunders Elsevier; 2012. p. 233–42.
8. Boudrieau RJ. Mandibular and maxillofacial fractures. In: Tobias KM, Johnston SA, editors. Veterinary surgery: small animal. Philadelphia: Elsevier Saunders; 2012. p. 1054–77.
9. Reiter AM, Lewis JR, Harvey CE. Dentistry for the surgeon. In: Tobias KM, Johnston SA, editors. Veterinary surgery: small animal. Philadelphia: Elsevier Saunders; 2012. p. 1037–53.
10. Smith MM, Legendre LF. Maxillofacial fracture repair using noninvasive techniques. In: Verstraete FJ, Lommer MJ, editors. Oral and maxillofacial surgery in dogs and cats. Philadelphia: Saunders Elsevier; 2012. p. 275–84.
11. Boudrieau RJ. Maxillofacial fracture repair using miniplates and screws. In: Verstraete FJ, Lommer MJ, editors. Oral and maxillofacial surgery in dogs and cats. Philadelphia: Saunders Elsevier; 2012. p. 293–308.
12. Schloss AJ, Marretta SM. Prognostic factors affecting teeth in the line of mandibular fractures. J Vet Dent 1990;7:7–9.
13. Marks SL. Enteral nutritional support. In: Verstraete FJ, Lommer MJ, editors. Oral and maxillofacial surgery in dogs and cats. Philadelphia: Saunders Elsevier; 2012. p. 43–54.
14. Manfra Marretta S. Maxillofacial surgery. Vet Clin North Am Small Anim Pract 1998;28:1285–96.
15. Manfra Marretta S. Maxillofacial fracture complications. In: Verstraete FJ, Lommer MJ, editors. Oral and maxillofacial surgery in dogs and cats. Philadelphia: Saunders Elsevier; 2012. p. 333–41.

16. Johnson AL. Management of specific fractures. In: Fossum TW, editor. Small animal surgery. St Louis (MO): Mosby Elsevier; 2007. p. 1015–142.
17. Matis U, Kostlin R. Symphyseal separation and fractures involving the incisive region. In: Verstraete FJ, Lommer MJ, editors. Oral and maxillofacial surgery in dogs and cats. Philadelphia: Saunders Elsevier; 2012. p. 265–74.
18. Cetinkaya MA, Yardimci C, Kaya U. Lingual arch bar application for treatment of rostral mandibular body fractures in cats. Vet Surg 2011;40:457–63.
19. Nicholson I, Wyatt J, Radke H, et al. Treatment of caudal mandibular fracture and temporomandibular joint fracture-luxation using a bi-gnathic encircling and retaining device. Vet Comp Orthop Traumatol 2010;23:102–8.
20. Swaim SF. Facial soft tissue injuries. In: Verstraete FJ, Lommer MJ, editors. Oral and maxillofacial surgery in dogs and cats. Philadelphia: Saunders Elsevier; 2012. p. 243–57.
21. Holmstrom SE, Fitch PF, Eisner ER. Endodontics. In: Holmstrom SE, Fitch PF, Eisner ER, editors. Veterinary dental techniques for the small animal practitioner. St Louis (MO): Saunders Elsevier; 2004. p. 339–414.
22. Boudrieau RJ. Maxillofacial fracture repair using intraosseous wires. In: Verstraete FJ, Lommer MJ, editors. Oral and maxillofacial surgery in dogs and cats. Philadelphia: Saunders Elsevier; 2012. p. 285–92.
23. Tsugawa AJ, Verstraete FJ. Maxillofacial fracture repair using external skeletal fixation. In: Verstraete FJ, Lommer MJ, editors. Oral and maxillofacial surgery in dogs and cats. Philadelphia: Saunders Elsevier; 2012. p. 309–19.
24. Verstraete FJ, Arzi B, Bezuidenhout AJ. Surgical approaches for mandibular and maxillofacial trauma repair. In: Verstraete FJ, Lommer MJ, editors. Oral and maxillofacial surgery in dogs and cats. Philadelphia: Saunders Elsevier; 2012. p. 259–64.
25. Boudrieau RJ, Kudisch M. Miniplate fixation for repair of mandibular and maxillary fractures in 15 dogs and 3 cats. Vet Surg 1996;25:277–91.
26. AONA AO North America Home Page. Available at: https://www.aona.org/. Accessed August 1, 2012.
27. DePuy Synthes. Synthes Global Internet. Available at: http://www.synthes.com/. Accessed August 1, 2012.
28. KLS Martin USA. KLS Martin USA: products. Available at: http://www.klsmartinusa.com/. Accessed August 1, 2012.
29. Manfra Marretta S. Cleft palate repair techniques. In: Verstraete FJ, Lommer MJ, editors. Oral and maxillofacial surgery in dogs and cats. Philadelphia: Saunders Elsevier; 2012. p. 351–61.
30. Hedlund CS, Fossum TW. Surgery of the digestive system. In: Fossum TW, editor. Small animal surgery. St Louis (MO): Mosby Elsevier; 2007. p. 339–530.
31. Reiter AM, Holt DE. Palate. In: Tobias KM, Johnston SA, editors. Veterinary surgery: small animal. Philadelphia: Elsevier Saunders; 2012. p. 1707–17.
32. Manfra Marretta S. Repair of acquired palatal defects. In: Verstraete FJ, Lommer MJ, editors. Oral and maxillofacial surgery in dogs and cats. Philadelphia: Saunders Elsevier; 2012. p. 363–72.
33. Beckman BW. Repair of secondary cleft palate in the dog. J Vet Dent 2011;28:58–62.
34. Stanley BJ. Tension-relieving techniques. In: Tobias KM, Johnston SA, editors. Veterinary surgery: small animal. Philadelphia: Elsevier Saunders; 2012. p. 1221–42.
35. Griffins LG, Sullivan M. Bilateral overlapping mucosal single-pedicle flaps for correction of soft palate defects. J Am Anim Hosp Assoc 2001;37:183–6.

36. Manfra Marretta S. Palatal defects. In: Harari J, editor. Small animal surgery secrets. Philadelphia: Hanley & Belfus; 2000. p. 347–50.
37. Holmstrom SE, Fitch PF, Eisner ER. Exodontics. In: Holmstrom SE, Fitch PF, Eisner ER, editors. Veterinary dental techniques for the small animal practitioner. St Louis (MO): Saunders Elsevier; 2004. p. 291–338.
38. Klokkevold PR. Localized bone augmentation and implant site development. In: Newman MG, Takei HH, Klokkevold PR, et al, editors. Carranza's clinical periodontology. St Louis (MO): Elsevier Saunders; 2012. p. 672–83.
39. Rocha L, Beckman B. Soft palate advancement flap for palatal oronasal fistulae. J Vet Dent 2010;27:132–3.
40. Manfra Marretta S, Grove TK, Grillo JF. Split palatal U-flap: a new technique for repair of caudal hard palate defects. J Vet Dent 1991;8:5–8.
41. Beckman BW. Split palatal U-flap for repair of caudal palatal defects. J Vet Dent 2006;23:267–9.
42. Smith MM. Island palatal mucoperiosteal flap for repair of oronasal fistula in a dog. J Vet Dent 2001;18:127–9.
43. Woodward TM. Greater palatine island axial pattern flap for repair of oronasal fistula related to eosinophilic granuloma. J Vet Dent 2006;23:161–6.
44. AVDC Nomenclature Committee. Recommendations Adopted by the AVDC Board. 2012. Available at: http://www.avdc.org/nomenclature.html. Accessed August 8, 2012.
45. Robertson JJ, Dean PW. Repair of a traumatically induced oronasal fistula in a cat with a rostral tongue flap. Vet Surg 1987;16:164–6.
46. Degner DA, Lanz OI, Walshaw R. Myoperitoneal microvascular free flaps in dogs: an anatomical study and a clinical case report. Vet Surg 1996;25:463–70.
47. Lanz OI. Free tissue transfer of the rectus abdominis myoperitoneal flap for oral reconstruction in a dog. J Vet Dent 2001;18:187–92.
48. Harvey CE, Emily PP. Oral surgery. In: Harvey CE, Emily PP, editors. Small animal dentistry. St Louis (MO): Mosby; 1993. p. 312–77.
49. Coles BH, Underwood LC. Repair of the traumatic oronasal fistula in the cat with a prosthetic acrylic implant. Vet Rec 1988;122:359–60.
50. Hale FA, Sylvestre AM, Miller C. The use of a prosthetic appliance to manage a large palatal defect in a dog. J Vet Dent 1997;14:61–4.
51. Smith MM, Rockfill AD. Prosthodontic appliance for repair of an oronasal fistula in a cat. J Am Vet Med Assoc 1996;208:1410–2.
52. Thoday KL, Charlton DA, Graham-Jones O, et al. The successful use of a prosthesis in the correction of a palatal defect in a dog. J Small Anim Pract 1975; 16:487–94.
53. Gardner DG. Epulides in the dog: a review. J Oral Pathol Med 1996;25:32–7.
54. Liptak JM, Withrow SJ. Cancer of the gastrointestinal tract: oral tumors. In: Withrow S, Vail D, editors. Small animal clinical oncology. St Louis (MO): Saunders Elsevier; 2007. p. 455–75.
55. Verstraete FJ. Mandibulectomy and maxillectomy. Vet Clin North Am Small Anim Pract 2005;35:1009–39, viii.
56. Kapatkin AS, Manfra Marretta S, Patnaik AK, et al. Mandibular swellings in cats: prospective study of 24 cats. J Am Anim Hosp Assoc 1991;27:575–80.
57. Krug W, Marretta SM, de Lorimier LP, et al. Diagnosis and management of Wegener's granulomatosis in a dog. J Vet Dent 2006;23:231–6.
58. DuPont GA, DeBowes LJ. Swelling and neoplasia. In: DuPont GA, DeBowes LJ, editors. Atlas of dental radiography in dogs and cats. St Louis (MO): Saunders; 2009. p. 182–94.

59. Lommer MJ, Verstraete FJ. Principles of oral oncologic surgery. In: Verstraete FJ, Lommer MJ, editors. Oral and maxillofacial surgery in dogs and cats. Philadelphia: Saunders Elsevier; 2012. p. 423–30.

60. Nemec A, Arzi B, Murphy B, et al. Prevalence and types of tooth resorption in dogs with oral tumors. Am J Vet Res 2012;73:1057–66.

61. White SC, Pharoah MJ. Principles of radiographic interpretation. In: White SC, Pharoah MJ, editors. Oral radiology principles and interpretation. St Louis (MO): Mosby Elsevier; 2009. p. 256–69.

62. Arzi B, Verstraete FJ. Clinical staging and biopsy of maxillofacial tumors. In: Verstraete FJ, Lommer MJ, editors. Oral and maxillofacial surgery in dogs and cats. Philadelphia: Saunders Elsevier; 2012. p. 373–80.

63. Liptak JM, Withrow SJ. Cancer of the gastrointestinal tract: intestinal tumors. In: Withrow S, Vail D, editors. Small animal clinical oncology. St Louis (MO): Saunders Elsevier; 2007. p. 491–503.

64. McEntee MC. Clinical behavior of nonodontogenic tumors. In: Verstraete FJ, Lommer MJ, editors. Oral and maxillofacial surgery in dogs and cats. Philadelphia: Saunders Elsevier; 2012. p. 387–402.

65. Chamberlain TP, Lommer MJ. Clinical behavior of odontogenic tumors. In: Verstraete FJ, Lommer MJ, editors. Oral and maxillofacial surgery in dogs and cats. Philadelphia: Saunders Elsevier; 2012. p. 403–10.

66. Lantz GC. Mandibulectomy techniques. In: Verstraete FJ, Lommer MJ, editors. Oral and maxillofacial surgery in dogs and cats. Philadelphia: Saunders Elsevier; 2012. p. 467–79.

67. Lantz GC. Maxillectomy techniques. In: Verstraete FJ, Lommer MJ, editors. Oral and maxillofacial surgery in dogs and cats. Philadelphia: Saunders Elsevier; 2012. p. 451–65.

68. Regezi JA, Sciubba JJ, Jordan RC. Cysts of the jaws and neck. In: Regezi JA, Sciubba JJ, Jordan RC, editors. Oral pathology: clinical pathologic correlations. St Louis (MO): Elsevier Saunders; 2012. p. 246–69.

69. Chamberlain TP, Verstraete FJ. Clinical behavior and management of odontogenic cysts. In: Verstraete FJ, Lommer MJ, editors. Oral and maxillofacial surgery in dogs and cats. Philadelphia: Saunders Elsevier; 2012. p. 481–94.

70. Verstraete FJ, Zin BP, Kass PH, et al. Clinical signs and histologic findings in dogs with odontogenic cysts: 41 cases (1995-2010). J Am Vet Med Assoc 2011;239: 1470–6.

71. Manfra Marretta S, Lommer MJ. Management of maxillofacial osteonecrosis. In: Verstraete FJ, Lommer MJ, editors. Oral and maxillofacial surgery in dogs and cats. Philadelphia: Saunders Elsevier; 2012. p. 519–24.

72. Boutoille F, Hennet P. Maxillary osteomyelitis in two Scottish terrier dogs with chronic ulcerative paradental stomatitis. J Vet Dent 2011;28:96–100.

73. Stepaniuk K. Bisphosphonate related osteonecrosis of the jaws: a review. J Vet Dent 2011;28:277–81.

74. Buelow ME, Manfra Marretta S, Barger A, et al. Lingual lesions in the dog and cat: recognition, diagnosis, and treatment. J Vet Dent 2011;28:151–62.

75. Buelow ME, Manfra Marretta S. Major glossectomy in the dog. J Vet Dent 2011; 28:210–4.

76. Marretta JJ, Garrett LD, Manfra Marretta S. Feline oral squamous cell carcinoma: an overview. Vet Med 2007;102:392–408.

77. Dennis MM, Ehrhart N, Duncan CG, et al. Frequency of and risk factors associated with lingual lesions in dogs: 1,196 cases (1995-2004). J Am Vet Med Assoc 2006;228:1533–7.

78. Brown DC. Small intestine. In: Tobias KM, Johnston SA, editors. Veterinary surgery: small animal. Philadelphia: Elsevier Saunders; 2012. p. 1513–41.
79. Lane JG. Surgical treatment of sialoceles. In: Verstraete FJ, Lommer MJ, editors. Oral and maxillofacial surgery in dogs and cats. Philadelphia: Saunders Elsevier; 2012. p. 501–10.
80. Temizsoylu MD, Avki S. Complete ventral ankyloglossia in three related dogs. J Am Vet Med Assoc 2003;223:1443–5.
81. Wiggs RB, Lobprise HB. Anatomy, diagnosis and management of disorders of the tongue. J Vet Dent 1993;10:16–23.
82. Seguin B. Surgical treatment of tongue, lip and cheek tumors. In: Verstraete FJ, Lommer MJ, editors. Oral and maxillofacial surgery in dogs and cats. Philadelphia: Saunders Elsevier; 2012. p. 431–49.
83. Dvorak LD, Beaver DP, Ellison GW, et al. Major glossectomy in dogs: a case series and proposed classification system. J Am Anim Hosp Assoc 2004;40:331–7.
84. Anderson GM. Soft tissues of the oral cavity. In: Tobias KM, Johnston SA, editors. Veterinary surgery: small animal. Philadelphia: Elsevier Saunders; 2012. p. 1425–38.
85. Smeak DD. Cheiloplasty. In: Verstraete FJ, Lommer MJ, editors. Oral and maxillofacial surgery in dogs and cats. Philadelphia: Saunders Elsevier; 2012. p. 511–4.
86. Pavletic MM. Facial reconstruction. In: Pavletic MM, editor. Atlas of small animal reconstructive surgery. Philadelphia: WB Saunders; 1999. p. 297–329.

Laser and Radiosurgery in Veterinary Dentistry

Jan Bellows, DVM, DAVDC, DABVP

KEYWORDS

- Laser • Radiosurgery • Oral surgery • CO_2 • Diode • Therapy laser

KEY POINTS

- The CO_2 and Diode lasers are most commonly used in veterinary dental surgery.
- Radiosurgery is useful for incising and excising oral tissues.
- Therapy low level lasers help to decrease oral inflammation.

LASER AND RADIOSURGERY IN VETERINARY DENTISTRY

The laser unit produces light of a single color wherein all light waves are coherent, which means that each wave is identical in physical size and shape. Basically a laser is concentrated light focused into an extremely small spot delivering a large amount of energy. This monochromatic, coherent wave of light energy emerges from the laser device as an efficient source of energy. When the laser light hits an object, it reflects, transmits, scatters, or is absorbed. The surgical laser can be adjusted to incise, excise, vaporize (ablate), cauterize, or amputate oral tissues. One important difference compared with scalpel surgery is that hemostasis can be provided while the tissue is being incised.

Lasers are named for the material contained within the center of the device, called the optical cavity. The core of the cavity is comprised of chemical elements, molecules, or compounds (the active medium), which can be a container of gas, a crystal, or a solid-state semiconductor. One popular laser in veterinary dentistry uses carbon dioxide as a gaseous active medium. Other devices are solid-state semiconductor wafers made with multiple layers of metals or solid rods of garnet crystal grown with various combinations of other elements. For simplicity the semiconductor lasers are called diodes, and the crystal lasers are designated with acronyms such as Nd:YAG (neodymium-doped yttrium, aluminum, garnet), Er,Cr:YSGG (erbium, chromium-doped yttrium, scandium, gallium, garnet), or Er:YAG (erbium-doped

All Pets Dental, 17100 Royal Palm Boulevard, Weston, FL 33326, USA
E-mail address: Dentalvet@aol.com

Vet Clin Small Anim 43 (2013) 651–668
http://dx.doi.org/10.1016/j.cvsm.2013.02.012
0195-5616/13/$ – see front matter © 2013 Elsevier Inc. All rights reserved.

yttrium, aluminum, garnet). This article will focus on the carbon dioxide (CO_2), diode, and therapy lasers and on radiosurgery as it applies to dentistry.

1. Diode and Nd:YAG wavelengths target the pigments in soft tissue and pathogens, and inflammatory and vascularized tissue.
2. CO_2 lasers interact with free water molecules in soft tissue and vaporize the intracellular water of pathogens.

Depending on the instrument's parameters and the optical properties of the tissue, the temperature will rise and various effects will occur. In general, most nonsporulating bacteria, including anaerobes, are readily deactivated at temperatures of 50°C. At 60°C, hemostasis can be obtained and inflammatory soft tissue present in periodontal disease can be removed. Soft tissue excisional or incisional surgery is accomplished at 100°C, wherein vaporization of intracellular and extracellular water causes ablation or removal of biologic tissue.

Differences in tissue content of substances such as water, protein, hemoglobin, and melanin can substantially influence the affect of a specific wavelength.

The cutting action depends on the type of laser and the targeted tissue. Generally, lasers operated in continuous mode cut comparably to a scalpel, whereas those in lower-pulsed modes (10–20 pulses/second) incise slower or rougher. For this reason, diode lasers used in contact mode often drag when making oral incisions.

CARBON DIOXIDE LASER (10,600 NM)

The water content of oral tissues absorbs the CO_2 wavelength (**Fig. 1**). CO_2 lasers are used in oral surgery for precise cutting or vaporizing soft tissue with hemostasis. Typically, "what you see is what you get" when using the CO_2 laser. Shallow thermal

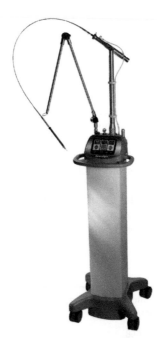

Fig. 1. Twenty-Watt CO_2 laser. (*Courtesy of* Aesculight Luxacare, Woodinville, WA, USA; with permission.)

necrosis zones of only 100 to 300 μm at incised tissue edges are typical. The diode laser commonly vaporizes several millimeters during oral procedures.

Inorganic components of teeth and bone also absorb at the CO_2 wavelength. High temperatures (>100°C) are required to truly vaporize hard tissue. Continuous-wave CO_2 lasers cannot ablate or cut calcified tissue without inducing severe charring and thermal injury to surrounding tissue, and should not be used for that purpose.

Modes used for dental applications include continuous wave and variations of the pulsed mode. For ablation of oral lesions, the superpulse mode is desirable because the pulse width is shorter than the thermal relaxation time of oral soft tissue, decreasing the lateral thermal damage.

For ablation of oral lesions, laser power is set between 10 and 15 W in continuous-wave mode or 20 W in a pulsed mode. Ablation laser beam spot size varies between 2 and 3 mm in diameter using the 0.4- to 0.8-mm tip size. Using paintbrush strokes (rastering), multiple applications of the laser are placed within the marginal outline. Moist gauze is used to wipe away the treated area of mucosa. When performed properly, only minimal charring is evident. Excessive heat conduction appears as charred tissue. Charring results from prolonged contact between the laser beam and the tissue and is usually caused by moving the handpiece too slowly across the lesion.

To use the CO_2 laser as a precise cutting instrument in oral surgery, the laser beam spot size at its focal point should be 0.2 to 0.3 mm from the tissue. Traction and countertraction of tissue with surgical sponges and tissue forceps facilitate incisional surgical technique (**Fig. 2**).

DIODE LASER

Diode lasers in the 800- to 980-nm range use contact mode optical fibers for cutting and vaporizing oral tissue. Diode laser energy penetrates deeper (1–3 mm) than CO_2 lasers. Diode lasers can be used for gingivectomy, gingival troughing, subgingival curettage, and other soft tissue procedures.

Frequent water irrigation is used as a heat sink to decrease thermal damage when using the diode laser in the oral cavity. Changes in tissue texture and color are best indicators of the diode's laser effect.

For contact incisional application, mechanical pressure is not necessary; the surgeon needs only sufficient force to guide the handpiece along the incision. The fiber can be used first in noncontact (free beam) and then placed in contact mode, but not vice versa. When the fiber is in contact mode, it should be kept in contact mode (**Fig. 3**).

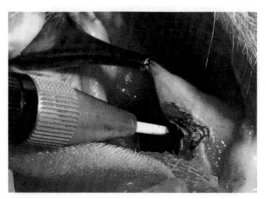

Fig. 2. CO_2 incising oral tissue.

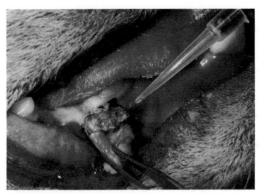

Fig. 3. Diode laser used in contact mode to excise oral mass.

LOW-LEVEL LASER THERAPY

The names to identify and differentiate therapeutic lasers from surgical lasers include soft, cold, low-intensity laser therapy, and low-level laser therapy (LLLT) (**Fig. 4**A).

The principle of using LLLT in dental procedures is to supply biostimulative light energy to the body's cells. Cellular photoreceptors (eg, cytochromophores and antenna pigments) can absorb low-level laser light and pass it on to mitochondria, which promptly produce the cell's fuel, ATP. The most popularly described treatment benefits of LLLT are analgesic effects and enhanced wound healing. In humans the analgesic effect is explained by the LLLT effect on enhanced synthesis of endorphin, decreased c-fiber activity, bradykinin, and altered pain threshold.

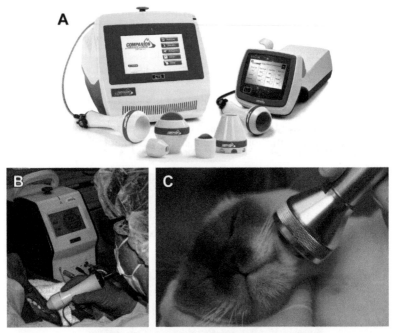

Fig. 4. (*A*) Low-level laser therapy units. (*Courtesy of* Companion Therapy, Newark, DE; with permission.) (*B*) Laser applied to the apex after root canal therapy. (*C*) Application of low-level laser therapy after full-mouth extraction stomatitis surgery.

POSTOPERATIVE THERAPY

The purpose of using LLLT as part of postoperative therapy is to provide patients with minimal pain and a shortened healing period. It can be applied to many dental procedures, including endodontics, periodontal treatments, and oral surgery.

For endodontics, 1 to 2 J of energy are applied from the wand-like probe to the periapical area (see **Fig. 4**B). For periodontal and operative surgery, the wand is focused directly over the operative area. These applications can occur in the immediate postoperative period or continued as once- or twice-weekly treatments when the patient has had more extensive surgical procedures (see **Fig. 4**C).

LASER SAFETY

The tooth pulp and periodontal ligament are sensitive to thermal injury, and can tolerate a rise in temperature for a short period of no more than a few degrees Celsius. The veterinarian using a laser in the oral cavity must be concerned with possible damage to sensitive oral structures, including the tooth pulp, periodontal ligament, and bone. The actual zone of damage that can be tolerated depends on the proximity and sensitivity of nearby tissue.

Lasers in the dental operating area have the potential to ignite materials on and around the surgical site. Examples of combustible materials include dry cotton swabs, gauze sponges, wooden tongue blades, alcohol wipes, and plastic instruments.

A potential fire danger in laser surgery of the oral cavity is the endotracheal tube. Special care must be taken to prevent the tube from coming in contact with the laser during surgery. Ignition of the endotracheal tube may produce a fire with a blowtorch effect inside the animal's airway. Premoistened gauze should be packed in the pharyngeal area to avoid injury. Unfortunately, oral procedures often are hemorrhagic, camouflaging the packed sponges. When premoistened gauze sponges are packed in the pharyngeal area, extreme care must be taken to ensure removal after the procedure. A tip is to appoint the surgical technician to count the number of sponges packed and removed during each procedure. Laser-safe endotracheal tubes are also available for use during laser surgery.

The plume or lased smoke is a by-product of laser surgery. The laser plume is primarily composed of vaporized water (steam); toxic substances, such as formaldehyde, hydrogen cyanide, and hydrocarbon particles; and cellular products. The smoke can be irritating to those exposed. A high-volume laser smoke evacuator should be used to remove the plume during oral procedures.

The following precautions should be taken when performing laser surgery:

- When the laser is in use, place a warning sign to alert those who enter the operatory.
- Ensure that everyone in the operatory wears shielded eyeglasses. With CO_2 lasers, clear prescription or plastic glasses can be worn.
- Shield nontarget areas. Wet gauze packs, especially around the endotracheal tube and caudal pharynx, are effective shields against the CO_2 laser beam effects. Wet gauze is effective because of the CO_2 laser energy's high absorption into water. Optical backstops consisting of moistened gauze may be placed below the target tissue to protect adjacent tissues from the CO_2 laser beam.
- Remove reflective metal materials from the immediate surgical area. Nonreflective surgical instruments are recommended.
- Use a vacuum evacuation system to draw off the plume cloud created when tissue vaporizes. If inhaled, the smoke plume may be irritating, infectious, or carcinogenic.

- Remove combustible materials, such as alcohol preps, flammable inhalant agents, oxygen, and drapes, from the immediate laser beam area.

RADIOSURGERY

A 4-MHz radiosignal energized surgical instrument can be used to produce a fine incision with minimal heat to incise, incise with coagulation, or only coagulate (**Fig. 5**). This technique is helpful for oral surgery, wherein proximity to underlying soft and hard tissue requires a delicate incision. Traditional electrosurgical machines that operate at lower frequencies of 1.5 to 2.5 MHz produce higher temperatures in tissue and are not recommended in proximity to underlying osseous tissue. High-frequency radiosurgery produces less tissue alteration and lateral heat to the surrounding tissue than does the low-frequency electrosurgical signal.

The clinician chooses the waveform that best meets the surgical objective.

- The fully filtered and rectified waveform produces 90% cutting and 10% coagulation. The fully filtered waveform is a pure continuous flow of high-frequency energy. The filter provides a continuous nonpulsating current, resembling a scalpel incision. The fully filtered and rectified waveform can be used for biopsy, frenectomy, mass removal, and surgery near bone.
- The fully rectified waveform produces 50% cutting and 50% coagulation. The fully rectified waveform can be used for gingivectomy, gingivoplasty, and troughing procedures for crown impressions. The fully rectified waveform should not be used when operating near bone.
- The partially rectified waveform produces 90% coagulation and 10% cutting with increased lateral heat and tissue shrinkage. Partially rectified waveforms should not be used near bone. Hemostasis can be accomplished using a unipole ball, broad-needle electrode, or bipolar forceps on vessels smaller than 2 mm in diameter.
- The fulguration waveform uses a half-wave current for coagulation and destruction of tissue. The electrode does not actually touch tissue, but rather coagulates through energy transferred to tissue. The fulguration waveform may be used for hemostasis near bone, removal and destruction of cyst remnants, and destruction of fistulous tracts. The electrode used is in the shape of a pencil or sphere and is positioned approximately 0.5 mm from the tissue surface.

Bipolar electrosurgery uses 2 equal-sized electrodes parallel to each other to make pinpoint coagulation an easy task. The waveform operates at a frequency of 4 MHz. Bipolar electrosurgery is especially useful when surgery is near dental hard tissue and bone.

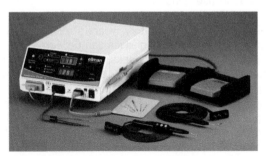

Fig. 5. Radiosurgery system. (*Courtesy of* Surgitron 4.0, Ellman International, Oceanside, NY, USA; with permission.)

The power setting determines the amount of energy transferred to the tissue. The setting should be high enough to prevent drag of the electrode through the tissue but not too high to create sparking. In one study, Silverman and colleagues[1] found that the char penetration was significantly less (0.158 mm) with radiosurgery compared with CO_2 laser (0.215 mm).

Electrode tips
- Diamond-shaped tips can be used for removing tissue that requires suturing. Diamond-shaped tips are commonly used for small biopsies. Only the bottom third of the electrode should penetrate the tissue, creating a V-shaped incision.
- Small elliptical loop tips can be used for gingival contouring and crown-lengthening procedures.
- Larger-loop tips can be used for gingivectomy and operculectomy.
- Triangle-shaped tips can be used for gingivoplasty and removal of the interproximal papilla.
- The Vari-Tip electrode (Ellman, Oceanside, NY) can be used in many applications (as seen in **Fig. 11**b and **Fig. 12**b). The Vari-Tip length is adjustable.
- Ball-shaped tips are used for gross coagulation.
- Pencil-point tips can be used for fine coagulation.
- Fulgurating tips are used for gross superficial destruction of tissue after biopsy, and for hemostasis during osseous surgery.

RADIOSURGICAL TECHNIQUES

Unlike with a scalpel blade, no pressure is required with radiosurgical techniques. The technique is as follows:

1. Hold the handpiece like a pen rather than a scalpel handle.
2. Move the electrode as rapidly as possible across the tissue in a brush-like stroke.
3. Keep the electrode perpendicular to the tissue surface.
4. Periodically remove buildup of charred coagulated tissue on the electrode tip.
5. Do not engage power to the electrode until the tip is in contact with the tissue.
6. Allow 8 seconds between cutting strokes in the same site to allow heat to dissipate.
7. Moisten the operative site with gauze soaked in sterile saline to reduce tissue resistance.

SMALL ANIMAL DENTAL LASER PROCEDURES
Periodontal Pocket Surgery

It is well accepted that periodontal disease is an inflammatory condition caused by the presence of bacteria. A recent study by Fontana and colleagues[2] on 40 rats with induced periodontal disease showed that a diode laser at 810-nm wavelength induced considerable bacterial elimination after laser energy application. In this study, bacterial samples were taken from periodontal pockets before and after subgingival laser irradiation. The microbiological analysis showed that bacteria such as *Prevotella* spp, beta-hemolytic streptococci, *Fusobacterium* spp, and *Pseudomonas* spp were significantly reduced.

An in vitro study by Kreisler and colleagues[3] on the proliferation rate of human periodontal ligament fibroblasts reported interesting findings on the biologic effects of a soft tissue laser. Human periodontal ligament fibroblasts were cultured and irradiated with an 809-nm wavelength diode laser. The rate of proliferation, determined by relative fluorescence units, was checked at 24, 48, and 72 hours after irradiation. The results indicated that cells in the test group (irradiated) showed a considerably higher proliferation activity than the controls. The differences were discernible up to a 72-hour observation time, and those differences were statistically significant. The same authors suggested that the laser treatment may be beneficial in regenerative periodontal therapy.

Clinical studies on humans with an 810-nm diode laser have been conducted and published by Moritz and colleagues.[4] Fifty patients with adult periodontitis were randomly subdivided into 2 groups. Subgingival bacteria samples were collected in all patients. Patients were treated either with laser or subgingival irrigations of hydrogen peroxide. After 6 months, values of the periodontal indices and further microbiologic samples were measured. The total bacterial count, and specific bacteria (eg, *Actinobacillus actinomycetemcomitans, Prevotella intermedia*, and *Porphyromonas gingivalis*), were assessed. The sites that received the subgingival laser treatment exhibited a much lower bacterial count. Furthermore, the reduction of values of bleeding on probing was 96.9% in the laser group compared with 66.7% in the control group. The authors concluded that diode laser treatment after scaling and root planing had a bactericidal effect and reduced inflammation.

The typical protocol for the use of a diode laser as an adjunct to conventional periodontal therapy involves ultrasonic scaling and root planing with horizontal strokes using a curette.

The diode laser can be used in the continuous or pulsed mode, and the average power can range from 0.8 to 1.0 W. The fiber-optic is inserted into the pocket to reach approximately 1.0 mm from the bottom of the defect. To prepare the laser for use, cleave and strip the fiber, attach the handpiece and cannula, and turn on the laser.

To begin sulcular debridement, insert the fiber in a vertical direction toward the bottom of the pocket with the laser tip oriented toward the soft tissue facing the pocket. Move the fiber in a horizontal and vertical fashion at a slow, moderate speed, keeping the fiber tip in contact with the epithelium and/or parallel to the root surface. A fine water spray can be used during the laser treatment for rinsing, and constant suction is required to aspirate the fumes that form during the ablation of the inflamed tissues. The amount of time to apply laser energy is proportional to the pocket depth (3 mm to 3 seconds, 4 mm to 4 seconds).

The CO_2 laser has also been shown to be effective in treating periodontal disease. In a study performed on Beagles with surgically induced furcation exposures, CO_2 laser treatment resulted in gingival growth of 1.2 mm and histologic evidence of new cementum formation.

When used in a defocused mode (≈ 4 mm spot size), the laser can provide precise surface vaporization and wound sterilization. It is indicated for removal of inflammatory or infectious lesions because the heat of the laser sterilizes both viral and bacterial particles.

Gingivoplasty

Gingivoplasty can be performed in cases of minimal lingually displaced canine teeth to remove gingival areas of mandibular canine tooth penetration. For the gingivoplasty, 8 to 10 W of superpulsed CO_2 laser energy in a defocused mode is used to vaporize sequential layers of tissue until the mandibular canine tooth is no longer impinging on the gingiva. The client should be advised that multiple re-treatments may be necessary if the teeth do not move, and because the vaporized impinged gingiva often regrows.

Gingivectomy

The CO_2 laser is versatile for precise incising or vaporizing of the gingiva. Higher CO_2 laser power (10–15 W) is used to remove moderate (<2 mm) amounts of hyperplastic gingiva. For thicker areas, the CO_2 laser may be used in a defocused or diverging mode for coagulation to help control bleeding after scalpel-blade gingivectomy (**Fig. 6**).

Gingival Hyperplasia

For the treatment of gingival hyperplasia, the CO_2 laser is set at 4 to 8 W in continuous mode and applied over the incised area after blade gingivectomy to shape the gingiva and aid hemostasis. The diode laser can also be used similar to a scalpel to remove hyperplastic gingival tissues (**Fig. 7**).

The radiosurgical unit is most useful in the treatment of gingival hyperplasia because of its incising and coagulation abilities. Hyperplastic tissue can be incised with either filtered or fully rectified waveforms. The filtered waveform is used in areas where the tissue is delicate and minimal tissue alteration is desired. The fully rectified waveform is used where the tissue is thick and fibrotic or in areas of hyperemia that require immediate hemostasis. The flexible fine wire electrode (Vari-Tip, Ellman) for is used for gingivoplasty set to a fully rectified filtered waveform. Gingivectomy can also be performed using a loop electrode set to a fully filtered and rectified waveforms. The incision angle should be set to be similar to the physiologic angle of the gingiva (30–40°). If

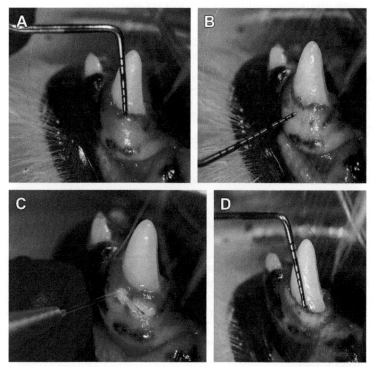

Fig. 6. (*A*) Checking pocket depth with periodontal probe. (*B*) Marking probing depth on attached gingiva. (*C*) Diode laser used to excise attached gingiva. (*D*) Postoperative appearance.

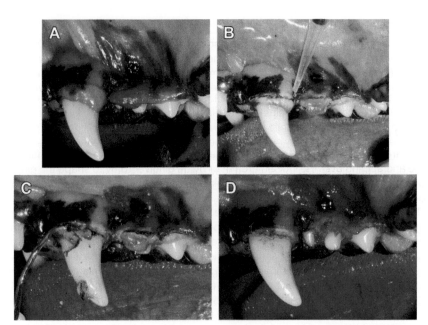

Fig. 7. (*A*) Gingival hyperplasia evident on the buccal surfaces of the canine tooth and first, second, and third premolars. (*B*) Diode laser used to excise excessive gingiva. (*C*) Curette used to remove hyperplastic gingiva. (*D*) Postoperative appearance.

necessary, bleeding vessels should be coagulated using a ball electrode with the partially rectified waveform setting. Excised tissue should be removed with a curette.

Flap Surgery

Flap surgery incisions can be performed with the diode, CO_2 laser, or radiosurgical unit. Human patients interviewed in one study reported less pain with laser surgery than with scalpel blade flap incisions.

A reverse bevel incision along the gingival margin can be made using a fine-wire radiosurgical electrode, as follows:

1. Make interdental incisions with the electrode.
2. Use a Freer or Molt elevator to separate the mucoperiosteal flap from the underlying bone.
3. Expose the flap and suture similarly to the non-scalpel blade procedure.

Operculectomy

Operculectomy removes overgrown dense fibrous tissue covering an impacted immature tooth to help eruption through removing the gingival obstruction.

Operculectomy can be performed with a laser to excise gingival tissue over an impacted tooth using 10 W of CO_2 laser energy with a 0.3 mm spot to incise a mucosal flap and expose the underlying crown. The diode laser and radiosurgical unit can also be used to expose the underlying crown (**Fig. 8**).

Tongue Lesion Surgery

Solitary and multiple tongue lesions can be excised using the CO_2 laser. A laser energy setting of 10 W with a spot/tip size of 0.4 mm is commonly used. Penetration into the

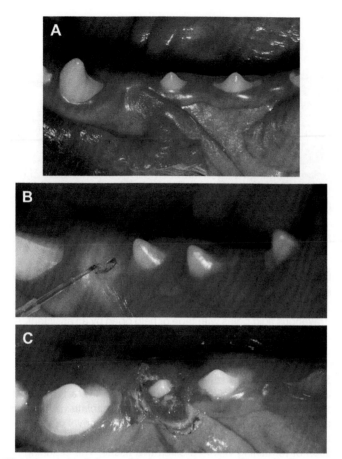

Fig. 8. (*A*) Clinically missing left mandibular first premolar. (*B*) CO_2 laser used to remove the gingiva over the partially erupted tooth. (*C*) Postsurgical appearance, crown exposed.

muscularis layer should be avoided. Absorbable sutures are generally placed if the postsurgical defect is greater than 3 mm (**Fig. 9**).

Gum Chewers Lesions

Removal of sublingual tissue folds (gum chewers lesions) can also be accomplished using the CO_2 laser. After excision, the laser power is decreased to 4 W with a defocused beam to seal small blood vessels. Sutures are not usually needed.

Feline Oropharyngeal Inflammation Therapy

CO_2 and diode laser ablation may be helpful as an adjunct therapy when proliferative caudal stomatitis is present and multiple extractions have been performed. After laser ablation, the inflammatory mass is replaced with fibrous less-reactive scar tissue. Laser treatment does not cure feline oropharyngeal inflammation and should not be recommended as monotherapy for this condition. Laser rastering will decrease the surface area for plaque bacteria to accumulate, lessening the antigenic load. Often monthly retreatment is necessary for the 3 months after extractions, followed by semiannual reevaluation and possible laser retreatment.

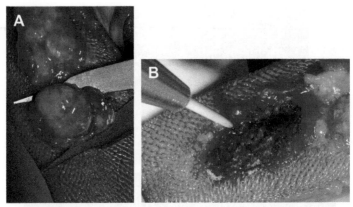

Fig. 9. (*A*) Gross debulking of an eosinophilic granuloma on a cat's tongue, (*B*) CO₂ laser ablation of the underling tissue for additional abnormality elimination and hemostasis.

An antiinflammatory dose of dexamethasone sodium phosphate is administered (0.1 mg/kg intravenously) before laser ablation to minimize oropharyngeal swelling. The patient is placed in sternal recumbency with the maxillae supported between 2 adjustable intravenous fluid poles with tape or held open by an assistant. After insuring adequate seal of the endotracheal cuff, a moistened gauze is wrapped around the endotracheal tube in the pharynx to prevent the laser from contacting it. A smoke evacuator is placed near the patient's mouth.

Four-quadrant regional anesthesia with long-acting 0.5% bupivacaine is administered. The CO_2 laser is set to 6 W in continuous mode delivered to a 0.8-mm ceramic tip used in focused (cutting) noncontact mode to thermoablate visible proliferative tissue of the caudal oral cavity (**Fig. 10**A–C). After gross removal of proliferative tissue, the wave-guide can be changed to accommodate a scanning handpiece capable of efficient ablation of remaining visible proliferative tissue. The scanning handpiece is used at a setting of 6 W in continuous mode. The tissue at the base of the excised portions is ablated layer by layer, which will usually create a char. Removal of char is recommended using saline-soaked cotton tipped applicators. This process is repeated multiple times until all visible proliferative tissue is removed. The remaining tissue shows a decreased tendency for spontaneous bleeding when touched with a gauze sponge. The treated surfaces are sprayed with 2 mg of lidocaine before extubation.

Laser therapy is performed at the initial extraction surgery to ablate inflamed gingiva (see **Fig. 10**D–K). Clinically, laser therapy seems to increase patient comfort, as evidenced by a prompt return to eating.

Oral Biopsy

Lasers can be used for excisional or incisional biopsies with controlled bleeding and improved visualization. Laser excision permits histologic evaluation and establishment of clean margins by a pathologist knowledgeable in laser-tissue interaction.

The CO_2 laser can incise soft tissue in a noncontact mode, making it particularly useful for biopsy on buccal and lingual surfaces. An excisional outline can be made rapidly, using repeated single pulses (5 W, 0.3-mm spot size) to circumscribe the desired target tissue. One edge of the incised margin can be elevated with forceps and the lesion undermined and harvested at the correct depth of dissection with the laser. With the beam defocused, the surgical wound is briskly "painted" in one pass

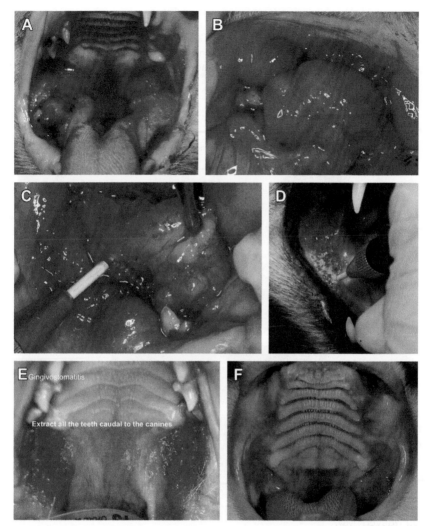

Fig. 10. (*A*) Marked caudal stomatitis. (*B*) Proliferative tissue contributing to plaque retention. (*C*) CO_2 laser used to debulk proliferative tissue. (*D*) Proper handpiece distance for ablation of inflamed tissue and as part of follow-up therapy. (*E*) Feline stomatitis and caudal mucositis. (*F*) Persistent inflammation 2 months after surgery. (*G*) Lasered areas in the caudal oral cavity. (*H*) Healed areas of inflammation 4 months postoperatively. (*I*) Caudal mucositis 1 year after full-mouth extraction. (*J*) CO_2 laser ablation. (*K*) Inflamed areas eliminated.

to seal off small lymphatics, blood vessels, and nerve endings. Sutures are not required unless the defect is greater than 8 mm. Radiosurgical units and diode lasers can also be used for oral biopsies (**Fig. 11**).

Oral Mass Surgery

The oral cavity is a common location for masses. The laser and radiosurgical unit allow relatively easy access to most of the lesions with excellent hemostasis (**Fig. 12**).

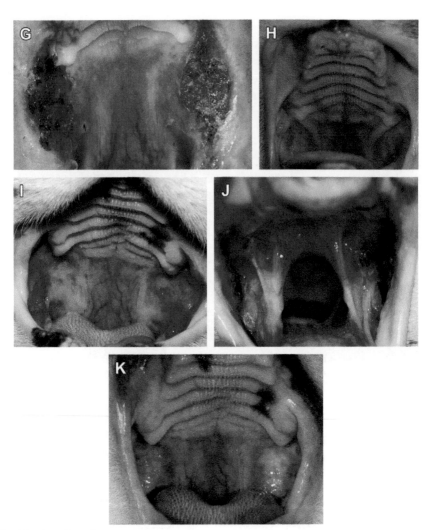

Fig. 10. (*continued*)

Laser use in oral cancer surgery provides advantages of hemostasis, decreased postoperative edema, and diminished infection. Additionally, because of the laser's ability to seal small blood vessels and lymphatics, there is a reduced likelihood of inducing tumor microemboli during the procedure.

Palliative treatment for nonresectable masses can also be accomplished using the laser and radiosurgical unit to debulk the mass before radiation therapy or to periodically decrease the tumor size to make the patient more comfortable.

Troughing for Crown Impressions

A trough is a channel created in the soft tissue around a crown preparation to allow space for placement of impression material. To create a trough, a thin layer of tissue from the sulcus is excised, exposing the crown margin preparation. If prepared

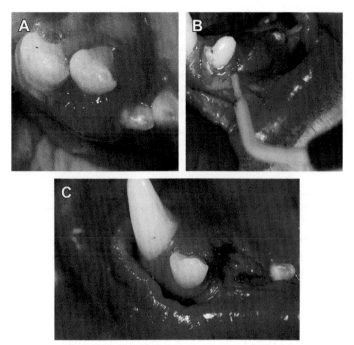

Fig. 11. (*A*) Oral mass surrounding a maxillary incisor. (*B*) Oral mass partially excised with radiosurgical unit after incisor extraction. (*C*) Postoperative appearance.

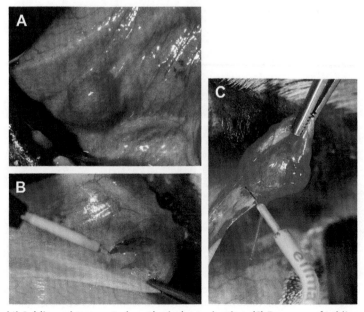

Fig. 12. (*A*) Sublingual mass noted on physical examination. (*B*) Exposure of sublingual mass with radiosurgical unit. (*C*) Fine dissection of the mass.

with a scalpel blade, the incised gingiva bleeds, generating additional surgical time for hemostasis and potential impression inaccuracy. The CO_2 or diode laser tip held in a near-parallel position to the tooth can form a trough. Care should be taken to avoid having the beam contact enamel or dentin (**Fig. 13**). The process is as follows:

1. Prepare the crown with the finish line at the gingival margin.
2. Place the CO_2, diode laser, or radiosurgical tip parallel to the tooth to prevent removal of excessive tissue height.
3. Move the tip from mesial to distal around the tooth to create the trough.
4. Irrigate the area postoperatively with 0.12% chlorhexidine.

Frenectomy

Frenectomy is used to loosen tight mandibular lips pressing debris against the gingiva overlying the mandibular canines. The process is as follows:

1. Dissect the frenulum toward the mandibular insertion with multiple stokes with the CO_2, diode, or radiosurgical unit using the Vari-Tip electrode in fully filtered waveform. Make the first incision vertically from the base of the bone where the frenulum attaches between the central incisors to the underside of the lip (**Fig. 14**).
2. Make a third or fourth horizontal releasing incision to remove the frenula from the oral cavity.
3. Suture the resultant defect with 4-0 or 5-0 absorbable suture on a cutting needle.

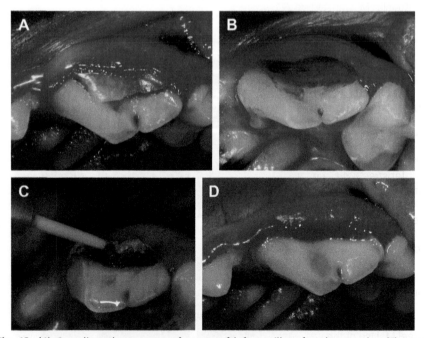

Fig. 13. (A) Complicated crown root fracture of left maxillary fourth premolar. (B) Large gingival defect remains after removal of the fractured segment. (C) CO_2 laser gingivectomy after root canal therapy. (D) Appearance 1 month after surgery before crown restoration, showing the defect eliminated.

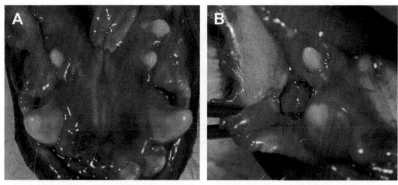

Fig. 14. (*A*) Tight frenulum causing periodontal disease of the mandibular canines and first premolars (*B*) CO_2 laser used to excise frenulum, releasing the contact.

REFERENCES

1. Silverman EB, Read RW, Boyle CR, et al. Histologic Comparison of Canine Skin Biopsies Collected Using Monopolar lectrosurgery, CO_2 Laser, Radiowave Radiosurgery, Skin Biopsy Punch, and Scalpel. Vet Surg 2007;36:50–6.
2. Fontana CR, Kurachi C, Mendonça CR, et al. Microbial reduction in periodontal pockets under exposition of a medium power diode laser: an experimental study in rats. Lasers Surg Med 2004;35(4):263–8.
3. Kreisler M, Christoffers AB, Al-Haj H, et al. Low level 809-nm diode laser-induced in vitro stimulation of the proliferation of human gingival fibroblasts. Lasers Surg Med 2002;30(5):365–9.
4. Andreas Moritz. Treatment of Periodontal Pockets with a Diode Laser. Lasers in Surgery and Medicine 1998;22:302–11.

FURTHER READINGS

Coleton S. Lasers in surgical periodontics and oral medicine. Dent Clin North Am 2004;48:937–62.
Crespi R, Covani U, Andreana S, et al. CO2 laser therapy in periodontal disease [abstract]. J Periodontol 1993;64:1103.
Crespi R, Covani U, Margarone JE, et al. Periodontal tissue regeneration in beagle dogs after laser therapy. Lasers Surg Med 1997;21:395–402.
Dederich DN. Laser/tissue interaction: what happens to laser light when is strikes tissue? J Am Dent Assoc 1993;124:57–61.
Fontana CR, Kurachi C, Mendonca CR, et al. Microbial reduction in periodontal pockets under exposition of a medium power diode laser: an experimental study in rats. Lasers Surg Med 2004;35:263–8.
Gutierrez T. Utilizing an 810 nm diode laser for bacterial reduction and coagulation as an adjunctive treatment of periodontal disease. Contemporary Oral Hygiene 2005;5:20–1.
Israel M. Use of the CO2 laser in soft tissue and periodontal surgery. Pract Periodontics Aesthet Dent 1994;6:57–64.
Karu TI. Photobiological fundamentals of low-power laser therapy. IEEE J Quantum Electronics 1987;23:1703–17.

Kreisler M, Christoffers AB, Willershausen B, et al. Effect of low-level GaAlAs laser irradiation on the proliferation rate of human periodontal ligament fibroblasts: an in vitro study. J Clin Periodontol 2003;30:353–8.

Lewis JR, Tsugawa AJ, Reiter AM. Use of CO_2 laser as an adjunctive treatment for caudal stomatitis in a cat. J Vet Dent 2007;24:240–9.

Mavrogiannis M, Thomason JM, Seymour RA. Lasers in periodontology. Dent Update 2004;31:535–47.

Moritz A, Gutknecht N, Doertbudak O, et al. Bacterial reduction in periodontal pockets through irradiation with a diode laser: a pilot study. J Clin Laser Med Surg 1997;15:33–7.

Moritz A, Schoop U, Goharkhay K, et al. Treatment of periodontal pockets with a diode laser. Lasers Surg Med 1998;22:302–11.

Ohshiro T, Calderhead RG. Low level laser therapy: a practical introduction. Chichester (England): John Wiley and Sons; 1988.

Pick RM, Pecaro BC, Silberman CJ. The laser gingivectomy. The use of the CO2 laser for the removal of phenytoin hyperplasia. J Periodontol 1985;56:492–6.

Pick RM, Pecaro BC. Use of the CO2 laser in soft tissue dental surgery. Lasers Surg Med 1987;7:207–13.

Raffetto N. Lasers for initial periodontal therapy. Dent Clin North Am 2004;48:923–36.

Research, Science and Therapy Committee of the American Academy of Periodontology. Lasers in periodontics. J Periodontol 2002;73:1231–9.

Sakurai Y, Yamaguchi M, Abiko Y. Inhibitory effect of low-level laser irradiation on LPS-stimulated prostaglandin E2 production and cyclooxygenase-2 in human gingival fibroblasts. Eur J Oral Sci 2000;108:29–34.

Silverman E, Read R. Histologic comparison of canine skin biopsies collected using monopolar electrosurgery, CO2 laser, radiowave radiosurgery, skin biopsy punch and scalpel. Vet Surg 2007;56:36–50.

Walsh LJ. The current status of low level laser therapy in dentistry. I. Soft tissue applications. Aust Dent J 1997;42:247–54.

Anesthesia and Pain Management for Small Animals

Brett Beckman, DVM, FAVD

KEYWORDS

- Veterinary dentistry • Anesthesia • Monitoring • Small animal • Pain management
- Analgesics • Periodontal disease

KEY POINTS

- Consideration should be given to analgesics as premedications to provide preemptive analgesia and lower the minimum alveolar concentrations of the inhalant.
- The potential risks of cardiac side effects and the lack of evidence of significant benefits make the routine preanesthetic administration of antimuscarinic agents no longer recommended in human and veterinary patients.
- Opioids are the basis for effective pain management in veterinary medicine.
- A complete understanding of nociception and the effect of chronic pain states on signal modulation is important in making appropriate decisions when choosing analgesics.
- Patients vary considerably in their analgesic needs based on individual pain tolerance, whether the procedure is regional or generalized, chronicity, existing pain behaviors, the invasiveness of the surgery, and the tissue management skills of the surgeon.

ANESTHESIA AND MONITORING

Anesthesia for oral surgery in dogs and cats requires special consideration and thorough planning to maximize patient safety. Well-trained technical staff capable of providing expedient delivery of a complete quality dental radiograph series and precision anesthesia monitoring are essential. Doctors need to be well versed in dental radiographic interpretation and competent and experienced in oral surgical techniques, most specifically in surgical extractions. The work flow from patient induction to recovery involves estimate generation and client communication with multiple staff members. Full mouth dental radiography often reveals unexpected disease, which requires long anesthetic procedures, making staff efficiency a major factor in patient safety. Complete knowledge of premedications, anesthetics, and analgesic agents combined with a thorough preoperative patient assessment and careful patient monitoring from induction to complete recovery all play essential roles in patient safety.

Florida Veterinary Dentistry and Oral Surgery, 11002 Nathan Court, Punta Gorda, FL 33952, USA
E-mail address: veterinarydentistry@gmail.com

Vet Clin Small Anim 43 (2013) 669–688
http://dx.doi.org/10.1016/j.cvsm.2013.02.006   **vetsmall.theclinics.com**

Patient Assessment

Preoperative assessment and planning should allow veterinarians to identify those patients at greatest risk of anesthetic complication. This assessment is not unlike any assessment in any patient anticipating anesthesia and should comprise a minimum database, including a signalment, history, physical examination, blood profile, urinalysis, and additional testing and imaging based on the individual health status of the patient. The American Society of Anesthesiologists (ASA) Patient Status Scale categorizes patients based on specific parameters.[1] The higher the ASA status, the greater risk for anesthetic complications necessitating intervention to avoid complications preoperatively. An excellent guideline to patient preoperative assessment can be found in the American Animal Hospital Association Anesthesia Guidelines for Dogs and Cats.[2]

Anesthetic Preparation

Dental procedures require specific instrumentation depending on the procedure being performed. Periodontal procedures, including mucogingival flaps and surgical extractions, comprise most intermediate to advanced procedures performed in the typical practice that is well equipped and trained to provide quality veterinary dental care. Equipment, patient preparation components, and instrument setup and testing before the procedure minimize or eliminate problems during the procedure that could compromise care or extend anesthesia times unnecessarily. Components involved in patient preparation include preoperative and induction drugs, catheters and emergency equipment, and medications. Equipment and instrumentation include all anesthetic delivery equipment, monitors, warming devices, fluids, suction, digital dental radiographic sensors, radiographic generators, imaging software, computers, high-speed delivery systems, handpieces, lighting, and surgical instrumentation. A knowledgeable anesthesia technician and a qualified dental technician should be constantly available to work cooperatively to provide patient premedication and induction as well as monitoring and maintenance of equipment and instrumentation intraoperatively.

Premedication

Proper planning and choice of premedication agents reduce patient stress, facilitate a smooth induction and recovery, minimize doses of concurrent induction and maintenance drugs, and support multimodal and preemptive pain management. Proper dental patient evaluation includes a thorough oral evaluation, periodontal probing, and full mouth dental radiography. Predictably, these diagnostics reveal unexpected disease that results in subsequent regional or generalized surgical manipulation of the oral cavity, making opioids an excellent choice as a primary premedication agent. Combining opioids with additional agents to enhance sedation and lower the dose of individual agents is a sound clinical decision in oral surgery patients.

Discussions of individual premedications and their properties are widespread within the veterinary literature; however, agents commonly combined with opioids to enhance the premedication experience for the patient and minimize inhalant requirements, enhancing patient safety, include acepromazine (Promace), dexmedetomidine (Dexdomitor), and midazolam (Versed). A detailed listing of premedication dosages and protocols can be obtained from the Veterinary Anesthesia Support Group.[3]

The premedication administration of antimuscarinics has historically been used to mitigate anesthesia-associated hypersalivation and the accumulation of excessive airway secretions. These agents produce tachycardia and secondary increased myocardial oxygen consumption, predisposing to the development of arrhythmias.[4] Low-dose atropine sulfate (Atroject) can also cause paradoxic bradycardia by blockade of sympathetic ganglionic M1 receptors.[5] The risk of cardiac side effects and the lack of proven benefits make the routine administration of antimuscarinics for premedication no longer recommended.

Induction

Induction and recovery represent the most critical phases of an anesthetic event resulting in dramatic hemodynamic and homeostatic changes. Chamber and mask induction enhance patient stress, cause environmental contamination, delay control of the patient's airway,[6] and increase the risk of anesthesia-related death.[7] Intravenous (IV) induction agents minimize or eliminate these concerns when combined with established premedication protocols.

Propofol is likely the most widely used induction agent in veterinary dentistry. Apnea and hypotension should be anticipated; however, the short duration of action renders these characteristics manageable. Not uncommonly, patients with cardiac disease undergo dental procedures. Etomidate (Amidate) is a safe alternative to propofol because of its minimal effects on the cardiovascular system. Other induction agents available in the United States include ketamine, midazolam, and tiletimine HCl/zolazepam HCl (Telazol) Two additional agents commonly used abroad are thiopental sodium (Pentothal) and alphaxalone (Saffan). A summary of induction agents, coinduction agents, and protocols for dogs and cats has been recently published.[8]

Preparation extends to induction, whereby endotracheal tubes, stylets, laryngoscopes, and lubricants are readily available to establish the patient's airway. After proper placement, endotracheal tube insufflation should effectively seal the airway, allowing for positive pressure ventilation and avoiding excess pressure on the tracheal mucosa. A proper cuff seal is important in veterinary dentistry. The most effective way to secure the tube for dental radiography and most oral procedures is by tying it around the patient's neck behind the ears.

Intubation through a lateral pharyngostomy may be appropriate for selective patients that require extensive surgery to the oral cavity or orthopedic procedures of the mandible or maxilla (**Fig. 1**). Major advantages include improved visualization within the operative field and the direct assessment of dental occlusion.

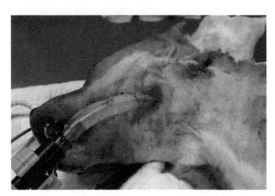

Fig. 1. Endotracheal intubation through lateral pharyngostomy for mandibular fracture repair, in a large breed dog. (*Photo Courtesy of* Luisito Pablo, DVM, Gainesville, FL.)

Monitoring

Recent estimates of mortality in small animal anesthesia seems to be of the order of 0.05% to 0.10% of healthy dogs and cats and 1% to 2% of debilitated dogs.[9] This mortality is substantially higher than reported in human anesthesia (0.02%–0.05%).[9] Strict patient monitoring is essential in avoiding anesthetic-related patient morbidity and mortality.

Veterinary practices now commonly use ancillary automated monitoring equipment to more accurately assess changes in cardiopulmonary function. However, it is important to consider the fallibility of electronic monitoring equipment, emphasizing the critical role of constant human assessment of anesthetic depth, cardiopulmonary function, body temperature, blood pressure, end-tidal carbon dioxide, and oxygen saturation in all patients undergoing an oral procedure.

Electrocardiography provides constant visual assessment of conduction abnormalities, arrhythmias, and heart rate.

Doppler ultrasonic blood flow monitoring represents a good alternative to direct cardiac auscultation and ensures auditory identification of the peripheral pulse. Adding a sphygmomanometer allows a relatively accurate noninvasive estimation of systolic blood pressure. Oscillometric blood pressure determination, although less reliable in small patients, has earned a role in effective patient monitoring.

Capnography represents a noninvasive monitoring tool for assessing expired carbon dioxide graphically over time. Deviations from normal values (40–50 mm Hg in lightly anesthetized patients) and wave form alterations can accurately identify critical changes in cardiopulmonary function requiring intervention and troubleshooting. This technology should be used in every veterinary oral surgical patient.

Although not as accurate and versatile as capnography, pulse oximetry plays a critical role in any dental operatory. A recent study showed a significant correlation between the use of pulse oximetry and the reduction of anesthesia-related death.[7]

Maintenance

The use of inhalant anesthetics represents the most convenient way to provide maintenance of anesthesia. Isoflurane (IsoFlo) and sevoflurane (SevoFlo) are the most commonly used inhalant agents. They offer a clear advantage when combined with appropriate premedication agents. In veterinary dental patients, nerve blocks can enhance the safety of inhalants, as can continuous rate infusions (CRIs). Both are discussed later in this article. The overrepresented small patient size encountered in veterinary patients with periodontal disease necessitates common use of a nonrebreathing system, particularly for patients less than 5 to 7 kg.[10]

Dental procedures require repeated manipulation of the patient to ensure efficient procurement of full mouth radiographs and access to the oral cavity for diagnostic evaluation and subsequent treatment of disease. Precautions must be taken to ensure that the patient's endotracheal tube is disconnected during movement to prevent cuff trauma to the trachea. Excessive head and neck manipulation can result in increased vagal tone and bradycardia and should be avoided. Careful cleaning of the caudal oral cavity with gauze and cotton-tipped applicators followed by a thorough visual evaluation of the entire oropharynx before extubation eliminates complications caused by aspiration.

Individual patient challenges increase anesthetic complications. Smaller patients are more predisposed to accidental drug overdose and hypothermia. Overweight cats have a significantly higher risk for perianesthetic complications.[11] Patient age, independent of patient physical status, has been identified as an important risk factor for anesthetic complications.[11] Patients with health status levels of ASA 3 to 5 are associated with anesthetic risk greater than 1%.[7]

The increasing complexity of a surgical procedure is associated with increased risk of anesthetic-related complications, including death. Increasing duration, independent of the type of surgical procedure, is associated with increased risk in small animals.[11] This aspect is of special interest in regard to patients undergoing dental procedures. Full mouth dental radiography provides extensive evaluation of occult disease, resulting in predictably long procedures. This observation underscores the practitioner's obligation to inform the entire staff to expect dental procedures of extended duration.

Hypothermia and hypotension are the most important factors affecting morbidity and mortality in small animal patients during anesthesia,[7] increasing significantly with duration.[12] Special consideration should be given to maintaining normal blood pressure and temperature in patients undergoing dental procedures.

All anesthetic agents, especially inhalants, can produce hypotension. Patients undergoing anesthetic episodes for dental procedures tend to be older because of the increased severity of periodontal disease in this population. Organ system compromise from decreased perfusion resulting from hypotension may be of considerable concern. Blood pressure should always be monitored to ensure early detection and appropriate treatment when pressure aberrations occur. Alteration in anesthetic depth crystalloids, colloids, and positive inotropes are common intervention strategies to maintain normotension.

Most patients presented for dental procedures are small dogs with periodontal disease and cats with periodontal disease or tooth resorption. The large surface area/body ratio in these patients predisposes them to hypothermia,[13] especially as anesthetic duration increases. Exacerbating factors include the need for an air/water coolant mechanism for burring bone and tooth when using high-speed dental delivery systems. Heat is also lost when the highly vascular oral cavity is held open for surgical access. Anesthetic requirements decrease with increasing hypothermia,[14] increasing the potential for inhalant overdose. Patient warming strategies can start in the preoperative period and should extend to the postoperative period. Warmed IV fluids, water-circulating and air-circulating devices, and patient extremity insulation are especially important in small dental patients. Heat supplements not designed for use in small animal patients should not be used, because they may cause significant thermal injury.[7] Hyperthermia is frequently associated with opioid administration, especially in cats, and is discussed in the section on analgesia.

Recovery

Fifty percent to 60% of anesthesia-related deaths in dogs and cats occur postoperatively, particularly in the first 3 hours of the postoperative period.[9] Strict observation of patients from extubation to unassisted standing ensures maximum patient safety. Preemptive analgesia and regional nerve blocks decrease or eliminate the need for additional analgesics in the immediate postoperative period. Even so, careful patient evaluation for pain behaviors is paramount, as discussed later in this article.

ANALGESIC CONCEPTS IN VETERINARY ORAL SURGERY
Nociception

The processing of noxious stimuli resulting in the brain's perception of pain is termed nociception.[14] Transduction, transmission, and modulation comprise the components of nociception.[15] A noxious stimulus (mechanical, chemical, or thermal) is changed into electrical energy by a peripheral nociceptor or free afferent nerve ending, resulting in transduction. The impulse is then transmitted from the region of oral damage through trigeminal afferent nerves. Modulation occurs when these fibers synapse with neurons in the nucleus caudalis in the medulla.[14] The function of the nucleus caudalis mimics that of the spinal cord dorsal horn, which modulates pain from areas other than the oral cavity.[16] Glutamate and substance P are proalgesic neuropeptides and activate pain signals by binding to their receptors on these neurons.[16] In an attempt to prevent this exacerbation of pain, endogenous opioids, serotonin, and norepinephrine descend from the higher centers.[16]

Central Sensitization

Inflammatory mediators are released from damaged oral tissue, including prostaglandins, potassium ions, hydrogen ions, adenosine triphosphate, bradykinin, and nerve growth factors.[15] Chronic oral pain involves perpetuation of this untreated inflammation, consequently producing changes in the neurons of the modulation center in the nucleus caudalis, resulting in a state called central sensitization or windup.[15,16] The increase in the sensitivity of these neurons exacerbates the frequency and intensity of nociception. Glutamate is a primary compound in this process, because it binds to the N-methyl-D-aspartate (NMDA) receptor to enhance windup.[15] NMDA receptor antagonists can therefore aid in management of central sensitization associated with oral pain states.

Preemptive Analgesia

Administration of analgesics before a painful stimulus to decrease pain after stimulus is termed preemptive analgesia. Established pain becomes difficult to control, necessitating providing pain management preoperatively.[15] Extended hospitalization, fluid support, additional analgesic requirements, and feeding assistance are likely consequences of inadequate preemptive analgesic patient management.

Multimodal Analgesia

Combining analgesics that act at different levels of the nociceptive pathway is termed multimodal analgesia. Peripheral inflammation, opioid receptors and NMDA receptors can be targeted by nonsteroidal antiinflammatory drugs (NSAIDs), opioids, and NMDA receptor antagonists, respectively, to produce balanced analgesia using multiple agents.

Preoperative Analgesic Considerations

The ideal preoperative protocol uses the concept of multimodal therapy to produce adequate sedation and preemptive analgesia. Multiple agents at low doses allow for a safer induction by decreasing the dose of the induction agent/s. Patients with chronic pain are a special consideration because they experience the exacerbated effects of increased intensity and frequency of ascending pain signals through the mechanism of central sensitization. A classic example of patients with chronic severe pain are dogs and more commonly cats with stomatitis. Preoperative constant rate infusions are an excellent means of delivering safe and effective low-dose analgesia to such patients.

When given with opioids, lidocaine has a sparing effect and decreases central hypersensitivity in significant pain states.[17] Dogs undergoing limb amputation receiving ketamine infusions were significantly more active on postoperative day 3 and showed significantly lower pain scores 12 and 18 hours after surgery than dogs that did not.[18] We commonly use the NMDA receptor antagonist ketamine in CRI with a μ agonist or partial μ agonist with or without lidocaine administered 2 to 24 hours before surgery. Calculations for loading doses, rates, and volumes of each component are completed on a CRI spreadsheet based on the agents chosen. These spreadsheets are made available for download from the Veterinary Anesthesia Support Group.[19]

Intraoperative Analgesic Considerations

Regional nerve blocks provide the bulk of analgesic management in the intraoperative period and are discussed extensively in this article. CRIs when used preoperatively are continued intraoperatively and extend for various durations throughout the postoperative period. Opioids decrease minimum alveolar concentration (MAC) safely and effectively in various veterinary species.[20–22] A low-dose delivery of morphine, lidocaine, and ketamine decreases isoflurane MAC in dogs without any adverse hemodynamic effects.[22]

Postoperative Analgesic Considerations

Patients vary considerably in their analgesic needs based on individual pain tolerance, whether the procedure is regional or generalized, chronicity, existing pain behaviors, the invasiveness of the surgery, and the tissue management skills of the surgeon. The Modified Glasgow Composite Pain Scale can be used to aid the practitioner in evaluating patients for postoperative pain (**Fig. 2**). In addition, frequent rechecks of patients with more chronic and painful conditions allow the practitioner to use palpation and visualize the healing process in damaged tissue to determine patient comfort levels.

Oral surgery patients can be accurately assessed for pain by extraoral and intraoral palpation. The response to manipulation of the oral cavity is evaluated during the initial preoperative awake oral examination and compared with patient response to similar manipulation postoperatively. Patients showing resistance to manipulation should receive strong consideration for alteration to the analgesic protocol. This strategy should be combined with continual behavioral evaluation by the pet guardian to determine if analgesics can be discontinued or additional agents added or duration of administration extended. Pain management recommendations for various oral conditions are described in **Table 1**. The ideal choice of analgesics allows many oral surgery patients to be discharged the day of surgery. Extended hospital stays are generally unnecessary if the proper analgesic management is maintained.

Specific Preparations to Ease Postoperative Administration

Oral surgery patients may be difficult for pet guardians to medicate postoperatively. Several agents are effective when given in alternative preparations that eliminate oral administration.

Long-Acting Fentanyl Transdermal Solution: Dogs

Recent approval of a long-acting fentanyl transdermal solution (Recuvyra) for dogs has mitigated the disadvantages of time of onset and variable effectiveness of fentanyl transdermal patches by providing a rapid-onset and long-acting agent for pain control in this species.[23] In a prospective, double-blind, positive-controlled multicenter noninferiority study,[24] long-acting fentanyl transdermal solution was found to be noninferior to buprenorphine injections every 6 hours over a 4-day period.

SHORT FORM OF THE GLASGOW COMPOSITE PAIN SCALE

Dog's name _____

Hospital Number _____ Date / / Time

Surgery Yes/No (delete as appropriate)

Procedure or Condition_____

_____

In the sections below please circle the appropriate score in each list and sum these to give the total score.

A. Look at dog in Kennel

Is the dog?

(i)

Quiet	0
Crying or whimpering	1
Groaning	2
Screaming	3

(ii)

Ignoring any wound or painful area	0
Looking at wound or painful area	1
Licking wound or painful area	2
Rubbing wound or painful area	3
Chewing wound or painful area	4

> In the case of spinal, pelvic or multiple limb fractures, or where assistance is required to aid locomotion do not carry out section **B** and proceed to **C**
> *Please tick if this is the case* ☐ then proceed to C.

B. Put lead on dog and lead out of the kennel.

When the dog rises/walks is it?

(iii)

Normal	0
Lame	1
Slow or reluctant	2
Stiff	3
It refuses to move	4

C. If it has a wound or painful area including abdomen, apply gentle pressure 2 inches round the site.

Does it?

(iv)

Do nothing	0
Look round	1
Flinch	2
Growl or guard area	3
Snap	4
Cry	5

D. Overall

Is the dog?

(v)

Happy and content or happy and bouncy	0
Quiet	1
Indifferent or non-responsive to surroundings	2
Nervous or anxious or fearful	3
Depressed or non-responsive to stimulation	4

Is the dog?

(vi)

Comfortable	0
Unsettled	1
Restless	2
Hunched or tense	3
Rigid	4

Total Score (i+ii+iii+iv+v+vi) = _____

Fig. 2. The Modified Glasgow Composite Pain Scale can be used to aid the practitioner in evaluating patients for postoperative pain.

Fentanyl Transdermal Patches: Cats

Fentanyl transdermal patches (Duragesic) minimize the need for an oral opioid for managing postoperative pain in cats undergoing oral surgical procedures. The onset of effect in cats is 6 to 12 hours.[25] This void between regional nerve block and

Table 1
Pain management recommendations for various oral conditions

Procedure	Agents (Recommended Postoperative Duration)
Endodontic therapy	Regional block ± NSAID (12–24 h)
Tooth extraction regional (fracture/intrinsically stained/malocclusion)	Regional block + NSAID (24–36 h) + tramadol (24–36 h)
Tooth extraction general (fracture/intrinsically stained/malocclusion)	Regional block + NSAID (24–36 h) + opioid (24–36 h)
Tooth extraction regional (periodontal/inflammatory)	Regional block + NSAID (24–36 h) + opioid (24–36 h) ± gabapentin (7 d–14 d)
Tooth extraction general inflammation (periodontal/inflammatory)	Regional block + NSAID (24–36 h) + opioid (36–48 h) + gabapentin (7 d–14 d)
Mandibulectomy/maxillectomy	Regional block + NSAID (24–36 h) + opioid (36–48 h) + gabapentin (7 d–14 d)
Jaw fracture acute	Regional block + NSAID (7–10 d) + opioid (7–10 d)
Jaw fracture chronic	Preoperative OLK CRI + regional block + NSAID (7–10 d) + opioid (7–10 d) + gabapentin (14–30 d)
Pain behavior any condition	Preoperative OLK CRI + regional block + NSAID (7–10 d) + opioid (7–10 d) + gabapentin (14–30 d)
Tooth extraction/stomatitis	Preoperative OLK CRI + regional block + NSAID (7 d: dogs) or robenacoxib (3 d: cats) + opioid (7–10 d) + gabapentin (14–60 d)

Amantidine or amitriptyline may be used instead of gabapentin. Robenacoxib is the only oral NSAID approved by the US Food and Drug Administration for cats that can be given on up to 3 consecutive days.
Abbreviation: OLK, opiod, lidocaine, ketamine.

analgesic premedication dissipation and the onset of action should be adequately covered with additional analgesics.

Buprenorphine Sustained Release

Buprenorphine is a partial agonist, making it less effective at the μ receptor than a pure agonist; however, it is a safe and effective analgesic used for mild to moderate pain control. Sustained-release buprenorphine (buprenorphine SR) has been used for amelioration of postsurgical pain in a variety of animals.[26] Buprenorphine SR has been shown to be as safe and efficacious as oral transmucosal buprenorphine in cats for ovariohysterectomy.[27] Expected duration of effect is 72 hours. It must be kept refrigerated and requires proper scheduled drug management. Care must be used in large animals because of significant sedation at the high end of the dose range.

Agents

Opioids

Opioid receptors are ubiquitous and particularly numerous in the central and peripheral nervous systems. The μ receptor is particularly abundant in somatic tissue, and stimulation of this receptor with endogenous and exogenous agents produces analgesia beyond that of other opioid receptor subtypes. Sedation accompanies analgesia and varies with the individual agents. This characteristic is considered positive when these agents are used as premedications for anesthesia. Opioids are considered the most effective and potent analgesics in veterinary medicine.

Functional classification of μ agonists provides insight into the relative effectiveness of opioid analgesics at producing an analgesic effect. Full μ agonists produce a maximum effect at the μ receptor and are recommended for severe to moderate pain. Common examples used in companion animals include morphine sulfate, hydromorphone (Dilaudid), and fentanyl. Partial agonists are less effective but still exert significant analgesia, making them good choices for moderate to mild pain. Buprenorphine is an effective example of this class. Agonists-antagonists such as butorphanol (Torbugesic) and nalbuphine and full antagonists like naloxone (Narcan) provide no appreciable effect at the μ receptor, making them beneficial as reversal agents for agonists and less effectively partial agonists should undesirable effects or overdose occur.

Opioid-induced respiratory depression is seldom significant in dogs and cat; however, hyperthermia is common, especially in cats.[28] Hypothermia is more common in the dog. Temperature should be monitored in all patients receiving opioids during the expected duration of effect of the individual agent. Hyperthermia in the cat may become significant and reversal may become necessary. Histamine release and subsequent hypotension accompanies IV injection of some opiates, particularly morphine, requiring slow IV or intramuscular administration. Opioids should be used with caution in patients with severe renal insufficiency, hypothyroidism, or Addison disease and in geriatric or debilitated patients. Defecation and vomiting can occur shortly after administration, followed by constipation, which is most common with morphine.

NSAIDs

Prostaglandins are proinflammatory compounds that are released from cells at the site of tissue injury. They play a major role in the perpetuation of inflammation and sensitize neurons to chemical, mechanical, and thermal stimuli.[29,30] NSAIDs inhibit cyclooxygenase 1 (Cox-1) and Cox-2 enzymes from breaking down arachidonic acid and producing prostaglandins. Selective Cox-2–sparing inhibitors and Cox-1–sparing NSAIDs are relatively safe agents in this class and minimize undesirable Cox-1 inhibition effects. This situation makes them effective agents for treating pain associated with inflammation.[31] Common examples are deracoxib (Deramaxx), carprofen (Rimadyl), firocoxib (Previcox), meloxicam (Metacam), robenecoxib (Onsior), and the Cox-1 sparing agent etodolac (Etogesic). Meloxicam is approved as a 1-time injectable in cats, whereas robenecoxib is approved for use preemptively and up to 3 days postoperatively. Similarly, 5-lipoxygenase (5-Lox) breaks down arachidonic acid–producing leukotrienes, which significantly enhances the inflammatory process. Tepoxalin (Zubrin) is a 5-Lox inhibitor and approved for use in dogs.

NMDA receptor antagonists

Central sensitization associated with oral pain occurs within the brainstem in the nucleus caudalis.[22] Inhibition or attenuation of central sensitization may be achieved with the use of NMDA receptor antagonists.[32] Ketamine (Ketaset) antagonizes the NMDA receptor in microdoses and can therefore be effectively administered as a component of a constant rate infusion. Amantadine (Symmetrel) is discussed in the section on reuptake inhibitors.

α₂ Agonists

Dexmedetomidine (Dexdomitor) is sedative and analgesic approved by the US Food and Drug Administration that provides reliable dose-dependent sedation, muscle relaxation, and anxiolysis. Recent studies have confirmed its safety and effectiveness as an analgesic CRI in dogs with ASA status I to II.[33–35] It enhances antinociception when combined with buprenorphine in the cat.[36]

Reuptake inhibitors

Amantadine is an antiviral medication that is used to treat Parkinson disease. It is a monoamine reuptake inhibitor and an NMDA receptor antagonist. It can be used as an adjunct to other common analgesics to treat chronic pain and central sensitzation.[37]

Amitriptyline (Elavil) is a tricyclic antidepressant and possesses several beneficial analgesic mechanisms, including the inhibition of serotonin and norepinephrine reuptake and NMDA receptor antagonism. It is most commonly used as an adjunct to other analgesics for chronic pain. This analgesic requires a detailed overview by the clinician before use because of numerous interactions with other compounds. Sedation and anticholinergic effects are common.

Tramadol (Ultram) is a popular serotonin and norepinephrine reuptake inhibitor with weak μ agonist activity, generally used in conjunction with NSAIDs or opioids for management of chronic and postoperative pain in dogs and cats. It is considered a safe and effective analgesic; however, its concurrent use with agents that could precipitate serotonin syndrome should be avoided. Serotonin syndrome is encountered when medications that increase serotonin levels in the body are given simultaneously. Signs are numerous and range from mild agitation to respiratory paralysis and death. Agents such as the selective serotonin reuptake inhibitors fluoxetine (Prozac) and paroxetine (Paxil) and the monoamine oxidase inhibitors amitraz (Preventic, ProMeris, Mitaban) and selegiline (Anipryl) should not be given concurrently with tramadol.

Agents with unestablished mechanisms

Gabapentin (Neurontin) has been shown in randomized placebo-controlled trials to reduce pain significantly in humans suffering from chronic, severe pain syndromes, including postherpetic neuralgia,[38,39] painful diabetic neuropathy,[40] and Guillain-Barré syndrome.[41] It has been used effectively in control of chronic pain in dogs and cats. Its mechanism of analgesic action is unknown.

Pregabalin (Lyrica) is similar to gabapentin because both are structural analogues of the inhibitory neurotransmitter γ-aminobutyric acid. It is 3 to 10 times more potent than gabapentin; however, it is considerably more expensive. Indications and efficacy have not been established for either agent.

REGIONAL NERVE BLOCKS FOR ORAL SURGERY IN DOGS AND CATS
Introduction

Painful surgical stimuli in veterinary patients require adequate anesthetic depths to eliminate patient movement and pain perception throughout the procedure. Companion animal oral surgery affords the practitioner an option to minimize anesthetic depth and maximize patient safety. Regional nerve blocks provide attenuation or elimination of sensory afferent signaling, resulting in significant reductions in inhalant requirements of patients undergoing oral surgery. Minimizing the MAC of an inhalant anesthetic has been shown to decrease the detrimental cardiovascular effects of the inhalant.[42–44] Minimizing inhalant requirements minimizes cardiovascular compromise and increases the safety of the anesthetic event.[45] A recent study in dogs cites a 23% decrease in MAC of isoflurane over controls after administration of an infraorbital nerve block using mepivicaine as the local agent.[5] Use of longer-acting agents such as bupivicaine provides the additional benefit of extended postoperative analgesia, minimizing the need for systemic analgesics in the immediate period postoperatively.

Instrumentation

Special instrumentation is not required to perform regional nerve blocks for companion animal oral surgery. Tuberculin in 3-ml and 6-ml syringes provides the volume capacity that spans patient size from small cats to large dogs. Common needle choices are 25-gauge, 5.87-mm (0.62-inch) for smaller patients and 22-gauge, 19.05-mm (0.75-inch) for larger patients. Smaller-gauge needles provide no benefit and often make confirmation of correct needle placement difficult because of their flexibility.

Agents

Bupivicaine is considered the agent of choice for regional nerve blocks for companion animal oral surgery either alone or in combination with lidocaine because of its safety and long duration of action. Safe and effective doses have been reported at 1 mg/kg of each agent combined in the same syringe. When using traditional concentrations of 2% lidocaine and 0.5% bupivicaine, a convenient maximum patient mixture can be drawn using 0.2 mL lidocaine:0.8 mL bupivicaine per 4.53 kg (10 pounds) as the maximum patient dose. Alone, bupivicaine may be used at 2 mg/kg as the maximum patient dose.

The volume of agent administration per site is dependent on patient size. The maximum total dose described earlier must always be observed. **Box 1** provides general recommendations of administration volumes of the lidocaine/bupivicaine mixture and bupivicaine as a sole agent.

Determination of the effectiveness of any dental nerve block is the observation of the patient's response to surgical manipulation of the region blocked after adequate time for the block to take effect. No studies exist in the veterinary literature concerning the onset of bupivicaine in the oral cavity of dogs or cats. In the human literature, studies using bupivicaine for inferior alveolar nerve blocks range from 6.24 ± 1.69 minutes[46] to 8.1 ± 2.7 minutes[47] to 12.6 ± 6.53[48] minutes to reach surgical sensory blockade. Despite the common practice of using mixtures of short-acting and long-acting local anesthetics in humans for peripheral blocks, studies using mixtures of lidocaine and bupivicaine are scant and none exists that describes mixing these agents for dental blocks. One study reported that mixing lidocaine and bupivicaine for sciatic and femoral nerve blocks shortened the mean onset at 15 minutes versus 30 minutes for bupivicaine alone and significantly shortened the sensory duration of the mixture at 12 to 13 hours versus bupivicaine alone at 19 to 22 hours (sciatic/femoral).[49] The time to surgical onset is shorter in the oral cavity than in peripheral nerves in these studies.

Box 1
Per site administration volume of local anesthetics

Feline/small dog up to 6 kg = 0.1 to 0.3 mL

Medium dog 6 to 25 kg = 0.3 to 0.6 mL

Large dog 26 to 40 kg = 0.8 to 1.2 mL

Extra large dog more than 41 kg = 1.4 to 1.6 mL

In our experience, companion animal patients predictably reach surgical sensory blockade in 8 minutes or less. Success after an adequate time to onset is determined by the lack of patient response to surgical insult. Increases in heart rate, respiration rate, and blood pressure under a light general anesthetic are indications that the block was unsuccessful. Although this situation is uncommon, administration of additional agent is warranted at this point if the volume to be administered is at or less than the recommended maximum total dose. Proper use of nerve blocks combined with adequate but minimal general anesthesia commonly results in the lack of response to major oral surgical insult but maintains a palpebral and swallowing reflex. It is not uncommon for patients maintained in this manner to start to ambulate on patient repositioning despite being motionless during the procedure, further confirming the success and underscoring the increased safety regional blocks provide.

Pain evaluation postoperatively starts on patient admission. Behavioral observation before and after premedication acts as a baseline for evaluating postoperative pain behaviors. In addition to patient observation, palpation and oral manipulation are excellent methods of assessment of nerve block effectiveness. The lack of response to firm extraoral and intraoral palpation are excellent indicators that regional blocks are successful.

Regional nerve blocks should not be attempted without proper training. Lecture and laboratory exposure using cadavers is indicated before local agent administration in live patients. Laboratory sessions generally use dyes that are injected into cadavers followed by dissection to confirm proper placement.

Rostral Maxillary (Infraorbital)

The infraorbital nerve block provides sensory blockade to the ipsilateral bone, tooth, and soft tissue from the maxillary third premolar rostral to the midline. It requires placement of the needle within the infraorbital foramen. The foramen resides just mesial to the mesiobuccal root of the maxillary fourth premolar (**Fig. 3**). To accomplish this block, the upper lip is raised to expose the arcade and soft tissue. This action raises the infraorbital neurovascular bundle dorsally. The needle is advanced palatal to the bundle and directly adjacent to the maxillary bone in a rostral to caudal direction (**Fig. 4**). The tip of the needle should advance 1 to 3 mm within the foramen, depending on patient size. Once the needle is in the desired location, aspiration should confirm that the needle is not in a vessel and the desired volume of agent is administered.

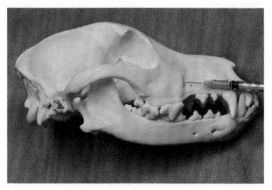

Fig. 3. Needle placement on a skull for the infraorbital nerve block. The infraorbital foramen resides just mesial to the mesiobuccal apex of the maxillary fourth premolar.

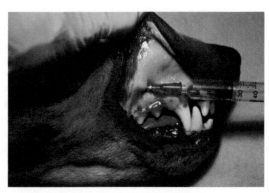

Fig. 4. Demonstration of proper technique on a cadaver specimen for the infraorbital nerve block. The needle is placed rostral to caudal direction and enters the infraorbital canal.

Caudal Maxillary (Maxillary)

The maxillary nerve block provides sensory blockade to the ipsilateral bone, tooth, and soft tissue of the entire ipsilateral oral cavity, including structures desensitized in the infraorbital nerve block and the teeth caudal to the third premolar, as well as the soft and hard palatal mucosa and bone. To accomplish this block, the mouth should be opened wide and the lip commissure retracted caudally (**Fig. 5**). Depending on patient size, the needle is advanced in a ventrodorsal direction 1 to 3 mm beyond the soft tissue directly caudal to the maxillary third molar (**Fig. 6**). Once the needle is in the desired location aspiration should confirm that the needle is not in a vessel and the desired volume of agent is administered.

Anatomic differences in skull conformation require alteration of agent placement for the caudal maxillary regional block in cats and small to medium brachycephalic dogs. In both instances the infraorbital canal length is attenuated versus the mesocephalic and dolicocephalic canine skull types. The infraorbital and pterygopalatine nerves are easily accessible by using the technique described for the rostral maxillary block. Therefore, the caudal maxillary block need not be used for small to medium brachycephalic dogs and the cat because the rostral block provides proper desensitization of the structures described earlier for the caudal maxillary block.

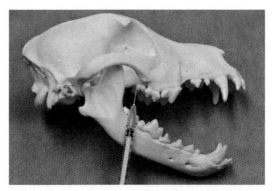

Fig. 5. Needle placement on a skull for the maxillary nerve block. The needle is advanced 1–3 mm beyond the soft palatal mucosa directly caudal to the central portion of second maxillary molar.

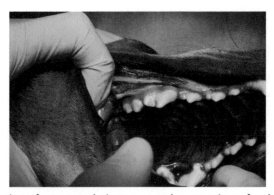

Fig. 6. Demonstration of proper technique on a cadaver specimen for the maxillary nerve block. The mouth is opened wide and the commissure retracted caudally to expose the region for facilitation of needle placement caudal to the second maxillary molar.

Rostral Mandibular (Mental)

The mental nerve block provides sensory blockade to the ipsilateral bone, tooth, and soft tissue from the mandibular second premolar rostral to the midline. It requires placement of the needle within the middle mental foramen. The foramen resides ventral to the mesial root of the mandibular second premolar one-third of the distance from the ventral to the dorsal mandibular body (**Fig. 7**). In the cat the foramen lies midway between the canine and third premolar in that there is no mandibular second premolar in this species. To accomplish this block, the mandibular labial frenulum is retracted ventrally and the needle inserted in a rostral to caudal direction at a slight downward inclination directly adjacent to the bone (**Fig. 8**). The needle passes into the foramen without meeting bone if performed correctly. The needle is advanced 1 to 3 mm within the foramen, depending on the size of the patient. Confirmation of correct needle placement is accomplished by lateral movement of the needle. If the needle is within the foramen resistance can be felt at the lateral wall of the foramen. If the needle does not enter the foramen, lateral movement results in visualization of the needle movement within the frenulum. Once the needle is in the desired location, aspiration should confirm that the needle is not in a vessel and the desired volume of agent is administered.

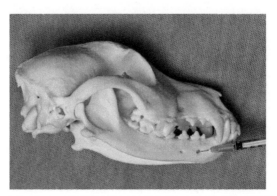

Fig. 7. Needle placement on a skull for the mental nerve block. The middle mental foramen resides ventral to the mesial root of the second mandibular premolar.

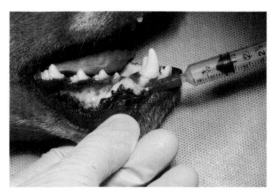

Fig. 8. Demonstration of proper technique on a cadaver specimen for the mental nerve block. The mandibular labial frenulum is retracted ventrally and the needle is directed at a slight ventral angle in a rostral to caudal direction directly into the foramen.

Because of the close approximation of the middle mental foramen to the apical extent of the surgical exposure using the vestibular approach to extraction of the mandibular canine tooth, we use the inferior alveolar nerve block when performing this procedure.

Caudal Mandibular (Inferior Alveolar)

The inferior alveolar nerve block provides sensory blockade to the ipsilateral bone, tooth, and soft tissue of the mandible from the molar to the midline. It requires placement of the needle ventral to the nerve before it enters the mandibular canal (**Fig. 9**). Palpation of the notch rostral to the angular process provides a regional landmark for needle placement (**Fig. 10**). In some dogs and many cats this notch cannot be palpated. In this case visualize an imaginary line coursing from the lateral canthus of the eye directly ventral and slightly caudal on the ventral mandible. While tilting the ipsilateral mandible dorsally, pass the needle through the skin at the caudal extent of the notch at a 45° angle (see **Fig. 11**). The tip of the needle should contact the lingual aspect of the mandible ventral and caudal to the mandibular foramen (**Fig. 10**).

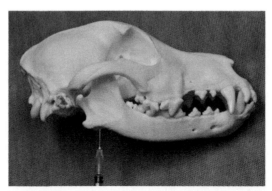

Fig. 9. The vestibular view of proper needle placement on a skull for the inferior alveolar nerve block. The mandibular foramen is located on the lingual aspect of the mandible, adjacent to the caudal portion of the notch rostral to the angular process.

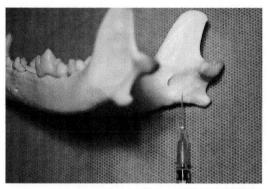

Fig. 10. The lingual view of proper needle placement on a skull for the inferior alveolar nerve block.

Although there exist anecdotal reports of patients experiencing considerable trauma from the carnassial teeth to the caudal portion of the tongue after administration of the inferior alveolar nerve block, this is uncommon. Patient observation from extubation to sternal recumbency prevents trauma to the patient from inadvertent self-mutilation of any kind. Proper administration of the agent does not affect the motor function of the tongue. Once the patient is sternal, the caudal tongue rests between the carnassial teeth, as it does in the awake patient. Lateral recumbency and lack of patient care during recovery are the logical events that lead to morbidity.

Knowledge of anesthesia and pain management is constantly evolving. The International Veterinary Academy of Pain Management (http://www.ivapm.org/) and the Veterinary Anesthesia Support Group (http://www.vasg.org/) are excellent resources that foster studies and share clinical experience, helping clinicians to provide timely and effective protocols for their patients. Research in the field is rapidly expanding, with hopes of developing new techniques, agents, and protocols to maximize analgesia and minimize side effects. It is beneficial for clinicians to remain current with this dynamic evolution to allow patients the safety and comfort to which they are entitled.

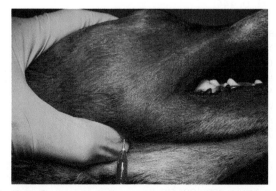

Fig. 11. Demonstration of proper technique on a cadaver specimen for the inferior alveolar nerve block. The needle enters the skin at a 45 degree angle to the mandibular body lingually to rest below the nerve prior to its entry into the mandibular canal.

ACKNOWLEDGMENTS

The author of this article Dr Brett Beckman would like to thank Dr Alessio Vigani for his contribution in this article.

REFERENCES

1. Muir WW. Considerations for general anesthesia. In: Tranquilli WJ, Thurmon JC, Grimm KG, editors. Lumb and Jones' veterinary anesthesia and analgesia. 4th edition. Ames (IA): Blackwell; 2007. p. 17–30.
2. Bednarski R, Grimm K, Harvey R, et al. AAHA anesthesia guidelines for dogs and cats. J Am Anim Hosp Assoc 2011;47:377–85.
3. Veterinary Anesthesia Support Group. Preanesthetic protocols. Available at: http://www.vasg.org/. Accessed August 23, 2012.
4. Meyer EC, Sommers K. Possible mechanisms of anti-cholinergic drug-induced bradycardia. Eur J Clin Pharmacol 1988;35(5):503–6.
5. Dyson D, Pettifer G. Evaluation of the arrhythmogenicity of a low dose of acepromazine: comparison with xylazine. Can J Vet Res 1997;61:241–5.
6. Tzannes S, Govendir M, Zaki S, et al. The use of sevoflurane in a 2:1 mixture of nitrous oxide and oxygen for rapid mask induction of anaesthesia in the cat. J Feline Med Surg 2002;2:83–90.
7. Brodbelt DC, Pfeiffer DU, Young LE, et al. Results of the confidential enquiry into perioperative small animal fatalities regarding risk factors for anesthetic-related death in dogs. J Am Vet Med Assoc 2008;233(7):1096–104.
8. Thurmon JC, Tranquilli WJ, Benson GJ, editors. Essentials of small animal anesthesia and analgesia. Hoboken (NJ): Wiley Blackwell; 2011. p. 286–7.
9. Brodbelt DC, Blissitt KJ, Hammond RA. The risk of death: the confidential enquiry into perioperative small animal fatalities. Vet Anaesth Analg 2008;35:365–73.
10. Hodgson DS. The case for non-rebreathing circuits for very small animals. Vet Clin North Am Small Anim Pract 1992;2:397–9.
11. Brodbelt DC, Pfeifer DU, Young L, et al. Risk factors for anaesthetic-related death in cats: results from the confidential enquiry into perioperative small animal fatalities (CEPSAF). Br J Anaesth 2007;99:617–23.
12. Muir WW, Hubbell JA, Skarda RT, et al. Handbook of veterinary pain management. 3rd edition. St Louis (MO): Mosby; 2002. p. 177–9.
13. Paddleford RR. Manual of small animal anesthesia. 2nd edition. Philadelphia: Saunders; 1999. p. 144.
14. Tranquilli WJ, Grimm KA, Lamont LA. Pain management for the small animal practitioner. Jackson (WY): Teton NewMedia; 2000. p. 6, 10.
15. Muir WW. Physiology and pathophysiology of pain. In: Gaynor JS, Muir WW, editors. Handbook of veterinary pain management. St Louis (MO): Mosby; 2002. p. 13–45.
16. Hargreaves KM, Hutter JW. Endodontic pharmacology. In: Cohen S, Burns RC, editors. Pathways of the pulp. St Louis (MO): Mosby; 2002. p. 665–81.
17. Koppert W, Weigand M, Neumann F, et al. Perioperative intravenous lidocaine has preventive effects on postoperative pain and morphine consumption after major abdominal surgery. Anesth Analg 2004;98:1050–5.
18. Wagner AE, Walton JA, Hellyer PW, et al. Use of low doses of ketamine administered by constant rate infusion as an adjunct for postoperative analgesia in dogs. J Am Vet Med Assoc 2002;221:72–5.
19. Veterinary Anesthesia Support Group. Drug delivery calculators. Available at: http://vasg.org/drug_delivery_calculators.htm. Accessed August 23, 2012.

20. Rowbotham M, Harden N, Stacey B, et al. Reduction of isoflurane MAC by fentanyl or remifentanil in rats. Vet Anaesth Analg 2003;30:250–6.
21. Criado AB, Gomez de Segura IA, Tendillo FJ, et al. Reduction of isoflurane MAC with buprenorphine and morphine in rats. Lab Anim 2000;34:252–9.
22. Muir WW III, Wiese AJ, March PA. Effects of morphine, lidocaine, ketamine, and morphine-lidocaine-ketamine drug combination on minimum alveolar concentration in dogs anesthetized with isoflurane. Am J Vet Res 2003;64:1155–60.
23. Kukanich B, Clark TP. The history and pharmacology of fentanyl: relevance to a novel, long-acting transdermal fentanyl solution newly approved for use in dogs. J Vet Pharmacol Ther 2012;35(Suppl 2):3–19.
24. Linton DD, Wilson MG, Newbound GC, et al. The effectiveness of a long-acting transdermal fentanyl solution compared to buprenorphine for the control of postoperative pain in dogs in a randomized, multicentered clinical study. J Vet Pharmacol Ther 2012;35(Suppl 2):53–64.
25. Riviere J, Papich M. Potential and problems of developing transdermal patches for veterinary applications. Adv Drug Deliv Rev 2001;50(3):175–203.
26. Roughan JV, Flecknell PA. Buprenorphine: a reappraisal of its antinociceptive effects and therapeutic use in alleviating post-operative pain in animals. Lab Anim 2002;36:322–43.
27. Catbagan DL, Quimby JM, Mama KR, et al. Comparison of the efficacy and adverse effects of sustained-release buprenorphine hydrochloride following subcutaneous administration and buprenorphine hydrochloride following oral transmucosal administration in cats undergoing ovariohysterectomy. Am J Vet Res 2011;72(4):461–6.
28. Niedfeldt RL, Robertson SA. Postanesthetic hyperthermia in cats: a retrospective comparison between hydromorphone and buprenorphine. Vet Anaesth Analg 2006;33(6):381–9.
29. Birrell GJ, McQueen DS, Iggo A, et al. PGI2-induced activation and sensitization of articular mechanonociceptors. Neurosci Lett 1991;124:5–8.
30. Mizumura K, Sato J, Kumazawa T. Effects of prostaglandins and other putative chemical intermediaries on the activity of canine testicular polymodal receptors studied in vitro. Pflugers Arch 1987;408:565–72.
31. McMahon SB, Bennett LH, Bevan S, et al. Inflammatory mediators and modulators of pain. In: McMahon SB, Koltzenburg M, editors. Wall and Melzack's textbook of pain. 5th edition. Philadelphia: Churchill Livingstone; 2006. p. 49–72.
32. Rusell IJ, Bieber CS. Myofascial pain and fibromyalgia syndrome. In: McMahon SB, Koltzenburg M, editors. Wall and Melzack's textbook of pain. 5th edition. Philadelphia: Churchill Livingstone; 2006. p. 3–34.
33. van Oostrom H, Doornenbal A, Schot A, et al. Neurophysiological assessment of the sedative and analgesic effects of a constant rate infusion of dexmedetomidine in the dog. Vet J 2011;190(3):338–44.
34. Valtolina C, Robben JH, Uilenreef J, et al. Clinical evaluation of the efficacy and safety of a constant rate infusion of dexmedetomidine for postoperative pain management in dogs. Vet Anaesth Analg 2009;36(4):369–83.
35. Uilenreef JJ, Murrell JC, McKusick BC, et al. Dexmedetomidine continuous rate infusion during isoflurane anaesthesia in canine surgical patients. Vet Anaesth Analg 2008;35(1):1–12.
36. Slingsby LS, Murrell JC, Taylor PM. Combination of dexmedetomidine with buprenorphine enhances the antinociceptive effect to a thermal stimulus in the cat compared with either agent alone. Vet Anaesth Analg 2010;37(2):162–70.

37. Gaynor JS. Other drugs used to treat pain. In: Gaynor JS, Muir WW, editors. Handbook of veterinary pain management. St Louis (MO): Mosby; 2002. p. 251–60.

38. Rowbotham M, Harden N, Stacey B, et al. Gabapentin for the treatment of postherpetic neuralgia: a randomized controlled trial. JAMA 1998;280:1837–42.

39. Rice AS, Maton S. Gabapentin in postherpetic neuralgia: a randomized, double blind, placebo controlled study. Pain 2001;94(2):215–24.

40. Pandey CK, Bose N, Garg G, et al. Gabapentin for the symptomatic treatment of painful neuropathy in patients with diabetes mellitus: a randomized controlled trial. JAMA 1998;280:1831–6.

41. Pandey CK, Bose N, et al. Gabapentin for the treatment of pain in Guillain-Barré syndrome: a double-blind, placebo-controlled, crossover study. Anesth Analg 2002;95:1719–23.

42. Muir WW III, Bednarski L, Bednarski R. Thiamylal and halothane-sparing effects of diazepam in dogs. J Vet Pharmacol Ther 1991;14:46–50.

43. Steffey EP, Baggot JD, Eisele JH, et al. Morphine-isoflurane interactions in dogs, swine, and rhesus monkeys. J Vet Pharmacol Ther 1994;17:202–10.

44. Jeong SM. Effects of electroacupuncture on minimum alveolar concentration of isoflurane and cardiovascular system in isoflurane anesthetized dogs. J Vet Sci 2002;3:193–201.

45. Snyder CJ, Snyder LB. Effect of mepivacaine in an infraorbital nerve block on minimum alveolar concentration of isoflurane in clinically normal anesthetized dogs undergoing a modified form of dental dolorimetry. J Am Vet Med Assoc 2013;242(2):199–204.

46. Pricco DF. An evaluation of bupivacaine for regional nerve block in oral surgery. J Oral Surg 1977;35:126–9.

47. Trieger N, Gillen GH. Bupivacaine anesthesia and postoperative analgesia in oral surgery. Anesth Prog 1979;26:20–3.

48. Stolf Filho N, Ranali J. Avaliação comparativa da bupivacaína e lidocaína em anestesia de pacientes submetidos a cirurgias de terceiros molares inferiores inclusos. Rev Assoc Paul Cir Dent 1990;44:145–8 [in Portuguese].

49. Cuvillon P, Nouvellon E, Ripart J, et al. A comparison of the pharmacodynamics and pharmacokinetics of bupivacaine, ropivacaine (with epinephrine) and their equal volume mixtures with lidocaine used for femoral and sciatic nerve blocks: a double-blind randomized study. Anesth Analg 2009;108(2):641–9.

Index

Note: Page numbers of article titles are in **boldface** type.

A

AAHA Dental Care Guidelines for Dogs and Cats, **453–463**
  abstract, 454
  client education and follow-up, 462–463
  dental procedures, 460–462
  facility requirements, 454
  introduction, 454
  materials, instruments, and equipment, 454–455
  nutrition, 463
  operator protection, 455–456
  patient assessment, 457–458
  planning dental cleaning and patient evaluation, 459–460
  postoperative management, 462
  recommendations and client education, 458–459
Age
  as factor in radiography of canine teeth, 516–517
α_2-Agonist(s)
  in oral surgery pain management
    in small animals, 678–679
American Animal Hospital Association (AAHA) Dental Care Guidelines for Dogs and
  Cats. *See* AAHA Dental Care Guidelines for Dogs and Cats
Analgesia/analgesics
  for oral surgery in small animals, 673–679
    α_2-agonists, 678–679
    buprenorphine sustained release, 677
    central sensitization, 674
    fentanyl transdermal patches, 676
    intraoperative considerations, 675
    long-acting fentanyl transdermal solution, 675
    multimodal, 674
    NMDA receptor antagonists, 678
    nociception, 673–674
    NSAIDs, 678
    opioids, 677–678
    postoperative considerations, 675
    preemptive, 674
    preoperative considerations, 674–675
    reuptake inhibitors, 679
Anamnesis
  in therapeutic decision making and planning in veterinary dentistry and oral surgery,
    472–473

Anesthesia/anesthetics
    for oral surgery in small animals, 591, **669–688**
        induction of, 671
        introduction, 669
        maintenance of, 672–673
        monitoring of, 672
        patient assessment prior to, 670
        patient preparation for, 670
        premedication, 670–671
        recovery from, 673
        regional nerve blocks, 679–685. *See also* Regional nerve blocks, for oral surgery
            in dogs and cats
Angled forceps
    for oral surgery in small animals, 596

    B

Barrier membranes
    for oral surgery in small animals, 605–606
Bisecting angle technique
    in canine dental radiography, 509–510
Bone plates and screws
    for oral surgery in small animals, 601–602
Bone replacement materials
    for oral surgery in small animals, 605
Buprenorphine sustained release
    for oral surgery in small animals, 677
Bur(s)
    for oral surgery in small animals, 592

    C

Carbon dioxide laser
    in veterinary dentistry, 652–653
Caries
    canine, 523–524
Cat(s)
    AAHA Dental Health Guidelines for, 453–463. *See also* AAHA Dental Care Guidelines
        for Dogs and Cats
    chronic gingivostomatitis in, 558–561
    dental radiography for, **533–554**. *See also* Dental radiography, feline
    full mouth extractions in, 583–584
    maxillofacial surgery in, **609–649**. *See also specific indications, e.g.,* Jaw fracture(s)
    oral surgery in, **609–649**. *See also specific indications, e.g.,* Jaw fracture(s)
        regional nerve blocks for, 679–685. *See also* Regional nerve blocks, for oral
            surgery in dogs and cats
Chisel(s)
    for oral surgery in small animals, 600
Computed tomography (CT)
    in small animals
        equipment for, 590

Contact mucositis
    in small animals, 561–562
Convergent roots
    canine, 529–531
Cotton-tipped applicators
    for oral surgery in small animals, 599
Crown impressions
    troughing for
        lasers in, 664–666
Curette(s)
    surgical
        for oral surgery in small animals, 599
Cutaneous diseases
    oral inflammation in small animals due to, 562–564
Cyst(s)
    dentigerous
        canine, 531
    odontogenic
        in dogs and cats
            management of, 636

D

Deciduous tooth
    persistent
        canine, 528
Dental cleaning
    in small animals
        equipment for, 592
Dental luxators
    for oral surgery in small animals, 591
Dental radiography
    canine, **507–532**
        developmental anomalies in, 526–531
            convergent roots, 529–531
            dentigerous cyst, 531
            dentin dysplasia, 528
            dilacerated roots, 528
            gemini tooth, 527
            impacted teeth, 531
            persistent deciduous tooth, 528
            radicular groove, 527
            supernumerary root, 527
            supernumerary tooth, 526–527
        indications for, 507–508
        introduction, 507
        normal anatomy, 511–517. See also Dog(s), teeth of, normal anatomy
        orientation, 510
        pathology in, 517–526
            caries, 523–524
            combined periodontal-endodontic disease, 520–522

Dental (*continued*)
    endodontic disease, 520
    neoplasia, 524–526
    periodontal disease, 517–519
    tooth resorption, 522–523
  patient positioning for, 509–510
  terminology associated with, 508–509
  tooth identification in, 508–509
 feline, **533–554**
  introduction, 533–534
  normal anatomy, 534–537
  pathology in, 538–553
    endodontic disease, 545–548
    neoplasia, 548–550
    orthopedic injury, 550–553
    periodontal disease, 542–545
    tooth resorption, 538–541
 for small animals, 495–504
  digital image handling and manipulation, 503–504
  equipment for, 589
  errors and artifacts, 502–503
  image sharing and compression, 504
  patient preparation and positioning for, 495
  procedures, 495–496
  of specific areas of oral cavity, 500–502
  techniques and positioning, 496–500
Dental service
  North American small animal
    standard of care in, **447–469**
Dental x-ray generators, 490–492
Dentigerous cyst
  canine, 531
Dentin dysplasia
  canine, 528
Diagnostic imaging techniques
  for small animals, 495–504
    dental radiography, 495–504, **507–554**. *See also* Dental radiography
    equipment for, 589–590
Diathermy
  for oral surgery in small animals, 603
Dilacerated roots
  canine, 528
Diode laser
  in veterinary dentistry, 653
Disinfection
  in oral surgery in small animals, 607
Dog(s)
  AAHA Dental Health Guidelines for, 453–463. *See also* AAHA Dental Care Guidelines
    for Dogs and Cats
  dental radiography for, **507–532**. *See also* Dental radiography
  maxillofacial surgery in, **609–649**. *See also specific indications, e.g.,* Jaw fracture(s)

oral surgery in, **609–649**. *See also specific indications, e.g.,* Jaw fracture(s)
    regional nerve blocks for, 679–685. *See also* Regional nerve blocks, for oral
        surgery in dogs and cats
teeth of
    normal anatomy, 511–517
        mandibular teeth, 515–516
        maxillary teeth, 512–514
        radiographic anatomy of tooth, 511–512
        radiographic changes with age, 516–517
Drain(s)
    for oral surgery in small animals, 604
Drape(s)
    for oral surgery in small animals, 592

E

Electrosurgery
    oral
        in small animals, 603–604
Elevator(s)
    for oral surgery in small animals, 591
    periosteal
        for oral surgery in small animals, 598
Endodontic disease
    canine, 520
    feline, 545–548
Endodontic files
    in dislodging partially mobile root tips, 583
Eosinophilic granuloma complex
    oral inflammation in small animals due to, 562–563
Epidermolysis bullosa acquisita
    oral inflammation in small animals due to, 564
Erythema multiforme
    oral inflammation in small animals due to, 563–564
Exodontics, **573–585**
    general principles, 574–579
    introduction, 573
    simple flap design in, 579
    surgical extractions, 579–584
        endodontic files to dislodge partially mobile root tips, 583
        feline full mouth extractions, 583–584
        peritome for extraction of deciduous canines, 583
        release for maxillary canine and maxillary fourth premolar extraction, 582–583
Extraction forceps
    for oral surgery in small animals, 591

F

Feeding tubes
    for oral surgery in small animals, 607
Feline chronic gingivostomatitis, 558–561

Feline full mouth extractions, 583–584
Feline oropharyngeal inflammation therapy
    lasers in, 661–662
Fentanyl transdermal patches
    for oral surgery in small animals, 676
Fentanyl transdermal solution
    long-acting
        for oral surgery in small animals, 675
Flap surgery
    lasers in, 660
Forceps
    for oral surgery in small animals
        angled forceps, 596
        extraction forceps, 591
        hemostatic forceps, 596
        pocket-marking forceps, 599
        thumb forceps, 594, 596
        tissue forceps, 596
Frenectomy
    lasers in, 666

G

Gemini tooth
    canine, 527
General Practice Standard of Care in Dentistry, 2013, 451–452
Gingival hyperplasia
    lasers in, 659–660
Gingivectomy
    lasers in, 659
Gingivectomy knives
    for oral surgery in small animals, 599
Gingivoplasty
    lasers in, 658
Gingivostomatitis
    feline chronic, 558–561
Gum chewer lesions
    surgery for
        lasers in, 661

H

Handpiece(s)
    for oral surgery in small animals, 592
Hemostatic agents
    topical
        for oral surgery in small animals, 606
Hemostatic forceps
    for oral surgery in small animals, 596
Home oral care
    after oral surgery in small animals, 607

I

Idiopathic inflammatory conditions
    oral inflammation in small animals due to, 558–562
        contact mucositis, 561–562
        feline chronic gingivostomatitis, 558–561
        plaque-reactive stomatitis, 561–562
Imaging equipment and techniques
    for small animals, **489–506**
        advanced 3-D imaging, 495
        dental x-ray generators, 490–492
        diagnostic imaging techniques, 495–504, **507–554**. *See also* Dental radiography
        intraoral receptors, 493–495
        introduction, 489–490
Impacted teeth
    canine, 531
Infectious conditions
    oral inflammation in small animals due to, 557–558
Inflammation
    oral
        in small animals, **555–571**. *See also* Oral inflammation, in small animals
Intraoral receptors, 493–495

J

Jaw fracture(s)
    in dogs and cats
        described, 609–611
        management of, 609–617
            noninvasive to minimally invasive, 611–612
            open/surgical, 612–615
            salvage problems in, 616–617

L

Laser(s)
    in veterinary dentistry, 604, **651–668**
        carbon dioxide laser, 652–653
        diode laser, 653
        introduction, 651–652
        low-level laser therapy, 654
        postoperative therapy with, 655
        procedures, 657–666
            feline oropharyngeal inflammation therapy, 661–662
            flap surgery, 660
            frenectomy, 666
            gingival hyperplasia, 659–660
            gingivectomy, 659
            gingivoplasty, 658
            gum chewers lesions management, 661
            operculectomy, 660
            oral biopsy, 662–663
            oral mass surgery, 663–664

Laser(s) (*continued*)
 periodontal pocket surgery, 657–658
 tongue lesion surgery, 660–661
 troughing for crown impressions, 664–666
 safety of, 655–656
Lesion(s). *See specific types, e.g.,* Odontogenic cyst
Lip(s)
 neoplasia of
 in dogs and cats
 management of, 641–645
Lip avulsions
 in dogs and cats
 management of, 641–645
Lip fold pyoderma
 in dogs and cats
 management of, 641–645
Long-acting fentanyl transdermal solution
 for oral surgery in small animals, 675

M

Mallet(s)
 for oral surgery in small animals, 600
Mandibular teeth
 canine
 normal anatomy, 515–516
Mass(es)
 oral
 in dogs and cats
 management of, 631–636
Maxillary canine(s)
 normal anatomy, 512–514
 surgical release for, 582–583
Maxillary fourth premolar extraction, 582–583
Maxillofacial surgery
 in dogs and cats, **609–649**. *See also specific indications, e.g.,* Jaw fracture(s)
Mayo bowl and bulb syringe
 for oral surgery in small animals, 600
Microsurgery
 oral
 in small animals, 606
Mucosal diseases
 oral inflammation in small animals due to, 562–564
Mucositis
 contact
 in small animals, 561–562
Mucous membrane pemphigoid
 oral inflammation in small animals due to, 564

N

Needle holders
 for oral surgery in small animals, 596

Neoplasia
    of canine oral cavity, 524–526
    of feline oral cavity, 548–550
    of lip
        in dogs and cats
            management of, 641–645
Neoplastic lesions
    oral inflammation in small animals due to, 566
NMDA receptor antagonists
    in oral surgery pain management in small animals, 678
Noncrushing tissue forceps
    for oral surgery in small animals, 596
Nonsteroidal anti-inflammatory drugs (NSAIDs)
    in oral surgery pain management in small animals, 678
North American small animal dental service
    standard of care in, **447–469**
NSAIDs. *See* Nonsteroidal anti-inflammatory drugs (NSAIDs)
Nutrition
    AAHA Dental Care Guidelines for Dogs and Cats on, 463

O

Odontogenic cyst
    in dogs and cats
        management of, 636
Operculectomy
    lasers in, 660
Opioid(s)
    in oral surgery pain management in small animals, 677–678
Oral and dental imaging equipment and techniques
    for small animals, **489–506**. *See also specific types and* Imaging equipment and
        techniques, for small animals
Oral biopsy
    equipment for, 591, 662–663
        lasers, 662–663
Oral inflammation
    in small animals, **555–571**
        described, 556–557
        idiopathic inflammatory conditions and, 558–562. *See also* Idiopathic inflammatory
            conditions, oral inflammation in small animals due to
        infectious conditions and, 557–558
        introduction, 555–556
        mucosal and cutaneous diseases and, 562–564
        neoplastic lesions and, 566
        reactive lesions and, 565
Oral lesions
    in dogs and cats
        management of, 636–645
            lip avulsions, 641–645
            lip fold pyoderma, 641–645
            lip neoplasia, 641–645

Oral (*continued*)
    odontogenic cysts, 636
    osteonecrosis, 637–640
    tongue lesions, 640–641
Oral masses
  in dogs and cats
    management of, 631–636
  surgery for
    lasers in
      in veterinary dentistry, 663–664
Oral surgery
  in dogs and cats, **609–649**. *See also specific indications, e.g.,* Jaw fracture(s)
  in small animals
    equipment for, **587–608**
      anesthesia (local and regional), 591
      angled forceps, 596
      barrier membranes, 605–606
      biopsy-related, 591
      bone plates and screws, 601–602
      bone replacement materials, 605
      chisel, 600
      cotton-tipped applicators, 599
      dental luxators, 591
      diagnostic imaging–related, 589–590
      diathermy, 603
      drains, 604
      drapes, 592
      electrosurgical, 603–604
      elevators, 591
      extraction forceps, 591
      feeding tubes, 607
      gingivectomy knives, 599
      handpieces, attachments, and burs, 592
      hemostatic forceps, 596
      introduction, 587
      lasers, 604
      mallet, 600
      Mayo bowl and bulb syringe, 600
      microsurgical, 606
      needle holders, 596
      noncrushing tissue forceps, 596
      oral examination–related, 588–589
      orthopedic pins, 601
      orthopedic wire, 600–601
      osteotome, 600
      periosteal elevators, 598
      pocket-marking forceps, 599
      power saws, 600
      powered systems, 592
      professional dental cleaning–related, 592
      radiosurgical, 603–604

    resin materials, 602
    retractors, 597–598
    rinsing solutions and culture medium, 604
    rongeurs, 598–599
    scalpel handle and blades, 594
    scissors, 594
    suction, 604
    surgical courettes, 599
    surgical loupe and headlamp, 587
    surgical marker pen and plastic ruler, 602
    surgical pack, 592–594
    suture material, 600
    swabs, 599
    tape, 602–603
    thumb forceps, 594, 596
    tissue forceps, 596
    topical hemostatic agents, 606
    towel clamps, 596
    wire twister and cutter, 601
    wooden dowel, 602
  home care after, 607
  sanitation, disinfection, and sterilization related to, 607
Oropharyngeal inflammation
  feline
    lasers in, 661–662
Orthopedic injury
  of feline oral cavity, 550–553
Orthopedic pins
  for oral surgery in small animals, 601
Orthopedic wire
  for oral surgery in small animals, 600–601
Osteoma
  of feline oral cavity, 549–550
Osteonecrosis
  in dogs and cats
    management of, 637–640
Osteotome
  for oral surgery in small animals, 600

P

Pain
  oral surgery in small animals and
    management of, **669–688**. See also Analgesia/analgesics, for oral surgery in small
      animals; Anesthesia/anesthetics, for oral surgery in small animals
Palatal/oronasal defects
  in dogs and cats
    described, 617–620
    management of, 617–631
      acquired defects, 624–631
      congenital defects of palate, 620–623

Palate
    congenital defects of
        in dogs and cats
            management of, 620–623
Parallel technique
    in canine dental radiography, 509
Pemphigus foliaceous
    oral inflammation in small animals due to, 564
Pemphigus vulgaris
    oral inflammation in small animals due to, 564
Periodontal disease
    canine, 517–519
    feline, 542–545
Periodontal-endodontic disease
    canine, 520–522
Periodontal pocket surgery
    lasers in
        in veterinary dentistry, 657–658
Periosteal elevators
    for oral surgery in small animals, 598
Peritome
    for extraction of deciduous canines, 583
Persistent deciduous tooth
    canine, 528
Physical examination
    in therapeutic decision making and planning in veterinary dentistry and oral surgery,
        473–479
Plaque-reactive stomatitis
    in small animals, 561–562
Pocket-marking forceps
    for oral surgery in small animals, 599
Power saw(s)
    for oral surgery in small animals, 600
Powered systems
    for oral surgery in small animals, 592

    R

Radicular groove
    canine, 527
Radiography
    dental. *See* Dental radiography
Radiosurgery
    in veterinary dentistry, 603–604, **651–668**
        described, 656–657
        introduction, 651–652
        techniques, 657
Reactive lesions
    oral inflammation in small animals due to, 565
Regional nerve blocks
    for oral surgery in dogs and cats, 679–685

    agents in, 680–681
    caudal mandibular, 684–685
    caudal maxillary, 682
    instrumentation in, 680
    introduction, 679–680
    rostral mandibular, 683–684
    rostral maxillary, 681
Resin materials
    for oral surgery in small animals, 602
Retractor(s)
    for oral surgery in small animals, 597–598
Reuptake inhibitors
    in oral surgery pain management
        in small animals, 679
Rinsing solutions and culture medium
    for oral surgery in small animals, 604
Rongeur(s)
    for oral surgery in small animals, 598–599
Root(s)
    convergent
        canine, 529–531
    dilacerated
        canine, 528

S

Sanitation
    in oral surgery in small animals, 607
Scalpel handle and blades
    for oral surgery in small animals, 594
Scissors
    for oral surgery in small animals, 594
Specialty Practice Dental Standard of Care, 2013, 450–451
Squamous cell carcinoma
    of feline oral cavity, 548–549
Sterilization
    in oral surgery in small animals, 607
Stomatitis
    plaque-reactive
        in small animals, 561–562
Suction
    for oral surgery in small animals, 604
Supernumerary root
    canine, 527
Supernumerary tooth
    canine, 526–527
Surgical curettes
    for oral surgery in small animals, 599
Surgical loupe and headlamp
    for oral surgery in small animals, 587
Surgical marker pen and plastic ruler
    for oral surgery in small animals, 602

Surgical pack
    for oral surgery in small animals, 592–594
Suture material
    for oral surgery in small animals, 600
Swab(s)
    for oral surgery in small animals, 599
Systemic lupus erythematosus
    oral inflammation in small animals due to, 564

T

Tape
    for oral surgery in small animals, 602–603
Teeth. See also specific types, e.g., Mandibular teeth
    impacted
        canine, 531
Therapeutic decision making and planning
    in veterinary dentistry and oral surgery, **471–487**
        anamnesis in, 472–473
        case examples, 479–485
        introduction, 471–472
        physical examination in, 473–479
        planning in, 485–487
        recording data in, 479
3-dimensional imaging
    advanced, 495
Thumb forceps
    for oral surgery in small animals, 594, 596
Tissue forceps
    for oral surgery in small animals, 596
Tongue lesions
    in dogs and cats
        management of, 640–641
            lasers in, 660–661
Tooth resorption
    canine, 522–523
    feline, 538–541
Topical hemostatic agents
    for oral surgery in small animals, 606
Towel clamps
    for oral surgery in small animals, 596

V

Veterinary dental advancement
    history of, 448–452
        general considerations in, 448–450
        General Practice Standard of Care in Dentistry, 2013, 451–452
        Specialty Practice Dental Standard of Care, 2013, 450–451
Veterinary dentistry and oral surgery
    therapeutic decision making and planning in, **471–487**. See also Therapeutic decision
        making and planning, in veterinary dentistry and oral surgery

W

Wire twister and cutter
    for oral surgery in small animals, 601
Wooden dowel
    for oral surgery in small animals, 602

X

X-ray generators, 490–492

Printed and bound by CPI Group (UK) Ltd, Croydon, CR0 4YY

03/10/2024

01040443-0011